Lung Cancer, Part I: Screening, Diagnosis, and Staging

Editors

JEAN DESLAURIERS
F. GRIFFITH PEARSON
FARID M. SHAMJI

THORACIC SURGERY CLINICS

www.thoracic.theclinics.com

Consulting Editor
M. BLAIR MARSHALL

May 2013 • Volume 23 • Number 2

ELSEVIER

1600 John F. Kennedy Boulevard ● Suite 1800 ● Philadelphia, Pennsylvania, 19103-2899

http://www.theclinics.com

THORACIC SURGERY CLINICS Volume 23, Number 2
May 2013 ISSN 1547-4127, ISBN-13: 978-1-4557-7340-4

Editor: Jessica McCool

Thoracic Surgery Clinics (ISSN 1547-4127) is published quarterly by Elsevier Inc., 360 Park Avenue South, New York, NY 10010-1710. Months of publication are February, May, August, and November. Business and editorial offices: 1600 John F. Kennedy Boulevard, Suite 1800, Philadelphia, PA 19103-2899. Periodicals postage paid at New York, NY, and additional mailing offices. Subscription prices are $335.00 per year (US individuals), $433.00 per year (US institutions), $159.00 per year (US Students), $416.00 per year (Canadian individuals), $547.00 per year (Canadian institutions), $216.00 per year (Canadian and foreign students), $443.00 per year (foreign individuals), and $547.00 per year (foreign institutions). Foreign air speed delivery is included in all Clinics' subscription prices. All prices are subject to change without notice. **POSTMASTER:** Send address changes to Thoracic Surgery Clinics, Elsevier Health Sciences Division, Subscription Customer Service, 3251 Riverport Lane, Maryland Heights, MO 63043. **Customer Service (orders, claims, online, change of address): Telephone: 1-800-654-2452 (U.S. and Canada); 314-447-8871 (outside U.S. and Canada). Fax: 314-447-8029. Email: journalscustomerservice-usa@elsevier.com (for print support); journalsonlinesupport-usa@elsevier.com (for online support).**

Reprints. For copies of 100 or more, of articles in this publication, please contact Commercial Rights Department, Elsevier Inc., 360 Park Avenue South, New York, NY 10010-1710. Tel: (212) 633-3812; Fax: (212) 462-1935; E-mail: reprints@elsevier.com.

Thoracic Surgery Clinics is covered in *MEDLINE/PubMed (Index Medicus)* and *EMBASE/Excerpta Medica*.

Printed and bound by CPI Group (UK) Ltd, Croydon, CR0 4YY

Transferred to digital print 2012

Contributors

CONSULTING EDITOR

M. BLAIR MARSHALL
Associate Professor of Surgery, Georgetown
University School of Medicine; Chief, Division
of Thoracic Surgery, Department of Surgery,
Georgetown University Medical Center,
Washington, DC

EDITORS

JEAN DESLAURIERS, MD, FRCS(C)
Professor of Surgery at Laval University,
Division of Thoracic Surgery, Institut
Universitaire de Cardiologie et de Pneumologie
de Québec (IUCPQ), Quebec City, Quebec,
Canada

**F. GRIFFITH PEARSON, MD, Bsc Med,
FRCS(Can), FACS**
Professor of Surgery Emeritus, Division of
Thoracic Surgery, Department of Surgery,
University Health Network - Toronto General
Hospital, University of Toronto, Toronto,
Ontario, Canada

FARID M. SHAMJI, MBBS, FRCS(C), FACS
Professor of Surgery, Division of Thoracic
Surgery, General Campus, The Ottawa
Hospital, Ottawa, Ontario, Canada

AUTHORS

DAVID G. BEER, PhD
Professor of Surgery and Radiation Oncology,
Section of Thoracic Surgery, Department of
Surgery; Co-Director, Cancer Genetics
Program, University of Michigan Health
System, Ann Arbor, Michigan

STEPHEN R. BRODERICK, MD
Division of Cardiothoracic Surgery,
Department of Surgery, Washington University
School of Medicine, St Louis, Missouri

AURÉLIE CAZES, MD, PhD
Department of Thoracic Pathology, Georges
Pompidou European Hospital, Paris-Descartes
University, Paris, France

JOEL DAVID COOPER, MD
Professor of Surgery, Division of Thoracic
Surgery, Department of Surgery, Hospital of
the University of Pennsylvania, University of
Pennsylvania School of Medicine, Philadelphia,
Pennsylvania

JEAN DESLAURIERS, MD, FRCS(C)
Professor of Surgery at Laval University,
Division of Thoracic Surgery, Institut
Universitaire de Cardiologie et de Pneumologie
de Québec (IUCPQ), Quebec City, Quebec,
Canada

CAROLYN DRESLER, MD, MPA
Medical Director, Tobacco Prevention and
Cessation Network, Arkansas Department of
Health, Little Rock, Arkansas

WILLIAM K. EVANS, MD, FRCPC
President, Juravinski Hospital and Cancer
Centre, Professor of Oncology, McMaster
University, Hamilton, Ontario, Canada

ELIZABETH FABRE-GUILLEVIN, MD
Department of Medical Oncology, Georges
Pompidou European Hospital, Paris-Descartes
University, Paris, France

MARCIO M. GOMES, MD, PhD
Assistant Professor, Department of Pathology
and Laboratory Medicine, The Ottawa Hospital,
University of Ottawa, Ottawa, Ontario, Canada

MEHDI HENNI, MD
Department of Radiation Oncology, Georges
Pompidou European Hospital, Paris-Descartes
University, Paris, France

SASHA JOSEPH, MD
Division of Medical Oncology, Department
of Medicine, New York University Langone
Clinical Cancer Center, New York, New York

ROBERT J. KORST, MD
Medical Director, Division of Thoracic Surgery,
Department of Surgery, The Daniel and Gloria
Blumenthal Cancer Center, Paramus; Director
of Thoracic Surgery, The Valley Health System,
Ridgewood, New Jersey

STEPHEN LAM, MD, FRCPC
Department of Integrative Oncology, British
Columbia Cancer Agency; Department of
Medicine, University of British Columbia,
Vancouver, British Columbia, Canada

FRANÇOISE LE PIMPEC BARTHES, MD, PhD
Department of General Thoracic Surgery,
Georges Pompidou European Hospital,
Paris-Descartes University, Paris, France

PIERRE MASSION, MD
Professor of Medicine, Ingram Professor of
Cancer Research; Professor of Cancer
Biology, Leader, Thoracic Program,
Vanderbilt-Ingram Cancer Center, Nashville,
Tennessee

ANNETTE McWILLIAMS, MB, FRCPC
Department of Integrative Oncology, British
Columbia Cancer Agency; Department of
Medicine, University of British Columbia,
Vancouver, British Columbia, Canada

PIERRE MORDANT, MD, PhD
Department of General Thoracic Surgery,
Georges Pompidou European Hospital,
Paris-Descartes University, Paris, France

MORIHITO OKADA, MD, PhD
Chairman and Professor, Department of
Surgical Oncology, Hiroshima University,
Minami-Ku, Hiroshima City, Hiroshima, Japan

HARVEY I. PASS, MD
Stephen A. Banner Professor of Thoracic
Oncology and Director, General Thoracic
Surgery; Vice-Chairman (Research),
Department of Cardiothoracic Surgery,
New York University Langone Medical Center,
New York, New York

UGO PASTORINO, MD
Head, Division of Thoracic Surgery, Istituto
Nazionale Tumori, Milan, Italy

G. ALEXANDER PATTERSON, MD
Division of Cardiothoracic Surgery,
Department of Surgery, Washington University
School of Medicine, St Louis, Missouri

**F. GRIFFITH PEARSON, MD, Bsc Med,
FRCS(Can), FACS**
Professor of Surgery Emeritus, Division of
Thoracic Surgery, Department of Surgery,
University Health Network - Toronto General
Hospital, University of Toronto, Toronto,
Ontario, Canada

MARC RIQUET, MD, PhD
Department of General Thoracic Surgery,
Georges Pompidou European Hospital,
Paris-Descartes University, Paris, France

JONATHAN M. SAMET, MD, MS
Department of Preventive Medicine, Keck
School of Medicine, University of Southern
California Institute for Global Health, University
of Southern California, Los Angeles, California

HARMANJATINDER S. SEKHON, MD, PhD
Assistant Professor, Department of Pathology
and Laboratory Medicine, The Ottawa Hospital,
University of Ottawa, Ottawa, Ontario, Canada

TAWIMAS SHAIPANICH, MD, FRCPC
Department of Integrative Oncology, British
Columbia Cancer Agency; Department of
Medicine, University of British Columbia,
Vancouver, British Columbia, Canada

FARID M. SHAMJI, MBBS, FRCS(C), FACS
Professor of Surgery, Division of Thoracic Surgery, General Campus, The Ottawa Hospital, Ottawa, Ontario, Canada

JOSEPH B. SHRAGER, MD
Professor of Cardiothoracic Surgery, Stanford University School of Medicine; Chief, Division of Thoracic Surgery, Thoracic Oncology Program Leader, Stanford Hospitals and Clinics; Va Palo Alto Health Care System, Stanford, California

CAROLINA A. SOUZA, MD, PhD
Associate Professor, Department of Diagnostic Imaging, The Ottawa Hospital, University of Ottawa, Ottawa, Ontario, Canada

NHA VODUC, MD, FRCPC
Assistant Professor, Division of Respirology, University of Ottawa, Ottawa, Ontario, Canada

DELPHINE WERMERT, MD
Department of Pneumology, Georges Pompidou European Hospital, Paris-Descartes University, Paris, France

KAZUHIRO YASUFUKU, MD, PhD
Director, Interventional Thoracic Surgery Program, University of Toronto; Assistant Professor of Surgery, Division of Thoracic Surgery, Toronto General Hospital, University Health Network, University of Toronto, Toronto, Ontario, Canada

Contents

> Tobacco smoking is the world's leading cause of avoidable premature mortality, reflecting the potent toxicity of tobacco smoke inhaled by smokers for decades. In the twentieth century, lung cancer was an early sentinel of the emergence of the still persisting epidemic of tobacco-caused disease. Smoking has declined in many countries, particularly the high-income countries, but low- and middle-income countries remain at risk because of the aggressive tactics of tobacco multinationals. The World Health Organization treaty, the Framework Convention on Tobacco Control, is a critical factor in countering these tactics and precipitating the end of the global epidemic of tobacco smoking.

> The epidemiology of lung cancer continues to evolve. Since the invention of a machine that could rapidly manufacture cigarettes in the 1880s, tobacco smoking has progressively been the major causative agent for the lung cancer epidemic. Until tobacco inhalation is ceased, globally, there will continue to be readily preventable lung cancers. Because cigarettes and other products the tobacco industry develops or modifies for inhalation are continually changing, the types of lung cancer could continue to change. There are other causes of lung cancer in people who never smoke, which include environmental and occupational. Enough is now known to implement strong policies that could eliminate most lung cancers.

> Tumor Board Conferences (TBCs) have been associated with higher adherence of staging and treatment to guidelines. The influence of TBCs on the rate of curative treatments has been established. Patients with lung nodules and tumors of unknown histology should not be presented before surgery, but every patient with malignant histology should be declared to the TBC coordinator and registered at the time of histologic confirmation. This approach allows physicians to deal rapidly with simple

cases on a systematic basis, to give more attention to the most complicated situations, and to offer every patient the benefit of a multidisciplinary approach.

Low-dose CT (LDCT) is effective in the early detection of lung cancer, providing higher resectability and long-term survival rates. The National Lung Screening Trial shows a statistically significant mortality reduction in LDCT compared with chest radiography. The efficacy and safety of annual LDCT screening in heavy smokers must be explored, and the magnitude of benefit compared with the cost of large-scale screening. Trials in Europe have different study designs and an observational arm. Strategies to reduce lung cancer mortality should combine early detection with primary prevention and innovative biologic approaches.

Indeterminate pulmonary nodules in asymptomatic individuals are common, and their incidence is expected to increase. Although evidence-based guidelines exist for the management of these lesions, they are not in complete agreement and are often not followed, resulting in inconsistent management. A dedicated program or clinic for the management of lung nodules would allow an institution to deliver evidence-based, standardized care for patients with indeterminate nodules, and should include multidisciplinary care, state-of-the-art technology and expertise, and a patient navigation system to provide a user-friendly service for both patients and referring physicians. A dedicated pulmonary nodule clinic has many potential advantages.

Bronchoscopy is a minimally invasive method for lung cancer diagnosis. Smaller and more maneuverable bronchoscopes with higher image resolution and an adequate biopsy channel are being developed. High-resolution multiplanar computed tomography (CT) is used to produce 3-dimensional virtual images of the bronchial tree. The target lesion can be confirmed by a mini-radial ultrasound probe and potentially other technologies such as optical coherence tomography. These tools may provide a safer alternative method to CT-guided transthoracic lung biopsy for peripheral lung lesions that are not pleural based.

Despite recent advances in treatment modalities, the survival rate of patients with lung cancer has not significantly improved. Therefore, new avenues are being explored in the era of evolving personalized patient management by early detection.

Cytology is now the mainstay to address the diagnostic needs of pulmonary malignancies. Cytology specimens deliver diagnostic results equivalent to tissue biopsies. Fine-needle aspirations are equally useful to perform diagnostic, predictive, and prognostic immunohistochemical markers and molecular analysis. This article reviews the main new technologies that produced this revolution. The new role of the cytopathologist in this time of interdisciplinary care is also discussed.

Lung adenocarcinoma, accounting for approximately 70% of non-small cell lung cancer, is becoming more frequently detected, and is a radiologically, histomorphologically, molecularly, and clinically heterogeneous tumor with a broad range of malignant behavior. Histologic subtyping is an important independent prognostic variable in lung adenocarcinoma. In the 2011 IASLC/ATS/ERS classification, the term bronchioloalveolar carcinoma is eliminated, adenocarcinoma in situ and minimally invasive adenocarcinoma are defined, and the term lepidic is resurrected. The impact of subtyping on patient survival according to the 2011 classification is independent of known prognostic factors, such as TNM stage. The role of clinical decision making for treating lung adenocarcinoma is predominantly based on subtyping similar to that of breast and prostate cancer.

Clinical Staging Strategies and Evaluation of Cardiopulmonary Function

Standardized clinical care pathways for the investigation of patients with lung cancer allow for a reduction in the time interval between suspicion of lung cancer and treatment, lower costs, increased patient satisfaction, and quality of care. It may also be associated with a modest increase in survival.

Integrated positron emission tomography (PET)/CT is routinely used for mediastinal nodal staging of non-small cell lung carcinoma in centers throughout the world. This modality is the most accurate noninvasive means by which to identify metastatic disease in mediastinal lymph nodes. This article reviews the evidence supporting the use of PET/CT and discusses the clinical applicability of this modality.

Although cervical mediastinoscopy has been considered the gold standard for mediastinal staging in non–small cell lung cancer, new minimally invasive endoscopic ultrasound technology, such as endobronchial ultrasound-guided transbronchial needle aspiration and endoscopic ultrasound fine-needle aspiration, have changed the practice of invasive staging. Based on the current evidence, minimally invasive endoscopic staging is the recommended choice in patients with high pretest probability of lymph node metastasis; however, all negative results should be verified by mediastinoscopy, especially in centers with low expertise. In patients with low pretest probability, mediastinoscopy may be omitted when adequate sampling is achieved with endoscopic modalities.

be considered for patients who have disseminated cancer, limited cardiopulmonary reserve, advanced chronologic and physiologic age, and those who decline treatment.

It can be difficult to determine whether a patient with more than a single, "solid" lung nodule suspicious for malignancy is suffering from synchronous primary tumors or intrapulmonary metastasis. For this reason, if resection can be performed an aggressive approach is often warranted after demonstrating no mediastinal nodal disease. Increasing evidence suggests that the survival of a patient with a single, invasive lepidic-predominant adenocarcinoma depends on the stage of the invasive tumor, not on the presumed multiple in situ tumors. A suggested clinical approach to each of these types of multifocal tumors, solid and lepidic, is proposed in this article.

THORACIC SURGERY CLINICS

Preface

Recent Advances in Screening, Diagnosis, and Staging of Lung Cancer: A Tribute to Robert J. Ginsberg

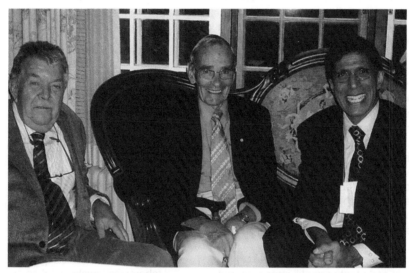

From left to right: Jean Deslauriers, MD, FRCS(C), F. Griffith Pearson, MD, Bsc Med, FRCS(Can), FACS, and Farid M. Shamji, MBBS, FRCS(C), FACS

Editors

On March 1st, 2003, the thoracic surgical community lost a valued member when Dr Robert J. Ginsberg died of the very disease that he spent a lifetime studying. He was a leader in the field of thoracic oncology and had a profound impact on the career and life of many of the authors of this 2-part issue on lung cancer. Indeed, most articles are written by thoracic surgeons and medical oncologists who not only possess detailed knowledge of the disease and comprehend it, but who were also friends or trainees of Dr Robert J. Ginsberg.

Lung cancer kills several million people annually and those numbers are more than breast, colon, and prostate cancer combined. This is due, for the most part, to cigarette smoking, which is constantly driven by the aggressive marketing strategies of the tobacco industry all over the world. As discussed by Dr Carolyn Dressler, other factors that may be as important as cigarette

smoking are environmental and occupational hazards. In China, for instance, the incidence of lung cancer has risen tremendously over the past 50 years, not only because of higher life expectancy for both men and women, but also in relation to heavy exposure to toxic fumes secondary to heating with coal and cooking with hot oils. In addition, a large proportion of Chinese men are heavy smokers and Asia has now become the focus of the advertising blitz of the tobacco companies.

Early diagnosis and strategies to expedite the investigation of patients suspected of having lung cancer are important issues because the disease will shift toward earlier stage and resection rates will increase. Indeed, low-dose computer tomography has proven effective in the early detection of lung cancer, providing both higher resectability rates and better long-term survival. As discussed by Dr Robert J. Korst, it is important to have dedicated pulmonary nodule clinics providing

Thorac Surg Clin 23 (2013) xiii–xiv
http://dx.doi.org/10.1016/j.thorsurg.2013.01.013
1547-4127/13/$ – see front matter © 2013 Published by Elsevier Inc.

thoracic.theclinics.com

evidence-based and standardized care as well as the use of state-of-the-art technology and expertise. In this new era where we are seeing a shift in lung cancer types from centrally located squamous carcinomas to more peripherally located adenocarcinomas, it is also important to subtype each tumor according to new international classifications and to learn how to treat them if they are multifocal. As discussed by Dr Harvey I. Pass, the use of biomarkers to tailor therapy and as prognostic factors is a rapidly expanding field.

Once the diagnosis of lung cancer has been made, clinical staging becomes an important issue, especially the documentation of the status of the mediastinal nodes. For this purpose, integrated positron emission tomography computed tomography is routinely used but its diagnostic accuracy for mediastinal nodes is insufficient. Bob Ginsberg was a master at mediastinoscopy but, currently, endobronchial ultrasound and endoscopic ultrasound are new minimally invasive technologies that have changed the practice of mediastinal staging. In the end, discussing all patients with documented lung cancer at multidisciplinary board conferences (Tumor Board Conferences) should be a national regulation because it leads to higher adherence to both staging and treatment guidelines.

It thus appears that the essential facts on lung cancer found in early texts are still important, but they have evolved and developed into a more refined science that must be well-known if one is to ensure that each lung cancer patient gets the best possible treatment.

Jean Deslauriers, MD, FRCS(C)
Division of Thoracic Surgery
Laval University
Institut Universitaire de Cardiologie et
de Pneumologie de Québec
2725 Chemin Sainte-Foy
Quebec City, Quebec G1V 4G5, Canada

F. Griffith Pearson, MD, Bsc Med, FRCS(Can),
FACS
RR #1
Mansfield, Ontario L0N 1M0, Canada

Farid M. Shamji, MBBS, FRCS(C), FACS
Division of Thoracic Surgery
General Campus
The Ottawa Hospital
501 Smyth Road, Room 6362
Box 708
Ottawa, Ontario, K1H 8L6, Canada

E-mail addresses:
jean.deslauriers@chg.ulaval.ca (J. Deslauriers)
fgpearson@hotmail.com (F.G. Pearson)
fshamji@ottawahospital.on.ca (F.M. Shamji)

Dedication
Tribute to Robert Jason Ginsberg (1940–2003)

Robert J. Ginsberg was a Canadian thoracic surgeon who became one of the most recognized world leaders in Thoracic Oncology. His success was the result of great leadership capability, drive, and innovative initiative, combined with his *exceptional* talent for obtaining loyal, enthusiastic support from colleagues from every level of status and experience. This leadership and organizational talent are exemplified by his coordination of the University of Toronto Group of Thoracic Surgeons, and their highly successful role in the (U.S.) National Institutes of Health–sponsored Lung Cancer Study Group (LCSG) trials and by the formation of the General Thoracic Surgical Club, of which he was a founding member. Dr Ginsberg served as the scientific program chairman for the first general thoracic surgery club meeting in 1988. That program featured the premeeting conference on clinical trials in lung cancer, which continues to be an important feature of that meeting to the present time **(Fig. 1)**.

Dr Ginsberg was born, raised, and largely educated in Toronto. He graduated with honors (AOA) from the University of Toronto Medical School in 1963 and obtained his Canadian Certificate of General Surgery in 1968. His leadership skills were demonstrated as an athlete in both high school and university, as he was the goalie for the Forest Hill High School hockey team and elected to be captain of the University of Toronto football team.

Following his general surgical training, Dr Ginsberg became the first chief resident in the newly created division of thoracic surgery at the Toronto General Hospital. He subsequently spent 1 year as a fellow at Baylor University in Dallas in the cardiothoracic service of Drs Donald Paulson and Harold Urschel. At the time, Dr Paulson was a world leader in the surgical staging and operative management of lung cancer. The following year, Dr Ginsberg served as the senior registrar at the University of Birmingham in England, where he acquired further experience in thoracic surgery. He worked with Dr Gordon Cummings, who generated Bob's lifelong interest in pulmonary function studies and their application for the selection and management of patients with resectable lung cancer.

Dr Ginsberg then returned to Canada to take a position as a thoracic surgeon at the Toronto Western Hospital in 1971 and served as Chief of that division from 1973 to 1981. Dr Ginsberg then joined the division of the thoracic surgery at the Toronto General Hospital as head of Thoracic Surgical Oncology from 1981 to 1984. Dr Ginsberg was then chosen to head a new and expanded division of thoracic surgery at the Mt. Sinai Hospital in Toronto, where he also served as Surgeon-in-Chief of that hospital.

In 1990, Dr Ginsberg left Canada to become Chief of Thoracic Surgery at Memorial Sloane-Kettering Cancer Center in New York. With his growing prominence in the field of thoracic surgery and oncology, he was much sought after as a visiting professor, lecturer, and participant in conferences and symposia. His curriculum vitae lists 65 such national and international presentations in his last 2 years at Sloane-Kettering Cancer Center.

Dr Ginsberg returned to Toronto in 2000 to assume the position of Professor of Thoracic Surgery and Chair of the Division of Thoracic Surgery for both the University of Toronto and the University Health Network.

Dr Ginsberg served as the President of the New York Society of Thoracic Surgery and the Canadian Association of Thoracic Surgeons. He was a member of many international organizations and served as a member of the editorial boards of 10 medical journals. He published 281 articles in scholarly journals and contributed chapters to 94 textbooks.

Although Dr Ginsberg's clinical and scientific contributions were indeed outstanding, what most distinguished him were his personal attributes. He was uncompromising in his standards and absolute in his honesty and integrity. Underneath his outward gruff and sometimes forbidding demeanor lay a sensitive, compassionate, and generous individual.

Robert Ginsberg was the epitome of the academic clinician—inquisitive, analytic, forever stimulating those around him to learn from experience. He clearly subscribed to the dictum of William Halsted that, "the hospital, the operating

Thorac Surg Clin 23 (2013) xv–xvii
http://dx.doi.org/10.1016/j.thorsurg.2013.01.017

thoracic.theclinics.com

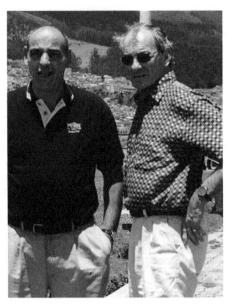

Fig. 1. Drs "Bob" Ginsberg (*left*) and Griff Pearson on the Equatorial line in Quito, Ecuador, in October 1999.

room and ward should be laboratories of the highest order." He was a remarkably unselfish individual, who sought neither fame, nor popularity, nor personal gain. That he failed in his attempt to shun personal fame and glory was clearly demonstrated by the international outpouring of affection shown for him at the testimonial in his honor given several weeks before his passing in 2003. To have attended that tribute and to have witnessed the large number of friends, colleagues, and admirers who came from every corner of the earth to express their admiration and friendship for him was truly unique and remarkable.

Dr Ginsberg's selflessness recruited enthusiastic and loyal support from all stations. A prime example of these qualities was provided on the occasion of the appointment of a new head of general thoracic surgery at Toronto General Hospital in 1978. When the previous head of the thoracic division there (one of us, FGP) had become surgeon-in-chief at the Toronto General Hospital, Dr Ginsberg was the "heir-apparent" for heading the thoracic division at that time. The other one of us (JDC) had been on staff since coming from the Massachusetts General Hospital in 1972 with the expressed intention of staying in Canada for about 5 years. When Dr Ginsberg learned that Dr Cooper would also like to be considered for the thoracic position and that if appointed was prepared to remain in Toronto for the subsequent 10 years (the usual term of a divisional chief), Dr Ginsberg appeared in Pearson's office and stated, "I wish to withdraw my name for this position." When asked why, his response was, "if

I take the job, Cooper will leave and *that would be a great loss for Toronto.*" Not only did Bob encourage Cooper's appointment, but within 1 year he agreed to join the division at the Toronto General Hospital and in his usual fashion was an energetic and enthusiastic team player, contributing to what has been called a "Division of Chiefs" (ie, Pearson, Ginsberg, Cooper, Todd, and Patterson). Indeed, when the initial, successful lung transplants were carried out by the thoracic surgical team, Bob Ginsberg chose to be the on-site coordinator at the time of the transplants. He would go back and forth between the adjacent operating rooms where the donor lung extraction was taking place in one, and the recipient lung removal was occurring in the other, keeping each team informed of the others' progress so as to minimize the ischemic time of the donor lung as much as possible.

His contribution to the Toronto Thoracic Surgical Group and their participation in "the NIH-LCSG multicenter North American randomized trials" (1977-1989) has already been mentioned. It is notable, however, that Ginsberg and a Medical Oncologist colleague (Michael Baker) wrote and submitted the successful Request for Proposal to the NIH from his then home hospital—the Toronto Western Hospital—not the Toronto General Hospital. Ginsberg subsequently became Principle Investigator for Toronto and remained so between 1979 and 1989, at which time the LCSG closed. The Toronto group was 1 of the 7 original, participating North American centers. Toronto entered almost half of the total number of patients in the trials. Once again, this remarkable volume was the result of Ginsberg's success in recruiting thoracic surgeons (and their patients) from the University of Toronto–affiliated hospitals. Ginsberg himself was a leader among the Principle Investigators from other participating American centers. He was the originator of the much quoted study on rates of mortality for some 2500 lung cancer resections entered in the trials during the first 3 years of study. Ginsberg proposed and wrote the protocol for the trial comparing lobectomy with lesser resection for stage 1, non-small-cell tumors.

In 2000, when Dr Ginsberg returned from New York to Toronto, it was once again to provide support to the Thoracic Division Chief at the Toronto General Hospital, Dr Shafique Keshavjee, known to us all as "Shaf." Shaf relates that as the University Chief of Thoracic Surgery, Dr Ginsberg "ran interference" for him, encouraging and helping in any way he could to assist Dr Keshavjee during his early years as the Toronto General Hospital Divisional Chief. Dr Keshavjee attributes his ability to grow and develop the current outstanding and unique clinical and research unit in thoracic surgery and lung transplantation at the University of Toronto to Dr Ginsberg's behind-the-scenes support.

Undoubtedly, his greatest pleasure was time spent with his family: his wife Charlotte, and their 3 children, Karen (pediatrician in New York City), Jordan (secondary school teacher in New York City), and David (restaurateur in Toronto). Many weekends and holidays were spent at the family cottage on Lake Simcoe, where Bob was constantly "adding or fixing something up." It was here that Charlotte and Bob had planned to retire. Bob and his wife were both experienced and enthusiastic world travelers. Bob was widely known for his love of good food, odd food, and fine restaurants. He was a formidable amateur chef.

Bob was a superb surgeon, teacher, and mentor. He took pride in his craftsmanship and he derived great satisfaction from the fellowship and teamwork he fostered at his own institution and in the cooperative multicenter clinical trials he supported. He left the credit for others. Those of us who had the privilege of working closely with Bob Ginsberg over a number of years have lost a distinguished colleague, an unwavering ally, and dear, irreplaceable friend.

F. Griffith Pearson, MD, Bsc Med, FRCS(Can), FACS
Professor of Surgery Emeritus
Division of Thoracic Surgery
Department of Surgery
University Health Network - Toronto
General Hospital
University of Toronto, 200 Elizabeth Street
Toronto, Ontario M5G 2C4, Canada

Joel David Cooper, MD
Professor of Surgery
Division of Thoracic Surgery
Department of Surgery
Hospital of the University of Pennsylvania
University of Pennsylvania School of Medicine
3400 Spruce Street, 6 White
Philadelphia, PA 19104, USA

E-mail address:
fgpearson@hotmail.com (F.G. Pearson)

Lung Cancer Prevention, Epidemiology, and Public Health

Tobacco Smoking
The Leading Cause of Preventable Disease Worldwide

Jonathan M. Samet, MD, MS

KEYWORDS

- Tobacco smoking • Lung cancer • Tobacco control

KEY POINTS

- Tobacco smoke is a rich and toxic mixture that causes disease through multiple mechanisms.
- The burden of disease caused by smoking is enormous, with more than 6 million premature deaths annually.
- To be effective, a package of tobacco-control measures is needed. Experience in high-income countries shows that tobacco control can be effective in reducing smoking.

INTRODUCTION

An overview of tobacco smoking represents an essential starting point for an issue on lung cancer. In the absence of tobacco smoking, there would be far fewer cases of lung cancer worldwide, and this typically fatal malignancy would be relatively uncommon and not the leading cause of cancer death in the world.[1] The increasing rate of lung cancer across the twentieth century and continuing into the twenty-first reflects the antecedent increase in cigarette smoking, initially in higher-income countries, particularly in North America and Europe, driven by the aggressive marketing and promotion of cigarettes by the tobacco industry. Lung cancer is not the only disease to be increased by smoking; the list includes many other cancers, cardiovascular disease, chronic obstructive pulmonary disease (COPD), and others. Not surprisingly, tobacco use is the leading cause of preventable death worldwide.[2]

This article, written for this tribute volume for Robert J. Ginsberg, MD FRCS(C), appropriately covers tobacco smoking including the profile of smoking worldwide, the mechanisms whereby it causes disease, and the resulting burden of disease. Dr Ginsberg contributed greatly to advancing the treatment of lung cancer. Another Canadian thoracic surgeon, Dr Evarts A. Graham, also made seminal contributions related to lung cancer and also died of this disease. Graham performed the first pneumonectomy for lung cancer in 1933 and then later teamed with a medical student, Ernst Wynder, at Washington University in St Louis, in performing one of the earliest case-control studies of smoking and lung cancer, published in 1950.[3] Since then, of course, numerous studies have linked smoking to lung cancer, and firm conclusions were reached 50 years ago that smoking causes lung cancer.[4]

This article begins with a brief historical overview of the rise of smoking and its identification as a cause of disease. Patterns of tobacco use worldwide are described, based on the most recent findings from the Global Adult Tobacco Survey (GATS) conducted by the World Health Organization (WHO) and the US Centers for Disease Control and Prevention, in collaboration with nations around the world.[5] Next, the mechanisms whereby smoking causes disease and the resulting disease burden are described. Lastly,

Department of Preventive Medicine, Keck School of Medicine, USC Institute for Global Health, University of Southern California, 2001 North Soto Street, Suite 330A, MC9239, Los Angeles, CA 90089-9239, USA
E-mail address: jsamet@med.usc.edu

Thorac Surg Clin 23 (2013) 103–112
http://dx.doi.org/10.1016/j.thorsurg.2013.01.009
1547-4127/13/$ – see front matter © 2013 Elsevier Inc. All rights reserved.

a snapshot is given of global efforts in tobacco control, with emphasis on the WHO's Framework Convention on Tobacco Control (FCTC).

HISTORICAL BACKGROUND

There is now an extensive body of literature describing the history of tobacco use, the rise of the tobacco industry, and the tactics that it used to sell its lethal products. This section offers a brief summary. For those wanting further information, 3 excellent books provide in-depth coverage: *Ashes to Ashes* by Richard Kluger (1996), *The Cigarette Century: The Rise, Fall, and Deadly Persistence of the Product That Defined America* by Allen Brandt,[6] and, most recently, *The Golden Holocaust* by Robert Proctor, which draws heavily on the industry documents.[7] Millions of pages of industry documents are available at the University of California, San Francisco, Legacy Tobacco Documents Library (http://legacy.library.ucsf.edu/).

Tobacco, a New World plant, was brought back to Europe by Columbus. In the Americas, the Native Americans used tobacco primarily for ceremonial and religious purposes, and it was apparently not used in a regular and potentially addictive way. After Columbus brought tobacco to Europe it was soon widely used, although largely in the form of snuff and pipe tobacco. Cigarettes were initially hand-rolled; in fact, Philip Morris was a tobacconist in London in the 1800s who made and sold cigarettes in his shop. The modern tobacco industry dates to the late 1800s, originating with the Duke family in the United States of North Carolina. James B. Duke purchased the rights to use the cigarette-making machine, developed by Bonsack, and quickly expanded the American Tobacco Company such that it sold most of the cigarettes consumed in the US by the start of the twentieth century. The highly successful strategies used by the industry to aggressively expand sales began at that time.[4,6,7] Because of its monopoly, the American Tobacco Company was dissolved under the US Sherman Antitrust Act in 1911.

In the United States cigarette smoking increased rapidly among men, beginning in the early twentieth century, and rose about 20 years later among women (**Fig. 1**). During these decades, smoking was generally considered to not adversely affect health, and the advertising and marketing campaigns of the tobacco industry were highly successful, such that by 1960 a majority of males in the United States and some other countries were cigarette smokers. Marketing targeted at women also was successful. Brands such as Virginia Slims were advertised with a marketing strategy targeting women, pushing the theme of "slimness" as being associated with cigarette smoking.[6,7]

By the mid-twentieth century, noncommunicable diseases (particularly lung cancer and coronary heart disease) were rapidly increasing, and investigations began on the causes of the increases. Earlier, clinical case reports and case series had

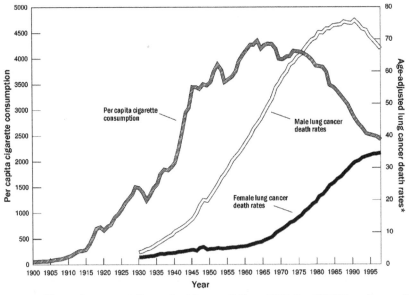

Fig. 1. Tobacco use and lung cancer mortality, United States, 1900 to 1997. Per 100,000 and age-adjusted to 1970 United States standard population. (*From* Hecht SS, Samet JM. Cigarette smoking. In: Rom WM, editor. Environmental and occupational medicine. 4th edition. Philadelphia: Wolters Kluwer/Lippincott Williams & Wilkins; 2007. p. 1521–51; with permission.)

called attention to the likely role of smoking and chewing tobacco as a cause of cancer. In their 1939 report on 7 cases of lung cancer treated with pneumonectomy, the surgeons Ochsner and De-Bakey commented on the possible role of smoking as a cause of lung cancer.[8] Based on a follow-up of families living in Baltimore in 1938, Pearl[9] reported that smokers did not live as long as nonsmokers.

More formal investigations, primarily using epidemiologic approaches and directed particularly at lung cancer and coronary heart disease, were initiated in the late 1940s and 1950s. Key initial observations that linked disease to smoking were made in epidemiologic studies performed to understand the changing patterns of disease, particularly the increase in lung cancer, coronary heart disease and stroke, and COPD, including chronic bronchitis and emphysema. There have been many landmark investigations of smoking and disease, including the case-control studies of lung cancer published as early as the 1940s and the cohort studies such as the Framingham study,[10] the British Physicians Study,[11] and the studies initiated by the American Cancer Society, with 2 involving 1 million Americans each.[12] These initial observations sparked complementary

laboratory studies on the mechanisms whereby tobacco smoking causes disease. The multidisciplinary approach to research on tobacco has been key in linking smoking to various diseases, and the observational evidence has been supported with an understanding of the mechanisms whereby smoking causes disease. By 1953, for example, Wynder and colleagues[13] had shown that painting the shaved skin of mice with cigarette-smoke condensate caused tumors. The 2010 report of the Surgeon General needed 700 pages to summarize the evidence on how smoking causes disease.[14]

By the late 1950s and early 1960s, the mounting evidence received formal review and evaluation by government committees, leading to definitive conclusions in the early 1960s. In the United Kingdom, the 1962 report of the Royal College of Physicians[15] concluded that smoking was a cause of lung cancer and bronchitis, and a contributing factor to coronary heart disease. In the United States, the 1964 landmark report of the Advisory Committee to the Surgeon General concluded that smoking was a cause of lung cancer in men and of chronic bronchitis.[16] Subsequent reports have led to a far longer list of diseases caused by smoking (**Fig. 2**).

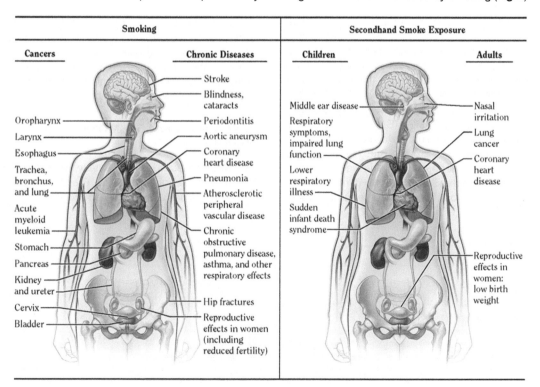

Fig. 2. Diseases caused by active smoking and by exposure to second-hand smoke. (*From* US Department of Health and Human Services. How tobacco smoke causes disease: the biology and behavioral basis for smoking-attributable disease. A report of the Surgeon General. Atlanta (GA): US Department of Health and Human Services, Centers for Disease Control and Prevention, National Center for Chronic Disease Prevention and Health Promotion, Office on Smoking and Health; 2010.)

The issue of passive smoking (ie, the inhalation of tobacco smoke from the smoking of others by nonsmokers) and health has a briefer history. Before the first epidemiologic studies in the late 1960s there had been scattered case reports, the Nazis had campaigned against smoking in public, and one German physician, Fritz Lickint, used the term "passive smoking" in his 1939 book.[17] In the 1960s the initial investigations focused on parental smoking and lower respiratory illnesses in infants; studies of lung function and respiratory symptoms in children soon followed.[18] The 1972 report of the Surgeon General was the first to call attention to passive smoking, referring to "public exposure to air pollution from tobacco smoke."[19] The first major studies on passive smoking and lung cancer in nonsmokers were reported in 1981[20,21] and by 1986 the evidence supported a conclusion that passive smoking was a cause of lung cancer in nonsmokers.[22–24] The list of diseases caused by passive smoking subsequently lengthened as well (see **Fig. 2**).

PATTERNS OF TOBACCO USE WORLDWIDE

Surveillance of causes is fundamental to disease control. In many countries, the prevalence of smoking is tracked regularly by performing surveys, typically of schoolchildren and general population samples. In the United States, for example, data are collected in multiple surveys such as the National Health Interview Survey (NHIS), the National Health and Nutrition Examination Survey (NHANES), and the Behavioral Risk Factor Surveillance System (BRFSS). The resulting data support the evaluation of interventions and the identification of groups with higher rates of smoking for tobacco-control initiatives.

Globally, a surveillance system is now in place as well, the Global Tobacco Surveillance System (GTSS), which includes a component directed at youth, the Global Youth Tobacco Survey (GYTS), and one directed at adults, the GATS. The first global report based on the GATS was published in 2012, drawing on findings from 14 low-income and middle-income countries and from the United States and the United Kingdom.[5] The findings showed a wide range of smoking prevalence among the 16 countries and far higher rates of smoking among men than women, although smoking among females approached that in males in several countries (**Fig. 3**). The percentages of former smokers also varied widely. In the United Kingdom and the United States, the majority of those who had ever smoked were former smokers at the time of the survey; by contrast, only 12% of ever smokers were former smokers in China and India. In total these GATS data, which covered most of the high-burden countries, documented tobacco use among about 850 million people. In 1999, the World Bank provided an estimate of about 1.1 billion smokers worldwide.[25]

The GYTS data collected from 13- to 15-year-olds in schools in most countries show that youth continue to smoke worldwide.[26] Even in this young age range smoking rates reach as high as 50%, and in many countries boys and girls are smoking with equal frequency. With diversification of the array of tobacco products available (eg, flavored cigars, electronic cigarettes, and snus), there is concern that these products will become a "gateway" to tobacco smoking as youth experiment with nicotine-containing products.

HOW DOES TOBACCO SMOKE CAUSE DISEASE?

Worldwide tobacco is used in many forms, classifiable as smoked or smokeless. There are several hundred million users of products other than

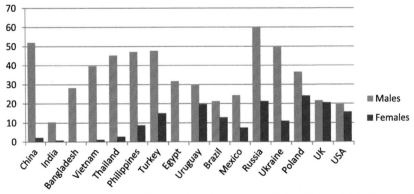

Fig. 3. Prevalence of current cigarette smoking in the 16 Countries of the Global Adult Tobacco Survey, adults 15+ years, 2008 to 2010. (*Data from* Giovino GA, Mirza SA, Samet JM, et al. Tobacco use in 16 countries with 4 billion population: the GATS collaborative group. Lancet 2012;380(9842):668–79.)

cigarettes and in some groups, for example women in India, various oral, smokeless products are much more widely used than either cigarettes or bidis (a locally made product comprising a hand-rolled cigarette with a leaf wrapper). These products also cause cancer and other health problems, although they do not increase the risk of lung cancer.

Tobacco smoke from manufactured cigarettes is generated by the burning of a complex organic material, tobacco, along with the various additives and paper, at a very high temperature.[14] This combustion produces an estimated 7000 compounds in the gaseous and particulate phases of the smoke, including numerous toxic components that can cause injury through inflammation and irritation, asphyxiation, carcinogenesis, and other mechanisms. Many of these compounds are well-known toxins, for example, benzene (a leukemogen), formaldehyde (an irritant and carcinogen), benzo[a]pyrene (a carcinogen), carbon monoxide and cyanide (asphyxiants), acrolein (an irritant), and polonium (a radioactive carcinogen). Cigarette smoke also contains metals and pesticides.

Active smokers inhale mainstream smoke (MS), the smoke drawn directly through the cigarette. This fresh smoke is inhaled without dilution, thus giving the smoker high doses of tobacco-smoke components. Typically a smoker takes 10 to 12 puffs from each cigarette, or about 240 puffs per day for smokers of 1 pack (20 cigarettes) daily. This pattern of smoking, if sustained for decades, results in remarkably high cumulative doses of toxic components in smoke.

Passive smokers (ie, nonactive smokers) inhale smoke that is often referred to as second-hand tobacco smoke (SHS), comprising a mixture of mostly side-stream smoke (SS) given off by the smoldering cigarette and some exhaled MS. SHS is diluted as the SS and exhaled MS mix with air and, consequently, concentrations of tobacco-smoke components in SHS are well below the levels in MS inhaled by the active smoker. Nonetheless, there are qualitative similarities between MS and SHS that support a generalization from the findings on the health risks of active smoking to those of passive smoking.[18,22] Recently, the term third-hand smoke has been used to refer to surface-deposited tobacco-smoke components, which persist in indoor environments and undergo chemical transformations.[27]

The MS inhaled by the smoker is an aerosol containing about 1×10^{10} small-diameter particles per milliliter.[28] Particles in this size range penetrate to the deepest portion of the lungs, reaching the bronchioles and the alveoli, where the majority is deposited. Once deposited, they release components, including nicotine, which cross the lung's

epithelium and enter the circulation. A variety of tobacco-smoke compounds and metabolites, including nicotine and cotinine, can be measured as biomarkers in blood and other biological matrices. Reactive gases in tobacco smoke, such as formaldehyde, are removed in the upper airways, whereas insoluble and unreactive gases, such as carbon monoxide, reach the alveoli where they diffuse into the bloodstream.

For decades, the yields of several components of tobacco smoke ("tar," carbon monoxide, and nicotine) have been measured with a machine, using a standard test protocol. During this test the smoke is separated into a vapor phase and a particulate phase, based on passage of the smoke through a filter. This filter retains 99.7% of particles with diameters of 0.3 μm and greater, and the retained material is referred to as "tar." The standardized machine-smoking conditions do not reflect the ways that smokers actually smoke, particularly for those newer cigarettes intended to have lower yields when assayed by a smoking machine and marketed with an implicit message of lowered risk to health. Smokers puff more deeply with such products than the machine settings, and the machine yields have little relationship to yields obtained by smokers. In several countries yields are no longer allowed to be shown on packages.

Both active and passive smokers absorb tobacco-smoke components through the lung's airways and alveoli and the mucosal surfaces of the upper airway, and many of these components then enter into the circulation and are distributed generally. There is also uptake of components, such as benzo[a]pyrene, directly into the cells that line the upper airway and the lung's airways. Some of the components undergo metabolic transformation into their active forms, and some evidence now indicates that metabolism-determining genes may affect susceptibility to tobacco smoke.[29] The genitourinary system is exposed to toxins in tobacco smoke through the excretion of compounds in the urine, including carcinogens. The gastrointestinal tract is exposed through direct deposition of smoke in the upper airway and the clearance of smoke-containing mucus from the trachea through the glottis into the esophagus. Not surprisingly, tobacco smoking has proved to be a multisystem cause of disease (see **Fig. 2**).

There is a substantial scientific literature on the mechanisms whereby complex tobacco-smoke exposure causes disease.[14] This body of research includes characterization of the many components in smoke, some having well-established toxicity. The toxicity of smoke has been studied by exposing animals to tobacco smoke and smoke condensate, in cellular and other laboratory systems for evaluating toxicity, and by assessing smokers for evidence of injury by tobacco smoke, using biomarkers such as tissue changes and levels of damaging enzymes and cytokines. This research points to several critical mechanisms, including oxidative injury and inflammation involved in the causation of lung disease and cardiovascular disease, increased blood coagulability that contributes to cardiovascular disease, multiple effects on the immune system that enhance the risk for infectious diseases, and carcinogenesis.

Fig. 4 provides a general schema for the causation of cancer by the carcinogens in tobacco smoke. There are both specific and nonspecific pathways through which smoking is thought to cause cancer. **Fig. 4** highlights the multiple processes that lead to uncontrolled cell growth and malignancy, and the multiple points in these processes at which tobacco-smoke components contribute to carcinogenesis. Emphasis has been given to DNA binding and mutations, but research also shows that tobacco smoke contributes to increased risk of cancer through epigenetic mechanisms.[14] For many tobacco-smoke carcinogens metabolic activation is needed, and genetic determinants of rates of activation may modify the risk of cancer in smokers.[14] Tobacco-specific carcinogens form adducts and lead to mutations in oncogenes and tumor-suppressor genes. Smoking has been found to specifically increase the frequency of DNA adducts of cigarette-smoke carcinogens such as benzo[a]pyrene and tobacco-specific nitrosamines in the lung and other organs, and to cause DNA damage and mutations in key oncogenes and tumor-suppressor genes. Recent research is more specifically characterizing the pathways through which smoking causes cancer.[14]

THE BURDEN OF SMOKING-CAUSED DISEASE

Active and passive smoking are causally associated with risk for numerous diseases and other adverse effects (see **Fig. 2**). **Table 1** provides estimates of risk for mortality from major causes of death associated with smoking. The estimates come from 2 epidemiologic studies performed by the American Cancer Society: Cancer Prevention Study (CPS) I (1959–1965) and CPS II (1982–1988). These studies document the strength of smoking as a cause of multiple diseases, the higher risks in men compared with women, and the rising risks in women, comparing the later with the earlier study. Risks for most smoking-caused diseases increase with the duration of smoking and the numbers of cigarettes smoked; the rising risks in women in the second study reflect the earlier onset of smoking and the heavier smoking of women in more recent birth cohorts.

These risks translate into a high burden of smoking-caused premature mortality and morbidity. As smoking became recognized as a substantial cause of disease, estimates were made of its contribution to the burden of morbidity and

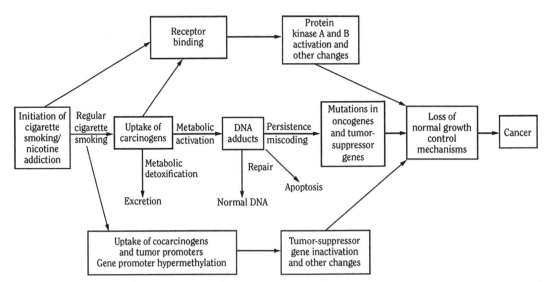

Fig. 4. From cigarette smoking to cancer through carcinogens in tobacco smoke. (*From* US Department of Health and Human Services. How tobacco smoke causes disease: the biology and behavioral basis for smoking-attributable disease. A report of the Surgeon General. Atlanta (GA): US Department of Health and Human Services, Centers for Disease Control and Prevention, National Center for Chronic Disease Prevention and Health Promotion, Office on Smoking and Health; 2010.)

Table 1
Age-adjusted relative risks of death from smoking-related diseases from the Cancer Prevention Study (CPS) I and CPS II

Disease Category (ICD-9 Code)	CPS I (1959–1965)				CPS II (1982–1988)			
	Males		Females		Males		Females	
	CS	FS	CS	FS	CS	FS	CS	FS
Neoplasms								
Lip, oral cavity, pharynx (140–149)	6.3	2.7	2.0	1.9	10.9	3.4	5.1	2.3
Esophagus (150)	3.6	1.3	1.9	2.2	6.8	4.5	7.8	2.8
Stomach (151)	1.8	1.7	1.0	1.0	2.0	1.5	1.4	1.3
Pancreas (157)	2.3	1.3	1.4	1.4	2.3	1.2	2.3	1.6
Larynx (161)	10.0	8.6	3.8	3.1	14.6	6.3	13.0	5.2
Trachea, bronchus, lung (162)	11.4	5.0	2.7	2.6	23.3	8.7	12.7	4.5
Cervix uteri (180)	—	—	1.1	1.3	—	—	1.6	1.1
Urinary bladder (188)	2.9	1.8	2.9	2.3	3.3	2.1	2.2	1.9
Kidney, other urinary (189)	1.8	1.8	1.4	1.5	2.7	1.7	1.3	1.1
Acute myeloid leukemia (204–208)	1.6	1.6	1.0	1.0	1.9	1.3	1.1	1.4
Cardiovascular diseases								
Ischemic heart disease (410–414)								
Age 35–64 y	2.3	1.6	1.8	1.7	2.8	1.6	3.1	1.3
Age ≥65 y	1.4	1.3	1.2	1.3	1.5	1.2	1.6	1.2
Other heart disease (390–398, 415–417, 420–429)	1.4	1.1	1.1	1.4	1.8	1.2	1.5	1.1
Cerebrovascular disease (430–438)								
Age 35–64 y	1.8	1.0	1.9	1.8	3.3	1.0	4.0	1.3
Age ≥65 y	1.2	1.0	1.0	1.1	1.6	1.0	1.5	1.0
Atherosclerosis (440)	3.1	2.0	1.9	1.5	2.4	1.3	1.8	1.0
Aortic aneurysm (441)	4.1	2.4	4.6	3.7	6.2	3.1	7.1	2.1
Other arterial disease (442–448)	3.1	2.0	1.9	1.5	2.1	1.0	2.2	1.1
Respiratory diseases								
Pneumonia, influenza (480–487)	1.8	1.6	1.0	1.0	1.8	1.4	2.2	1.1
Bronchitis, emphysema (490–492)	8.8	10.2	5.9	5.9	17.1	15.6	12.0	11.8
Chronic airways obstruction (496)	5.5	9.6	5.1	5.3	10.6	6.8	13.1	6.8
Perinatal conditions								
Short gestation/low birth weight (765)	—	—	1.8	—	—	—	1.8	—
Respiratory distress syndrome (769)	—	—	1.8	—	—	—	1.3	—
Other respiratory conditions in newborns (770)	—	—	1.8	—	—	—	1.4	—
Sudden infant death syndrome (798.0)	—	—	1.5	—	—	—	2.3	—

Results are presented for persons 35 years or older unless otherwise indicated.
Abbreviations: CS, current smokers; FS, former smokers; ICD-9, International Classification of Diseases, 9th revision.

mortality within specific countries and then globally. A variety of methods have been developed for this purpose, all making a comparison between the existing burden of disease and that which would have occurred in the absence of smoking.[30,31] The estimates of attributable deaths and the costs associated with active and passive smoking are enormous, and have offered a strong rationale for aggressive tobacco control.

Worldwide, the adverse health consequences of tobacco use make it the world's leading cause of preventable morbidity and mortality. Estimates made for 2015 by the WHO project an estimated mortality burden of more than 6 million deaths per year.[2] Although deaths from lung cancer exceed 1 million, the largest contributors are cardiovascular and respiratory diseases. By region, tobacco annually kills more than 1 million in East Asia and the Pacific; 897,000 in Europe and Central Asia; 250,000 in Latin America; 121,000 in the Middle East and North Africa; 879,000 in South Asia; and 135,000 in sub-Saharan Africa. In the future, without effective tobacco control the burden will increase greatly in the low-income and middle-income countries. By 2025, China could experience 2 million tobacco-related deaths annually.[32]

There is also a substantial burden of disease globally from SHS exposure. In 2004, an estimated 40% of children, 33% of men, and 35% of women were exposed to SHS. Combining these exposure figures with the risks for diseases caused by SHS produced the following estimates of deaths worldwide: 379,000 from ischemic heart disease, 165,000 from lower respiratory infections, 36,900 from asthma, and 21,400 from lung cancer; 603,000 deaths in total.[33]

THE GLOBAL EFFORT IN TOBACCO CONTROL

Tobacco control has had a lengthy evolution that has been closely linked to the evolution of the evidence on the health effects of active and passive smoking.[34] The initial findings on lung cancer were followed by efforts to educate the public about the risks of smoking, with the expectation that they would stop. In the United States, the 1964 Surgeon General's report led to pack warnings and the banning of tobacco advertising on television. The finding that passive smoking caused lung cancer motivated the implementation of smoking bans in public places and workplaces, and initiated a change in social norms around smoking that moved smoking from being viewed as acceptable to unacceptable. As noted by Surgeon General Koop in the preface to the 1986 report, "the right of smokers to smoke ends where their behavior affects the health and well-being of others…" Approaches to smoking cessation became more effective when nicotine was identified as addictive, nicotine replacement therapy and other pharmacologic approaches were introduced, and stronger behavioral approaches were advanced. Research and experience also documented the need to raise taxes, to use aggressive countermarketing to denormalize smoking, and to protect children from the reach of the tobacco industry. Most importantly, decades of evidence shows that a multicomponent strategy is needed that both targets nonsmokers to keep them from smoking and encourages and supports smokers to quit. The success of an aggressive multifaceted strategy in New York City is exemplary.[35]

Many nations have implemented tobacco-control programs. Most importantly there is now the FCTC, ratified and in force for most nations of the world, although not for the United States and Indonesia. Many universal elements of national tobacco-control policy are core provisions of the FCTC. Key provisions include a comprehensive ban on tobacco advertising, promotion, and sponsorship; a ban on misleading descriptors such as "light"; and a mandate to place rotating warnings that cover at least 30% of tobacco packaging and encouragement for even larger, graphic warnings. The FCTC also urges countries to implement smoke-free workplace laws, address tobacco smuggling, and increase tobacco taxes. The FCTC has now been in place for more than 5 years, and progress is slowly being made in implementing its components.[36]

Building on the FCTC process, the WHO released its first Report on Control of the Tobacco Epidemic, entitled MPOWER, in 2008.[37] MPOWER is a comprehensive tobacco-control strategy intended to provide a programmatic counterpart to the FCTC. MPOWER includes 6 key tobacco-control measures including Monitoring the epidemic, Protecting nonsmokers from exposure to SHS, Warning smokers of the health effects of smoking with strong, effective health warnings, Enforcing advertising bans, and Raising the price of tobacco products. The WHO is tracking implementation of MPOWER and coverage of the world's population by its provisions. To date its reach is still limited, although increasing coverage of the world's population by its elements can be anticipated.[38] Fortunately, global tobacco control has benefited greatly from funding from the Bloomberg Family Foundation and the Bill and Melinda Gates Foundation, first made available in 2007 and now slated to continue through 2016. These funds have supported capacity building in tobacco control, policy advocacy, regulation, and surveillance.

SUMMARY

Tobacco smoking is the world's leading cause of avoidable premature mortality, reflecting the potent toxicity of tobacco smoke inhaled by smokers for decades. Lung cancer was a sentinel of the emergence of the still persisting epidemic of tobacco-caused disease. Fortunately, smoking has declined in many countries, particularly the high-income countries, but the low-income and middle-income countries remain at risk because of the aggressive tactics of the multinational tobacco companies. The FCTC is a critical factor in countering these tactics, and is working toward ending the tragic global epidemic of tobacco smoking.

REFERENCES

1. Jemal A, Bray F, Center MM, et al. Global cancer statistics. CA Cancer J Clin 2011;61(2):69–90.
2. Mathers CD, Loncar D. Projections of global mortality and burden of disease from 2002 to 2030. PLoS Med 2006;3(11):e442.
3. Horn L, Johnson DH, Evarts A. Graham and the first pneumonectomy for lung cancer. J Clin Oncol 2008; 26(19):3268–75.
4. Kluger R. Ashes to ashes: America's hundred-year cigarette war, the public health, and the unabashed triumph of Philip Morris. New York: Alfred A. Knopf; 1996.
5. Giovino GA, Mirza SA, Samet JM, et al. Tobacco use in 16 Countries with 4 billion population: the GATS collaborative group. Lancet 2012;380(9842):668–79.
6. Brandt AM. The cigarette century: the rise, fall, and deadly persistence of the product that defined America. New York: Basic Books; 2007.
7. Proctor R. Golden holocaust: origins of the cigarette catastrophe and the case for abolition. Berkeley (CA): University of California Press; 2011.
8. Ochsner M, DeBakey M. Primary pulmonary malignancy. Treatment by total pneumonectomy; analyses of 79 collected cases and presentation of 7 personal cases. Surg Gynecol Obstet 1939;68:435–51.
9. Pearl R. Tobacco smoking and longevity. Science 1938;87(2253):216–7.
10. Dawber TR. The Framingham study. The epidemiology of atherosclerotic disease. Cambridge (MA): Harvard University Press; 1980.
11. Doll R, Hill AB. The mortality of doctors in relation to their smoking habits. A preliminary report. Br Med J 1954;1:1451–5.
12. U.S. Department of Health Human Services, Public Health Service, National Cancer Institute. Changes in cigarette-related disease risks and their implication for prevention and control. In: Burns DM, Garfinkel L, Samet JM, editors. Bethesda (MD): U.S. Government Printing Office; 1997 (NIH Publication No. 97–4213).
13. Wynder EL, Graham EA, Croninger AB. Experimental production of carcinoma with cigarette tar. Cancer Res 1953;13:855–64.
14. U.S. Department of Health and Human Services. How tobacco smoke causes disease: the biology and behavioral basis for smoking-attributable disease. A report of the Surgeon General. Atlanta (GA): U.S. Department of Health and Human Services, Centers for Disease Control and Prevention, National Center for Chronic Disease Prevention and Health Promotion, Office on Smoking and Health; 2010.
15. Royal College of Physicians of London. Smoking and health. Summary of a report of the Royal College of Physicians of London on smoking in relation to cancer of the lung and other diseases. London: Pitman Medical Publishing Co, LTD; 1962.
16. U.S. Department of Health Education and Welfare. Smoking and health. Report of the Advisory Committee to the Surgeon General. Washington, DC: U.S. Government Printing Office; 1964. DHEW Publication No. [PHS] 1103.
17. Proctor RN. Cancer wars. How politics shapes what we know and don't know about cancer. New York: Basic Books; 1995.
18. U.S. Department of Health and Human Services. The health consequences of involuntary exposure to tobacco smoke. A report of the Surgeon General. Atlanta (GA): U.S. Department of Health and Human Services, Centers for Disease Control and Prevention, Coordinating Center for Health Promotion, National Center for Chronic Disease Prevention and Health Promotion, Office on Smoking and Health; 2006.
19. U.S. Department of Health Education Welfare. The health consequences of smoking. A report of the Surgeon General. Atlanta (GA): U.S. Government Printing Office; 1972.
20. Hirayama T. Non-smoking wives of heavy smokers have a higher risk of lung cancer: a study from Japan. Br Med J (Clin Res Ed) 1981;282(6259):183–5.
21. Trichopoulos D, Kalandidi A, Sparros L, et al. Lung cancer and passive smoking. Int J Cancer 1981; 27(1):1–4.
22. U.S. Department of Health and Human Services. The health consequences of involuntary smoking. A report of the Surgeon General. Washington, DC: U.S. Department of Health and Human Services, Public Health Service, Office on Smoking and Health; 1986. 32676. DHHS Publication No. (CDC) 87–8398.
23. National Research Council, Committee on Passive Smoking. Environmental tobacco smoke: measuring exposures and assessing health effects. Washington, DC: National Academy Press; 1986. 32676.
24. International Agency for Research on Cancer. IARC monographs on the evaluation of the carcinogenic risk of chemicals to humans: tobacco smoking. Lyon (France): World Health Organization; 1986. IARC; -32676.
25. Jha P, Chaloupka FJ. Curbing the epidemic: governments and the economics of tobacco control. Washington, DC: World Bank; 1999.
26. Eriksen M, Mackay J, Ross H. The tobacco atlas. 4th edition. Atlanta (GA): American Cancer Society, World Lung Foundation; 2012.
27. Matt GE, Quintana PJ, Destaillats H, et al. Thirdhand tobacco smoke: emerging evidence and arguments for a multidisciplinary research agenda. Environ Health Perspect 2011;119(9):1218–26.
28. Hoffmann D, Hecht SS, Cooper CS, et al. Advances in tobacco carcinogenesis. Handbook of experimental pharmacology. Heidelberg (Germany): Springer-Verlag; 1990. p. 63–102.
29. International Agency for Research on Cancer. Tobacco smoke and involuntary smoking. IARC

monograph 83. Lyon (France): International Agency for Research on Cancer; 2004.

30. U.S. Department of Health and Human Services. The health consequences of smoking. A report of the Surgeon General. Atlanta (GA): U.S. Department of Health and Human Services, Centers for Disease Control and Prevention, National Center for Chronic Disease Prevention and Health Promotion, Office on Smoking and Health; 2004.

31. Peto R, Lopez AD, Boreham J, et al. Mortality from tobacco in developed countries: indirect estimation from national vital statistics. Lancet 1992;339(8804): 1268–78.

32. Jha P. Avoidable global cancer deaths and total deaths from smoking. Nat Rev Cancer 2009;9(9): 655–64.

33. Oberg M, Jaakkola MS, Woodward A, et al. World-wide burden of disease from exposure to second-hand smoke: a retrospective analysis of data from 192 countries. Lancet 2011;377(9760):139–46.

34. Wipfli H, Samet JM. Global economic and health benefits of tobacco control: part 2. Clin Pharmacol Ther 2009;86(3):272–80.

35. Frieden TR, Mostashari F, Kerker BD, et al. Adult tobacco use levels after intensive tobacco control measures: New York, 2002-2003. Am J Public Health 2005;95(6):1016–23.

36. Samet JM, Wipfli HL. Globe still in grip of addiction. Nature 2010;463(7284):1020–1.

37. World Health Organization. WHO report on the global tobacco epidemic, 2008: the MPOWER package. Geneva (Switzerland): World Health Organization; 2008.

38. World Health Organization. WHO report on the global tobacco epidemic, 2011: Warning about the dangers of tobacco. Geneva (Switzerland): World Health Organization; 2011.

The Changing Epidemic of Lung Cancer and Occupational and Environmental Risk Factors

Carolyn Dresler, MD, MPA*

KEYWORDS

- Smoking • Changing histology • Gender differences

KEY POINTS

- Smoking is the key causative agent for most lung cancers globally; 70% occur in developing economies from growing tobacco use.
- Types of cigarettes can influence the changes seen in histology, with a shift being seen from squamous cell to more adenocarcinomas.
- As more women smoke around the world, more women are developing lung cancer and most of these are adenocarcinomas.
- There remain a substantial number of lung cancers that occur from environmental and industrial exposures.
- Stronger policies, based on well-established evidence, could dramatically decrease the number of deaths from lung cancer globally.

INTRODUCTION

Lung cancer has become the epidemic it is because of the tobacco industry and their marketing of progressively more addictive products. There are other causes of lung cancer, but they are responsible for a substantial minority of cases and do not seem to be an increasing cause of disease. To decrease the morbidity and mortality from lung cancer, one must first definitively address the manufacturing and marketing of a product that, when used as intended, kills.

The rates of lung cancer are variable and predictable based primarily on tobacco use prevalence, as discussed in Samet's article elsewhere in this issue. Currently, lung cancer is the leading cause of cancer death in most developed countries, where tobacco use prevalence has been highest for the longest. In the United States, Canada, most western European countries, and Australia, lung cancer is the leading cause of cancer death in men and increasingly so in women.

CHANGES IN LUNG CANCER RATES OVER TIME

In the United States, the death rate from lung cancer was less than 5 per 100,000 in 1919, and rose during the next 65 to 70 years. It was not until the early 1990s that the lung cancer death rate reached a plateau at more than 90 per 100,000 and subsequently began to decline for men (**Fig. 1**A).[1] Lung cancer death rate for women, however, continued to rise through the 1990s, and seem to be currently at a plateau or starting to decrease (see **Fig. 1**B). Western countries tend to have the highest age-standardized mortalities (2008): United States, 24.1; Canada, 24.9; Denmark, 30; Hungary, 26.2; United Kingdom, 20.8; and China, 18.3. In men, the age-standardized rates are much higher (2008): United States, 38.2; Canada, 26.2; Russia, 50.6; Poland, 61.8; Uruguay, 48.4; Croatia, 56.3; Korea, 37.9; Japan, 29.2; and China 39.6 (304,020 deaths per year in China alone).[2] The number of deaths in the lung cancer epidemic is appalling,

Tobacco Prevention and Cessation Network, Arkansas Department of Health, 4815 West Markham Street, Little Rock, AR 72205, USA
* 4419 Renn Street, Rockville, MD 20853-2747.
E-mail address: carolyn_dresler@ksg03.harvard.edu

Thorac Surg Clin 23 (2013) 113–122
http://dx.doi.org/10.1016/j.thorsurg.2013.01.015
1547-4127/13/$ – see front matter © 2013 Elsevier Inc. All rights reserved.

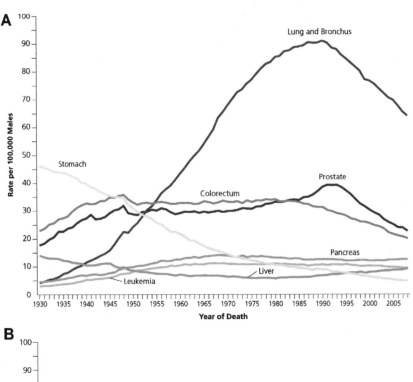

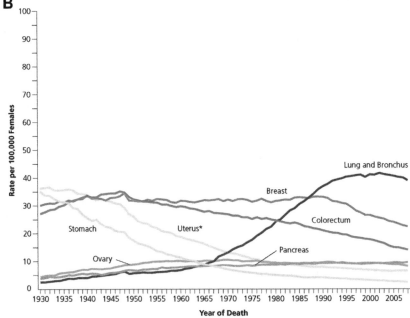

Fig. 1. (*A*) Cancer death rates in males, 1930 to 2008 (age adjusted to 2000 US standard population). (*B*) Trends in cancer death rates in women, 1930 to 2008 (age adjusted to 2000 US standard population). (*From* Siegel R, Maishadham D, Jemal A. Cancer statistics, 2012. CA Cancer J Clin 2012;62:10–29; with permission.)

especially when one considers the perspective that lung cancer takes more lives in the United States than breast, prostate, and colorectal cancers combined, and that most lung cancer deaths are preventable. Additionally, it is critical to examine the lung cancer epidemic in different racial or ethnic groups within a country, because their rates may vary significantly from the majority population. In the United States, Hispanics, who have historically smoked at much lower rates, also have lower rates of lung cancer (**Fig. 2**).[3] In Hispanic women in the United States, breast cancer remains the largest cause of cancer death, whereas in white women, lung cancer has been the leading cause of cancer death for more than a decade. These variations by gender, race, and ethnicity are usually predictable

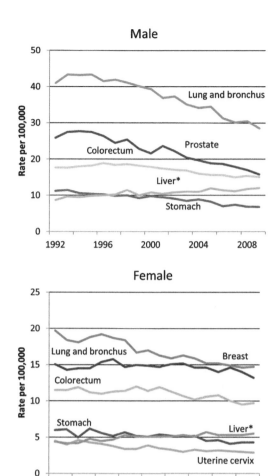

Male

(Graph: Rate per 100,000 vs year 1992–2008, lines labeled Lung and bronchus, Colorectum, Prostate, Liver, Stomach)*

Female

(Graph: Rate per 100,000 vs year 1992–2008, lines labeled Lung and bronchus, Breast, Colorectum, Stomach, Liver, Uterine cervix)*

Year of death

*Includes intrahepatic bile duct.

Fig. 2. Trends in cancer death rates in Hispanics in the United States, 1992 to 2009. (*From* Siegel R, Maishadham D, Jemal A. Cancer statistics for Hispanics/Latinos, 2012. CA Cancer J Clin 2012;62: 283–98; with permission.)

by examining their respective rates of smoking prevalence.

Unfortunately, lung cancer globally is often diagnosed at an advanced stage in older individuals who often harbor additional comorbidities, rendering most patients with lung cancer unresectable and incurable. The 5-year survival rate for all patients with lung cancer in the United States is a mere 16%, and this has only changed slightly from a 13% survival rate noted in 1975 to 1977.[4] In other countries, the variability in 5-year survival can be quite dramatic ranging from 4.6 in Malta, 8.2 in Scotland, 16.3 in Belgium, and 21 for females in South Korea.[5,6] Globally, the rates are lower in men at approximately 14%, and higher in women at around 18%.[7] Despite advances in many aspects of medical care, lung cancer cures

remain elusive. Therefore, the greatest potential for impact on reducing the number of lung cancer deaths on an epidemiologic level seems to be with control of risk and prevention, with advances in treatment of this deadly disease adding little.

Lopez and colleagues[8] developed a descriptive model that correlates the rise of the prevalence of cigarette smoking with the rise in the death rate caused by smoking-related illnesses with an approximately 20- to 25-year lag period (**Fig. 3**). This model becomes even stronger when gender is taken into account, because smoking rates vary significantly by gender through time. The Lopez model predicts that death rates caused by tobacco-induced illnesses occur at a rate of roughly 50% of the smoking rate given the 20- to 25-year lag (eg, for a population with a 60% smoking rate, 30% of the deaths 20 years later will be secondary to smoking). The model is then broken down into stages. Stage I represents the initiation of cigarettes into a society with low smoking rates, particularly in males, and very low death rates caused by smoking. Stage II demonstrates a rapid rise in smoking prevalence in men to its peak with an increase in the death rate. Smoking rates in women are just starting to increase with few resultant deaths. Stage III demonstrates a decline in smoking in men, but women still have a continued rise in smoking. The deaths in men continue to rise, following the 20- to 25-year lag from the peak in smoking, whereas the deaths in women are beginning to increase. In Stage IV there is a decrease in male and female smoking prevalence rates, with also declining death rates. Countries categorized in Stage 4 include Western Europe including the United Kingdom, Canada, and Australia. Examples in Stage 3 include Eastern and Southern Europe. Examples for Stage 2 are China, Southeast Asia, and Latin America and for Stage 1, Sub-Saharan Africa. **Fig. 4** demonstrates lung cancer mortality in several countries, and from it one can estimate the status of the preceding tobacco use epidemic.[9] GLOBOCAN is a tremendous resource provided by the International Agency for Research on Cancer (IARC) for incidence and mortality globally for all cancers, including lung cancer. For an interactive resource that provides graphs and maps with interactive incidence and mortality rates see http://globocan.iarc.fr/factsheets/cancers/lung. asp. **Fig. 4** demonstrates the trends in global lung cancer mortality rates in several countries.[2] Note the shape of the curves that describe the preceding smoking prevalence curves.

Not only is the tobacco industry responsible for the huge lung cancer epidemic that continues to grow in most parts of the world, but it is also

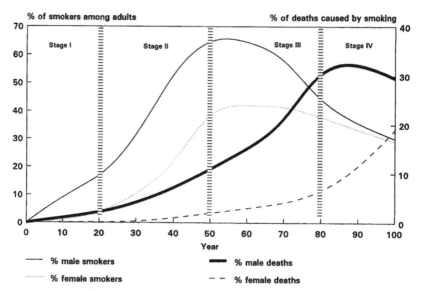

Fig. 3. The Lopez descriptive model associates changes in smoking rates and subsequent changes in death rates caused by smoking-related diseases. (*From* Lopez AD, Collishaw NE, Piha T. A descriptive model of the cigarette epidemic in developed countries. Tobacco Control 1994;3:242–7; with permission.)

probably responsible for the changing or variable histology seen in many countries. In the United States, the predominant histology in men had been squamous cell carcinoma until the early 1990s; in women adenocarcinoma has been the predominant cell type, with a dramatic rise in cancer deaths in the 1970s. Women in the United States began smoking significantly more in the 1950s, resulting in the increase in lung cancers seen a couple of decades later (see **Fig. 1**B).

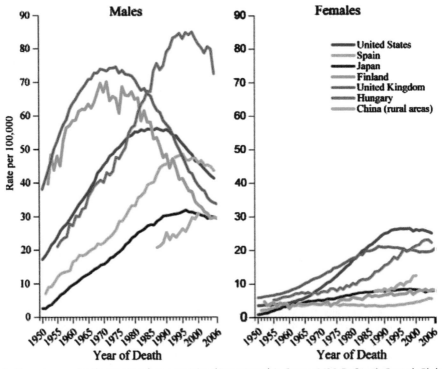

Fig. 4. Global lung cancer death rates in a few countries. (*From* Jemal A, Center MM, DeSantis C, et al. Global patterns of cancer incidence and mortality rates and trends. Cancer Epidemiol Biomarkers Prev 2010;19(8):1893–907; by permission from the American Association for Cancer Research.)

Coincident with this increased uptake in smoking by women was increased targeting of women by the tobacco industry, in addition to the changing construction of cigarettes. In the 1950s, increased reporting of the link between smoking and lung cancer was published and the tobacco industry began placing filters onto cigarettes creating the impression of a "safer" cigarette.[10,11] Women have predominantly smoked filtered cigarettes, because across the globe, filtered cigarettes were the ones marketed to women, and over time, the same is true for men (**Fig. 5**). At present, more than 90% of cigarettes smoked in the United States are cigarettes with filters.[12] This is important because filtered cigarettes result in more adenocarcinoma than squamous cell lung cancer.[13,14] The mechanism is still being determined in the transparent scientific literature, but the tobacco industry has highly engineered their product to deliver the addictive drug, nicotine, deep into the alveoli for the most rapid and efficient absorption. It is probably a combination of the type of filter and the engineering of the remainder of the cigarette, along with all of the chemicals added to the product that influences the resultant histology of the lung cancer. However, the result is similar around the world: as the tobacco epidemic progresses, more men and subsequently women smoke filtered cigarettes resulting in decreases of squamous cell and small cell lung cancer as the proportion of filtered cigarettes dominate the market with an increase in adenocarcinoma (**Fig. 6**).[15]

The association between rising and falling smoking rates and lung cancer rates is powerful, and if tobacco control could rapidly and significantly decrease smoking rates, lung cancer rates should more dramatically decrease. The predicted fall in lung cancer rates from decreased smoking has been supported by an observational study of lung cancer incidence in the San Francisco-Oakland area, and its change relative to enactment of the California tobacco control program.[16] In 1988, the California tobacco control program was initiated, and demonstrated a significant decrease in cigarette consumption over time with associated decreases in lung cancer, significantly different than lung cancer rates in the remainder of the United States.

ENVIRONMENTAL RISK FACTORS

Sources of air pollution have been implicated in lung cancer risk, but certain factors, such as living in an urban environment, are difficult to define and to quantify. It is also difficult to exclude the role of secondhand tobacco smoke (SHS). One of the earliest occupational risk studies showed that roofers exposed to coal tar fumes had a 50% increased lung cancer risk after 20 years, and 150% increased risk after 40 years, which could not be attributed to smoking status.[17] Cooking with coal, particularly in poorly ventilated rooms, has been attributed as a major cause of lung cancer in never-smoking women in China.[18] Data from 2008 demonstrate that the lung cancer death rate in women in China in women is approximately 18.3 per 100,000 compared with 24.1 per 100,000 in the United States. However, the number of deaths differs: 71,032 in the United States and

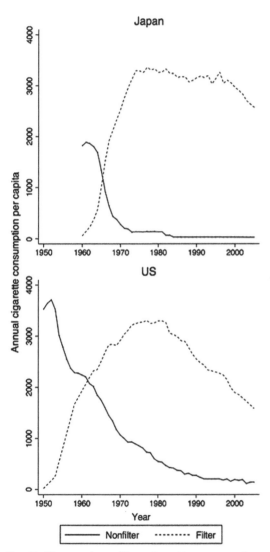

Fig. 5. Filter and nonfilter cigarette consumptions over time in Japan and the United States. (*From* Ito H, Matsuo K, Tanaka H, et al. Nonfilter and filter cigarette consumption and the incidence of lung cancer by histologic type in Japan and the United States: analysis of 30-year data from population-based cancer registries. Int J Cancer 2011;128(8):1918–28; with permission.)

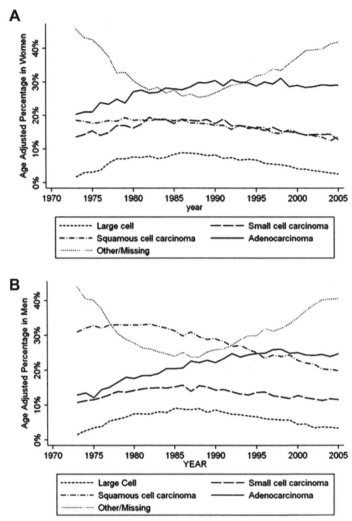

Fig. 6. Age-adjusted percentages of common histologic subtypes of lung cancer in (*A*) women and (*B*) men. (*From* Egleston BL, Meireles SI, Flieder DB, et al. Population-based trends in lung cancer incidence in women. Semin Oncol 2009;36:506–15; with permission.)

148,793 in China.[2] This lung cancer death rate in women in China occurs in an environment where women smoke approximately 3%, yet have high exposure to contamination from indoor coal or other cooking fumes.

A recent systematic review of biomass fuel and coal use was published. The odds ratio (OR) for exposure to coal smoke as a result of cooking was 1.83 (95% confidence interval [CI], 1.60–2.06) compared with biomass fuel with an OR of 1.50 (95% CI, 1.17–1.94). Women were at greater risk than men and effects were more prominent for the development of adenocarcinoma compared with squamous cell or unspecified cell types.[19]

An excellent recent review of respiratory cancers and occupational exposure has summarized several studies, including volumes 1 to 77

(1972–2001) of the IARC relative to lung cancer carcinogens (**Table 1**).[20]

The attributable fractions for occupational exposure causation of lung cancer vary from 5% to 40% in men and 2% to 4% in women.[20] The major occupational carcinogens responsible for causing lung cancer are asbestos, arsenic, beryllium, cadmium, chromium, diesel fumes, nickel, and silica.[21,22] These occupational carcinogens can also cause lung cancer in the general population. Asbestos, silica, and nickel-chromium exposures have been shown to have a population attributable fraction for lung cancer of 18.1%, 5.7%, and 7%, respectively.[23] Although the data are not completely clear, studies have demonstrated silica to be associated with squamous and small cell carcinoma more than with adenocarcinoma. In

Table 1
Group I occupational lung cancer carcinogens with sufficient evidence

Asbestos	Ionizing Radiation	Radon
Beryllium	Coal tar and pitches	Crystalline silica
Bis (chloromethyl) ether, chloromethyl methyl ether	PAHs: benzo(a)pyrene	Talc containing asbestiform fibers
Cadmium and cadmium compounds	Nickel compounds	Secondhand smoke
Chromium (VI) compounds	Soots	Exposure circumstances: aluminum production; coal gasification; hematite mining (radon); iron and steel founding; painter; tin miners
Arsenic		

Data from Brown T, Darnton A, Fortunato L, et al. British Occupational Cancer Burden Study Group. Occupational cancer in Britain – respiratory cancer sites: larynx, lung and mesothelioma. Br J Cancer 2012;107:S56–70.

addition, as has been known with asbestos, the risk for lung cancer is synergistically higher if there is also a history of smoking with silica exposure. Relative risks (RR) for occupational exposures to silicas have been estimated from 1.32 to 1.41, with small variations depending on whether the study was a cohort or case-control. Increased RR (2.37; 95% CI, 1.98–2.84) was seen in patients who also had a diagnosis of silicosis.[20] With silica being one of the most common occupational exposures, it is particularly important for these workers, predominantly in construction jobs, to be aware of their risk for lung cancer (and of course, to not smoke).[21]

Asbestos is still a well-recognized occupational carcinogen, despite significant efforts to decrease its use and exposure. Serpentine (chrysotile) and amphiboles (crocidolite, amosite, tremolite) are the forms of asbestos that cause cancer, although the amphiboles are probably more causative. It is estimated that there is a 1:1 ratio of lung cancer to mesothelioma, although the data are quite variable and depend on degree of exposure and probably the type of asbestos fibers.[20] Although there is a synergistic effect on cancer risk, if there is both smoking and asbestos exposure and the mechanism is not yet clear, asbestos remains a carcinogen as an independent agent.[24]

A more ubiquitous environmental carcinogen that has been implicated in the development of lung cancer in nonsmokers is exposure to elevated levels of indoor radon. A naturally occurring gas, radon is emitted from the earth as a degradation product of uranium.[24] It percolates up through the soil, and can become concentrated in indoor structures, particularly in underground areas or those with poor ventilation. Exposure to radon can occur either in a workplace or home. Occupational exposure to radon causing lung cancer is estimated to be low: less than 14% of the radon-attributable

deaths occurred from radon in the workplace.[20] Radon exposure is estimated to be the causal agent of lung cancer for cases in the Unites States in never-smokers at 2100 to 2900 cases per year.[25] Even though these numbers are low compared with the number caused by tobacco, radon exposure is one of the major causes of lung cancer in people who do not smoke. Although radon and its decay products, such as polonium-210 and polonium-214, cause lung cancer in nonsmokers, the combined exposure of radon, its by-products, and cigarette smoking has a combined effect greater than additive risk, and reflects multiplicative risk.[26]

Studies, including an international review by IARC, have demonstrated that diesel fuel and diesel engine emissions increase the risk of lung cancer in a causal manner with an OR of 1.8 (95% CI, 1.2–2.6)[27,28] In addition, it seems that smoking combined with diesel fume exposure results in a synergistic risk of lung cancer and that squamous cell is the most common histology.

Arsenic has long been recognized as a carcinogen.[24,29] Epidemiologic evidence from Chile has demonstrated the significant risk of lung cancer from arsenic in the drinking water.[30] Thus, environmental exposure from drinking water besides occupational exposure from mining, such as copper mining, can increase the risk for cancer, predominately squamous cell, from arsensic exposure in a dose-related manner.[30–32] As with the other environmental or occupational carcinogens, smoking seems to increase the risk for lung cancer from arsenic exposure.

SECONDHAND SMOKE

Cigarette smoking is the most notorious risk factor for the development of lung cancer, with a RR of a smoker developing lung cancer approximately

12 to 15 times that of the nonsmoker. However, lifelong never-smokers, without other recognized exposures to carcinogens, do develop lung cancer leading researchers to evaluate other potential risk factors that could account for its development. Mainstream smoke is that which is actively drawn in by a smoker. SHS or environmental tobacco smoke is defined as passive inhalation of either the exhaled smoke from an active smoker or passive inhalation of "sidestream" smoke, the product of a lit cigarette smoldering but not previously inhaled. Cigarette smoke contains gaseous carcinogens and particulate matter carcinogens (eg, "tar"). It is intuitive that cigarette smoke, which contains thousands of chemicals and dozens of carcinogens including polyaromatic hydrocarbons, N-nitrosamines, benzene, arsenic, and acetaldehyde, can lead to the development of lung cancer. No safe level of SHS has been determined.[33] The occupational exposure at work of SHS was assessed. A meta-analysis of 35 cases-controls and 5 cohort studies demonstrated RR in nonsmokers of 1.15 (95% CI, 1.04–1.28) for women and 1.29 (95% CI, 0.93–1.78) for men.[34] Most of this exposure is in service sector employees. Certain nonsmokers were at increased risk, such as flight attendants from the era when smoking on airplanes was permitted. Bartenders have known SHS exposure, with elevated levels of carcinogens in their blood.[35] Perhaps the best studied cohort of secondhand smokers is the nonsmoking spouses of men who smoke. Meta-analysis of innumerable studies have indisputably demonstrated that there is no safe level of SHS, with women having an excess risk of 20% and 30% for men for the development of lung cancer when exposed to spousal smoking. In addition, the evidence is clear that risk increases with increased exposure to SHS.[36]

The occurrence of lung cancer has a well-recognized familial clustering established in linkage studies. Cancer registries from Utah, Sweden, and Iceland have clearly established the increased risk. Meta-analyses have demonstrated an increased OR of 1.63 (95% CI, 1.31–2.01) if there is a family member who had lung cancer, and this increases substantially as more family members are diagnosed with lung cancer.[37] The patients with lung cancer within this analysis were significantly more likely to have a history of smoking. Studies have demonstrated an increased familial risk for developing lung cancer without smoking exposure, but the evidence is less clear.

Lung cancer occurs in people who have never smoked and had no clear exposure to an identified carcinogen. Thun and colleagues[38] completed a thorough analysis of self-reported never-smokers in 13 cohorts and 22 cancer registry datasets and concluded the following: never-smoking men have higher death rates than women; women and men incidence rates are similar across all ages greater than 40 years; Asians living in Asia and African Americans have higher death rates than Europeans; and women do not have a higher or increasing incidence than men. These are important findings, because much discussion and publications in recent years have suggested alternative information. It is critical to understand that there can be an increasingly proportion of people with lung cancer who have never smoked, as the proportion of people with lung cancer who have smoked decreases. This increasing proportion does not indicate that more people (including women) who have never smoked are increasingly being diagnosed with lung cancer. That said, as the tobacco use epidemic is decreasing in more western economies, the number of people with lung cancer who have never smoked will become a larger proportion of the whole, and their lung cancer must be better understood and treated. Lung cancer not caused by tobacco has a different genomic profile than that caused by tobacco, and predictably should be treated differently. It is important for clinicians and researchers to understand the differences between the various causative carcinogens (known or unknown) to best determine appropriate therapy.

Despite the known and proved carcinogenic risk of tobacco exposure, most lifelong smokers do not develop lung cancer, and conversely there are infrequent lifelong never-smokers who develop lung cancer in the absence of identifiable carcinogenic exposure. The complex interrelationships between smoking and other environmental carcinogens are becoming better defined and have been shown to have synergistic, not simply additive impact on the development of lung cancer. It will be intriguing to understand the future of lung cancer in China. At present, this most populous country in the world has a huge number of men who have smoked, and are at risk for a tobacco-related lung cancer. However, the women, who currently have a low smoking rate of approximately 3%, still have a very large risk for lung cancer from as yet unclear etiology (although environment risks seem to be prominent, as previously mentioned). Although tobacco is by far the most attributable risk for lung cancer, it is not the only one. Enough is now known to substantially decrease the incidence of lung cancer through strong tobacco control, but there is still much to learn about how to prevent the remaining risk factors. By evaluating and understanding these relationships, perhaps future efforts at identifying high-risk individuals may lead to earlier detection, and by appreciating the risk of SHS and other environmental carcinogens, future efforts to reduce exposure may gain support in the battle against this deadly disease.

SUMMARY

Over the past 100 years, the rise of lung cancer from an otherwise rare disease to the most common cause of cancer death in men, and in many countries, in women, has been striking. Tobacco control is a key component to reduce the burden of lung cancer on society, but the development of lung cancer is not uniform in all smokers, and it does develop in some lifelong never-smokers. Focusing only on tobacco control addresses one environmental issue, but neglects other well-studied factors and individual patient characteristics. The development of lung cancer can certainly be better understood by more thoroughly appreciating the complex intertwined relationship of environmental factors and host factors, such as the heterogeneity of genetic and molecular differences, which lead to variable risks of developing lung cancer. If there is a true desire to rapidly decrease the number of deaths from lung cancer, all societies should aggressively implement evidence-based tobacco control policies. At least these very preventable deaths can be eliminated in the near future.[16]

REFERENCES

1. Siegel R, Maishadham D, Jemal A. Cancer statistics, 2012. CA Cancer J Clin 2012;62:10–29.
2. International Agency for Research on Cancer Globocan 2008. Available at: http://globocan.iarc.fr/factsheets/cancers/lung.asp. Accessed October 15, 2012.
3. Siegel R, Maishadham D, Jemal A. Cancer statistics for Hispanics/Latinos, 2012. CA Cancer J Clin 2012; 62:283–98.
4. Surveillance Epidemiology and End Results. providing information on cancer statistics to help reduce the burden of this disease on the U.S. population. National Cancer Institute: U.S. National Institutes of Health. Available at: http://seer.cancer.gov/faststats/index.php. Accessed February 5, 2013.
5. Verdecchia A, Francisci S, Brenner H, et al, EUROCARE-4 Working Group. Recent cancer survival in Europe: a 2000-02 period analysis of EUROCARE-4 data. Lancet Oncol 2007;8(9):784–96.
6. Jung KW, Park S, Kong HJ, et al. Cancer statistics in Korea: incidence, mortality and survival in 2006-7. J Korean Med Sci 2010;25:1113–21.
7. Youlden DR, Cramb SM, Baade PD. The international epidemiology of lung cancer: geographical distribution and secular trends. J Thorac Oncol 2008;3(8):819–31.
8. Lopez AD, Collishaw NE, Piha T. A descriptive model of the cigarette epidemic in developed countries. Tobac Contr 1994;3:242–7.
9. Jemal A, Center MM, DeSantis C, et al. Global patterns of cancer incidence and mortality rates and trends. Cancer Epidemiol Biomarkers Prev 2010; 19(8):1893–907.
10. Wynder EL, Graham EA. Tobacco smoking as a possible etiologic factor in bronchiogenic carcinoma; a study of 684 proved cases. JAMA 1950; 143(4):329–36.
11. Doll R, Hill AB. Smoking and carcinoma of the lung: preliminary report. Br Med J 1950;2(4682):739–48.
12. Ito H, Matsuo K, Tanaka H, et al. Nonfilter and filter cigarette consumption and the incidence of lung cancer by histological type in Japan and the United States: analysis of 30-year data from population-based cancer registries. Int J Cancer 2011;128(8):1918–28.
13. Stellman SD, Muscat JE, Thompson S, et al. Risk of squamous cell carcinoma and adenocarcinoma of the lung in relation to lifetime filter cigarette smoking. Cancer 1997;80:382–8.
14. Thun MJ, Lally CA, Flannery JT, et al. Cigarette smoking and changes in the histopathology of lung cancer. J Natl Cancer Inst 1997;89:1580–6.
15. Egleston BL, Meireles SI, Flieder DB, et al. Population-based trends in lung cancer incidence in women. Semin Oncol 2009;36:506–15.
16. Barnoya J, Glantz S. Association of the California tobacco control program with declines in lung cancer incidence. Cancer Causes Control 2004;15:689–95.
17. Hammond EC, Selikoff IJ, Lawther PL, et al. Inhalation of benzpyrene and cancer in man. Ann N Y Acad Sci 1976;271:116–24.
18. Lan Q, He X, Shen M, et al. Variation in lung cancer risk by smoky coal subtype in Xuanwei, China. Int J Cancer 2008;123:2164–9.
19. Kurmi OP, Arya PH, Lam KB, et al. Lung cancer risk of solid fuel smoke exposure: a systematic review and meta-analysis. Eur Respir J 2012;40(5):1228–37.
20. Brown T, Darnton A, Fortunato L, et al, British Occupational Cancer Burden Study Group. Occupational cancer in Britain: respiratory cancer sites: larynx, lung and mesothelioma. Br J Cancer 2012;107:S56–70.
21. Driscoll T, Nelson DI, Steenland K, et al. The global burden of disease due to occupational carcinogens. Am J Ind Med 2005;48:419–31.
22. Alberg A, Samet JM. Epidemiology of lung cancer. Chest 2003;123(Suppl 1):21S–49S.
23. De Matteis S, Consonni D, Lubin JH, et al. Impact of occupational carcinogens on lung cancer risk in a general population. Int J Epidemiol 2012;41(3):711–21.
24. Samet JM, Avila-Tang E, Boffetta P, et al. Lung cancer in never smokers: clinical epidemiology and environmental risk factors. Clin Cancer Res 2009;15(18):5626–45.

25. National Research Council. Committee on Health risks of exposure to radon, Board on Radiation effects Research and Commission on Life Sciences Health effects of exposure to radon (BEIR IV). Washington, DC: National Academy Press; 1999.

26. Lubin JH, Boice JD Jr. Lung cancer risk from residential radon: metaanalysis of eight epidemiologic studies. J Natl Cancer Inst 1997;89:49–57.

27. Pintos J, Parent ME, Richardson L, et al. Occupational exposure to diesel engine emissions and risk of lung cancer: evidence from two case-control studies in Montreal, Canada. Occup Environ Med 2012;69(11):787–92.

28. Benbrahim-Talla L, Baan RA, Grosse Y, et al. IARC Working Group. Carcinogenicity of diesel-engine and gasoline-engine exhausts and some nitroarenes. Lancet Oncol 2012;13:663–4.

29. Pershagen G, Wall S, Taube A, et al. On the interaction between occupational arsenic exposure and smoking and its relationship to lung cancer. Scand J Work Environ Health 1981;7:302–9.

30. Ferreccio C, Gonzalez C, Milosavljevic V, et al. Lung cancer and arsenic concentrations in drinking water in Chile. Epidemiology 2000;11(6):673–9.

31. Martinez DV, Becker-Santos DD, Vucic EA, et al. Induction of human squamous cell-type carcinomas by arsenic. J Skin Cancer 2011;2011:454157.

32. Martinez VD, Vucic EA, Lam S, et al. Arsenic and lung cancer in never-smokers: lessons from Chile. Am J Respir Crit Care Med 2012;185(10):1131–2.

33. U.S. Department of Health and Human Services. The health consequences of involuntary exposure to tobacco smoke: a report of the Surgeon General. Secondhand smoke what it means to you. U.S. Department of Health and Human Services, Center for Disease Control and Prevention, Coordinating Center for Health Promotion, National Center for Chronic Disease Prevention and Health Promotion, Office on Smoking and Health, 2006.

34. Zhong L, Goldberg M, Parent ME, et al. Exposure to environmental tobacco smoke and the risk of lung cancer: a meta-analysis. Lung Cancer 2000;27:3–18.

35. MacLure M, Katz RBA, Bryant MS, et al. Elevated blood levels of carcinogens in passive smokers. Am J Public Health 1989;79:1381–4.

36. International Agency for Research on Cancer. IARC Monographs on the evaluation on carcinogenic risks to humans, tobacco smoke and involuntary smoking, vol. 83. Lyon (France): International Agency for Research on Cancer; 2004.

37. Lissowska J, Foretova L, Dąbek J, et al. Family history and lung cancer risk: international multicentre case-control study in Eastern and Central Europe and meta-analyses. Cancer Causes Control 2010;21: 1091–104.

38. Thun MJ, Hannan LM, Adams-Campbell LL, et al. Lung cancer occurrence in never-smokers: an analysis of 13 cohorts and 22 cancer registry studies. PLoS Med 2008;5(9):e185. http://dx.doi.org/10.1371/journal.pmed.0050185.

Should All Cases of Lung Cancer be Presented at Tumor Board Conferences?

Marc Riquet, MD, PhD[a],*, Pierre Mordant, MD, PhD[a],
Mehdi Henni, MD[b], Delphine Wermert, MD[c],
Elizabeth Fabre-Guillevin, MD[d], Aurélie Cazes, MD, PhD[e],
Françoise Le Pimpec Barthes, MD, PhD[a]

KEYWORDS

- Lung cancer • Multimodality treatment • Multidisciplinary team

KEY POINTS

- Tumor Board Conferences (TBCs) were established more than a decade ago to deal with the increasing complexity of cancer care.
- Because the organization of TBCs varies greatly among centers and regions, national regulation is mandatory to ensure a homogeneous quality of care.
- These meetings have been associated with higher adherence of both staging and treatment to current guidelines. The influence of TBCs on the rate of curative treatments is also established.
- In the particular case of non–small cell lung cancer, it is recommended that patients with lung nodule and tumor of unknown histology should not be presented before surgery.
- Every patient with malignant histology should be declared to the TBC coordinator, registered at the time of the histologic confirmation, and discussed only if either the treatment or the patient does not fit the standard guidelines.

INTRODUCTION: NATURE OF THE PROBLEM

Also known as multidisciplinary cancer conferences, Tumor Board Conferences (TBCs) are cancer case reviews organized by members of multidisciplinary teams or clinics according to different care systems. They are an established part of cancer care in the United States and are required for the accreditation of centers delivering cancer care by the US Commission on Cancer and the American College of Surgeons. In Canada, where few hospitals have developed case conferences, Wright and colleagues[1] described in 2007 the process of creating a province-wide standards document for TBCs, the importance of which was recently emphasized.[2] In France, where they are also required in order to be accredited, they have been obligatory since 2006, and 100% of patients who have cancer must be presented at TBCs. The goal is to provide each patient with best care and management and to avoid disparity and inequality between regions, sometimes even within a region, of the same state. All types of cancer, including lung cancer, are included. However, this approach is time-consuming and guidelines now exist in all Western countries to ensure best treatment

[a] Department of General Thoracic Surgery, Georges Pompidou European Hospital, Paris-Descartes University, 20 rue Leblanc, Paris 75015, France; [b] Department of Radiation Oncology, Georges Pompidou European Hospital, Paris-Descartes University, 20 rue Leblanc, Paris 75015, France; [c] Department of Pneumology, Georges Pompidou European Hospital, Paris-Descartes University, 20 rue Leblanc, Paris 75015, France; [d] Department of Medical Oncology, Georges Pompidou European Hospital, Paris-Descartes University, 20 rue Leblanc, Paris 75015, France; [e] Department of Thoracic Pathology, Georges Pompidou European Hospital, Paris-Descartes University, 20 rue Leblanc, Paris 75015, France
* Corresponding author. Department of General Thoracic Surgery, Georges Pompidou European Hospital, 20 rue Leblanc, Paris 75015, France.
E-mail address: marc.riquet@egp.aphp.fr

Thorac Surg Clin 23 (2013) 123–128
http://dx.doi.org/10.1016/j.thorsurg.2013.01.003
1547-4127/13/$ – see front matter © 2013 Elsevier Inc. All rights reserved.

choices. In France, 30,000 new cases of lung cancers occur each year.[3] Some cases are easy to solve by following state-of-the-art guidelines, which questions the necessity and benefits of presenting all cases of lung cancer at TBCs.

HISTORICAL NOTES AND HIGHLIGHTS

TBCs have existed for a long time in university hospitals in many regions in France and were already commonly available in Paris when the first author began as a resident in 1973 (Marc Riquet, personal data, 1973). They were common practice in surgery but also in chest medicine; cases of lung cancer were presented in the presence of thoracic surgeons, pulmonologists, and radiation oncologists; medical oncologists were not implicated in multimodality treatments at that time. Different types of TBCs had also already been functioning in the cancer center Institut Gustave-Roussy since the 1960s.[3] However, there was a disparity between regions and care centers, which led in 2003 to the first Cancer Plan of the French Government, generalizing TBC practice in all health sectors of the territory.

In the United States, the concepts of cancer centers, to facilitate and centralize patient care, education, and research, evolved after passing of the National Cancer Act in 1971[4]; many community hospitals with no mission for laboratory-based research or education had created cancer centers focusing on patient care, before TBCs were established as part of cancer care and accreditation of cancer centers. Evidence has existed that participation in clinical trials and referral to specialist centers confers survival advantage for patients with certain types of cancer, such as non–small cell lung cancer (NSCLC).[5] Recommendations on practice organization in managing lung cancer were established in 2003,[6] including a multidisciplinary approach, referral pattern, management decisions, timetable, communication, and ongoing care. Recommendations about a multidisciplinary approach were that (1) all cancer units, treatment facilities, and centers should have a multidisciplinary lung cancer conference that meets on a regular and continuing basis, and (2) multidisciplinary lung cancer teams should consider establishing a multispecialty lung cancer clinic. Dillman and Chico[4] reported that survival improved significantly in patients treated at an integrated community cancer center compared with historical survival and patients from the SEER (Surveillance Epidemiology and End Results) registry. However, the situation evolved differently in other countries.

In England, survival rates were lower than the European average across a range of cancer types in the late 1980s and early 1990s. The first major step was the publication of the Calman-Hine Report in 1995, which set out the key principles governing the provision of high-quality care and highlighted the importance of specialist multidisciplinary teams.[7] In 1999, cancer was declared to be a priority, leading to the publication of the National Health Service Cancer Plan in 2000, and to subsequent improvements in lung cancer management, including multidisciplinary team working.[8] Beattie and colleagues[9] reported the Irish results of the National Cancer Plan (Campbell report, 1996), which established that North Ireland should have 1 cancer center. The percentage of all new cases of patients who have lung cancer who were discussed at TBC increased from 19% in 1996 to 64% in 2006. This increase was associated with an overall increase in patients presented at TBCs involving thoracic surgeons, and a 50% increase in the proportion of surgical resection between the first and last group.

In Australia, Conron and colleagues[10] found that there was no equal access to lung cancer multidisciplinary clinics across the different states. Proposed measures aimed at increasing the awareness of the benefits of multidisciplinary lung cancer care through education, establishing satellite clinics in regional areas with links to fully resourced TBCs, and developing infrastructure that allows teleconferencing and electronic transfer of data.

OUTCOMES AND PROGNOSIS

Specialties involved in TBCs include pulmonology, thoracic surgery, medical oncology, radiation oncology, pathology, and radiology. Valuable contributions also come from nursing, social work, psychology, psychiatry, pastoral care, and palliative care. Sometimes, other surgical specialties may be required (eg, neurosurgery, plastic surgery, vascular and cardiac surgery).

Effects of TBCs on NSCLC Management

In 2005, Forrest and colleagues[11] reported that the introduction of a multidisciplinary team was associated with an increase in the proportion of patients being staged, presenting with stage IIIb disease and receiving chemotherapy, which was associated with a doubling of survival in patients with (inoperable) stage III disease. However, some centers had chosen to organize a multidisciplinary thoracic oncology clinic rather than TBCs. The retrospective comparison of multidisciplinary thoracic oncology clinics and weekly TBCs failed to show any difference regarding timeliness of diagnostic and treatment decisions,[12] suggesting that TBCs could be a valuable alternative to multi-disciplinary clinics.

A few years later, Coory and colleagues[13] performed a systematic international review of multidisciplinary team meetings in the management of lung cancer. Searches were performed between 1984 and 2007 and 16 studies were found, but their clinical heterogeneity rendered statistical pooling impossible. Only 2 studies reported an improvement in survival; both were before-and-after designs, providing weak evidence of any causal association. Another study reported in 2009 by Bydder and colleagues[14] suggested that patients with inoperable NSCLC who had been discussed at a multidisciplinary meeting could have better survival than those whose case was not discussed. However, these studies provide only low level of evidence, and the influence of TBCs on overall survival is still to be confirmed through a prospective design.

In the systematic review by Coory and colleagues,[13] 6 studies reported a significant modification in management of patients, with an increase in the proportion of patients undergoing surgical resection, chemotherapy, or radiotherapy with curative intent. More recently, Boxer and colleagues[15] reported a large series including 504 patients who were presented at TBCs and 484 patients who were not. A similar proportion of patients underwent surgery in both groups; however, a significantly greater proportion of patients in the TBC group received radiotherapy, chemotherapy, and referrals to palliative care. TBC discussion did not have an impact on survival.

Concordance of TBCs with State-of-the-Art Guidelines

In the survey conducted by Stinchcomb and colleagues[16] to compare physician beliefs against the evidence-based guidelines, most physicians found the evidence-based guidelines beneficial. Nevertheless, practice beliefs differ from the guidelines in selected areas, including screening for lung cancer, use of postoperative radiotherapy, and benefits of chemotherapy for stage IV disease.

Assuming the positive role of evidence-based guidelines on clinical practice and patient outcome, many studies have questioned the concordance between TBC recommendations and related guidelines. In a retrospective study, Conron and colleagues[10] found a high rate of adherence to international guideline recommendations concerning timely lung cancer diagnosis, staging, and treatment implementation. In a prospective study, Vinod and colleagues[17] confirmed that the overall adherence to guidelines was high, with a reported rate of

71%. The TBC did not recommend guideline treatments for patients older than 70 years, Eastern Cooperative Oncology Group performance status of 2 or higher, and stage III NSCLC. The primary reasons for this were physician decision (39%), co-morbidity (25%), and technical factors (22%). Individual factors that may preclude guideline treatment cannot be accounted for by guidelines.

In a recent large retrospective study, Freeman and colleagues[18] compared the experiences of 535 patients before and 687 patients after the formation of a TBC. Patients with NSCLC were evaluated for completeness of staging, multidisciplinary evaluation before the initiation of therapy, time from pathologic diagnosis to treatment, multimodality therapy, and adherence to national treatment guidelines. After the initiation of a TBC, the number of patients receiving a complete staging evaluation (79% vs 93%, $P<.0001$), multidisciplinary evaluation before therapy (62% vs 96%, $P<.0001$), and adherence to the National Comprehensive Cancer Network treatment guidelines (81% vs 97%, $P<.0001$) all increased significantly, whereas mean days from diagnosis to treatment significantly decreased (29 vs 17 days, $P<.0001$). Among patients undergoing surgical resection, the proportion of patients undergoing induction therapy increased from 10% to 21% ($P<.0005$), and the proportion of stage IIIA NSCLC also increased significantly from 12% to 20% ($P = .0079$).

Side Effects of TBCs

In France, 30,000 new cases of lung cancers occur each year.[3] It has been estimated that each patient may be presented between 3 to 5 times at TBC.[3] This situation accounts for about 120,000 TBCs reassembling between 4 and 8 specialists, which is a mean of 720,000 consultations, representing about 14 million Euros per year, without taking into account other costs such as secretarial costs, mailing, and so forth. In Grenoble University Hospital (France) in 2008, the total TBC activity represented the equivalent of 3 fully employed doctors.[19]

Aside from these important costs, TBCs have often been accused of delaying the surgical management of patients with NSCLC. In France, Abbo and colleagues[20] studied the influence of TBCs on the timing of surgery. The investigators retrospectively reviewed all patients operated on for primary lung cancer in their institution in 2010. A total of 141 patients were included in the study, with 86 cases (61%) presented at TBC before surgery and 55 cases (39%) presented after. The mean time between first imaging and treatment initiation was 70 days, but it was significantly shorter when the cases were presented after surgery

(55 days) than before (79 days, $P<.0001$). Both groups were otherwise similar regarding American Association of Anaesthetists score, performance status, comorbidities, tumor stage, and preoperative FEV_1 (forced expiratory volume in 1 second).

The timing of management is a crucial issue that suffers from heterogeneity in its definition and determinants. Regarding the definition, Ouwens and colleagues[21] considered it a main criterion that the diagnostic course should be completed within 21 calendar days, and that the patients should begin therapy within 35 calendar days, from the time of the first visit to the pulmonologist. Freeman and colleagues[18] reported that in the United States, the delay from diagnosis to treatment significantly decreased to 17 days after initiation of the TBC, whereas in France, the data reported by Abbo and colleagues[20] suggested the opposite. Whatever the influence of TBC on the timing of management, its influence on survival should be studied independently. Many studies failed to show the prognostic influence of the timing of management on overall survival in patients with NSCLC.[22–26] These data have been recently questioned by the positive results of the National Lung Screening Trial,[27] which suggest that earlier diagnosis and shorter management could result in better survival for patients with NSCLC. Despite this lack of scientific evidence, many harmful examples of procrastination can be cited in clinical practice, and both the psychological issues sustained by patients and the competition among surgical centers clearly favor a shorter delay from first imaging to initiation of treatment.

Psychological issues may also concern the medical staff participating in a TBC. In particular, the difficult role played by nonclinical specialties, combining both a high degree of stress and a low degree of reward, has been recently outlined. Among cancer care professionals, high levels of emotional exhaustion were particularly apparent in team leaders and nurses, but feelings of low levels of personal accomplishment were prevalent in histopathologists and radiologists.[28]

TBCs can also be effective from an educational point of view. In 2009, Fischel and Dillman[29] developed an effective lung cancer program in their community hospital. Stressing the benefits of the TBC, the investigators include its educational aspects, given that each specialty can help to educate the other attendees regarding specific information or insight from their unique point of view. As new data, techniques, and procedure become available, the TBC is able to integrate these into the already established guidelines based on recent literature and personal knowledge. Establishing a journal club to review articles

on subjects related to lung cancer care is an effective way to update all members involved, bringing in outside doctors who may not have time to attend the weekly meetings and building camaraderie among team members.

COMMENTS AND CONTROVERSIES
Indications of TBCs

Regarding patients with NSCLC, the main controversies concern the indication of TBC, because some patients undergo surgery with no previous diagnosis, some patients with limited tumors do not require adjuvant treatment after complete resection, and some patients with metastatic tumors need treatment usually considered as standard.

Should all lung nodules and tumors of unknown histology be presented before surgery?

The answer is clearly no. The role of the TBC is not to replace the meetings organized by the departments of thoracic surgery or chest medicine. Conron and colleagues[10] found that members of a lung cancer TBC were involved in the diagnosis and management of a wide range of benign and malignant pulmonary, pleural, and mediastinal disease. In the absence of previous malignancy, the management of pulmonary nodules is under the responsibility of the chest clinician, thoracic surgeon, and radiologist. Medical and radiation oncologists have neither the formation nor the time to hear about every pulmonary nodule before histologic diagnosis.

Should all histologically confirmed NSCLC be presented before surgery?

This question is still debated. Wright[1] stated that all new cancer cases, inpatient and ambulatory, and the proposed treatment plan should be forwarded to the TBC coordinator. However, not all cases forwarded to the TBC coordinator need to be discussed at the TBC. The individual physician and the TBC Chair can determine which cases are discussed in detail at the TBC.

In France, all histologically confirmed NSCLC should be declared and registered by the TBC coordinator before treatment.

- If the treatment is considered as standard by updated recommendations (ie, surgical resection for cT1N0M0 tumor), and if the patient is fit enough to benefit from it (ie, patients with acceptable predictive postoperative FEV_1 and no cardiac comorbidities), the case is registered, but the decision is taken with no further discussion. This registration is important, because it allows both the surgical team to double check for completeness of preoperative explorations, and the oncological team to prepare the discussion of the case that will be organized after the postoperative course and the definitive pathology staging.

• If there is no standard treatment (ie, clinical stage IIIA- N2 disease), if the patient is not fit enough to benefit from the standard treatment (ie, they have severe respiratory failure), or if either the patient or their physician wants to consider other options, the case is registered, presented by the physician in charge, and the decision is taken after multidisciplinary discussion. This discussion allows the organization of multimodal strategies incorporating induction, surgical, and adjuvant treatments. This discussion is also important for considering the inclusion of the patient in prospective therapeutic trials.

Some exceptions can be anticipated, albeit detailed in neither regulatory documents nor scientific articles. These exceptions follow the need for urgent treatment before the date of the next TBC. Surgical (videothoracoscopy for malignant pleuritis associated with stage IV NSCLC), medical (chemotherapy for superior vena cava syndrome), and radiation oncology (radiation of unstable spine metastases) can be affected. The decision to initiate treatment before the TBC can be made by the physician in charge of the patient, with the support of the TBC coordinator. The case is then discussed a posteriori to confirm the adequacy of management.

Should all histologically confirmed NSCLC be presented after surgery?

The answer is clearly yes. Again, if the treatment is considered as standard and the patient is fit enough to benefit from it, the case is registered, the decision is taken without discussion, and the postoperative management can be scheduled. If there is no standard treatment, if the patient is not fit enough to benefit from it, or if either the patient or their physician wants to consider other options, the case is registered, presented by the physician in charge, and the decision is taken after multidisciplinary discussion.

Responsibility for the Final Decision and Potential Secondary Deviation

Osarogiagbon and colleagues[30] evaluated patient outcomes after discussion in a thoracic TBC. There was no concordance between TBC recommendations and final management in 37% of patients. The

only demographic factors significantly associated with receipt of discordant care were health insurance status and race, and 60% of all discordant care could be attributed to clinicians' decisions. Patients who received concordant care had significantly shorter delay to onset of definitive therapy ($P<.002$), longer overall survival ($P<.004$), and longer progression-free survival ($P<.02$).

However, further studies are mandatory to better understand the reason for deviation from the TBC decision. At the end of the process, the responsibility for the final decision lies with the physician in charge of the patients, as the only physician who is aware of the whole situation, including the patient's wishes, psychology, social context, and the particular relation between patient and doctor. Therefore, secondary deviations are acceptable if they are decided reasonably and explained correctly to the patient and the members of the TBC.

SUMMARY

The increasing complexity of lung cancer care led to the spread of multidisciplinary TBCs more than a decade ago. These meetings have been associated with higher adherence of both staging and treatment to current guidelines. The impact of TBCs on the timing of management and overall survival remains unknown, but their influence on the rate of curative treatments is established.

In the particular case of NSCLC, it could be suggested that patients with lung nodules and tumors of unknown histology should not be presented before surgery, but that every patient with malignant histology should be declared to the TBC coordinator and registered at the time of histologic confirmation. If the treatment is standard and the patient is fit enough to benefit from it, the decision is taken without further discussion. If the treatment is not standard, or if the patient cannot benefit from the standard treatment, or if for any reason the patient or their clinician wants to consider other options, the case is discussed on a multidisciplinary basis.

This approach allows physicians to deal rapidly with simple cases on a systematic basis, to give more attention to the most complicated situations, and to offer every patient the benefit of a multidisciplinary approach, including proposal of symptomatic care, coordination of multimodal treatments, and inclusion in clinical trials.

REFERENCES

1. Wright FC, De Vito C, Langer B, et al, the Expert Panel on Multidisciplinary Cancer Conferences

Standards. Multidisciplinary cancer conferences: a systematic review and development of practice standards. Eur J Cancer 2007;43:1002–10.

2. Ellis PM. The importance of multidisciplinary team management of patients with non-small-cell lung cancer. Curr Oncol 2012;19:S7–15.

3. Depierre A. La réunion de concertation pluridisciplinaire. La Lettre du Pneumologue 2006;9:168–70.

4. Dillman RO, Chico SD. Cancer patient survival improvement is correlated with the opening of a community cancer center: comparison with intramural and extramural benchmarks. J Oncol Pract 2005;1:84–92.

5. Davis S, Wright PW, Schulman SF, et al. Participants in prospective randomised clinical trials for resected non-small cell lung cancer have improved survival compared with non participants in such trials. Cancer 1985;56:1710–8.

6. Alberts MA, Bepler G, Hazelton T, et al. Practice organization. Chest 2003;123:332S–7S.

7. Howard RA. The Calman-Hine report: a personal retrospective on the UK's first comprehensive policy on cancer services. Lancet Oncol 2006;7:336–46.

8. Griffith C, Turner J. United Kingdom National Health Service. Cancer Services Collaborative "Improvement Partnership", redesign of cancer services. A national approach. Eur J Surg Oncol 2004;30:1–86.

9. Beattie G, Bannon F, McGuigan J. Lung cancer resection rates have increased significantly in females during a 15-year period. Eur J Cardiothorac Surg 2010;38:484–90.

10. Conron M, Phuah S, Steinfort D, et al. Analysis of multidisciplinary lung cancer practice. Intern Med J 2007;37:18–25.

11. Forrest LM, McMillan DC, McArdle CS, et al. An evaluation of a multidisciplinary team, in a single centre, on treatment and survival in patients with inoperable non-small-cell lung cancer. Br J Cancer 2005;93:977–8.

12. Riedel RF, Wang X, Cormack M, et al. Impact of a multidisciplinary thoracic oncology clinic on the timeliness of care. J Thorac Oncol 2006;1:692–6.

13. Coory M, Gkolia P, Yang IA, et al. Systematic review of multidisciplinary teams in the management of lung cancer. Lung Cancer 2008;60:14–21.

14. Bydder S, Nowak A, Marion K, et al. The impact of case discussion at a multidisciplinary team meeting on the treatment and survival of patients with inoperable non-small cell lung cancer. Intern Med J 2009; 39:838–48.

15. Boxer MM, Vinot SK, Shafiq J, et al. Do multidisciplinary team meetings make a difference in the management of lung cancer? Cancer 2011;117: 5112–20.

16. Stinchcombe TE, Detterbeck MD, Lin L, et al. Beliefs among physicians in the diagnostic and therapeutic approach to non-small cell lung cancer. J Thorac Oncol 2007;2:819–26.

17. Vinod SK, Sidhom MA, Delaney GP. Do multidisciplinary meetings follow guideline-based care? J Oncol Pract 2010;6:276–81.

18. Freeman RK, Van Woerkom JM, Vyverberg A, et al. The effect of a multidisciplinary thoracic malignancy conference on the treatment of patients with lung cancer. Eur J Cardiothorac Surg 2010;38:1–5.

19. Guillem P, Bolla M, Courby S, et al. Evaluation des reunions de concertation pluridisciplinaire en cancérologie: quelles priorités pour quelles ameliorations? Bull Cancer 2011;98:989–98.

20. Abbo O, Rivera C, Berjaud J, et al. Impact de la date de réunion de concertation pluridisciplinaire sur les délais de prise en charge des patients opérés pour cancer bronchopulmonaire primitif. Chirurgie thoracique Cardio-Vasculaire 2012;16(1):7–10.

21. Ouwens MM, Hermens RR, Termeer RA, et al. Quality of integrated care for patients with non-small cell lung cancer: variations and determinants of care. Cancer 2007;110:1782–90.

22. Bozcuk H, Martin C. Does treatment delay affect survival in non-small cell lung cancer? A retrospective analysis from a single UK centre. Lung Cancer 2001;34:243–52.

23. Aragoneses FG, Moreno N, Leon P, et al, Bronchogenic Carcinoma Cooperative Group of the Spanish Society of Pneumology and Thoracic Surgery (GCCB-S). Influence of delays on survival in the surgical treatment of bronchogenic carcinoma. Lung Cancer 2002;36:59–63.

24. Quarterman RL, McMillan A, Ratcliffe MB, et al. Effect of preoperative delay on prognosis for patients with early stage non-small cell lung cancer. J Thorac Cardiovasc Surg 2003;125(1):108–13.

25. Myrdal G, Lambe M, Hillerdal G, et al. Effect of delays on prognosis in patients with non-small cell lung cancer. Thorax 2004;59(1):45–9.

26. Salomaa ER, Sällinen S, Hiekkanen H, et al. Delays in the diagnosis and treatment of lung cancer. Chest 2005;128(4):2282–8.

27. National Lung Screening Trial Research Team, Aberle DR, Adams AM, Berg CD, et al. Reduced lung-cancer mortality with low-dose computed tomographic screening. N Engl J Med 2011;365(5):395–409.

28. Catt S, Fallowfield L, Jenkins V, et al. The informational roles and psychological health of members of 10 oncology multidisciplinary teams in the UK. Br J Cancer 2005;93(10):1092–7.

29. Fischel RJ, Dillman RO. Developing an effective lung cancer program in a community hospital setting. Clin Lung Cancer 2009;10:239–43.

30. Osarogiagbon RU, Phelps G, McFarlane J, et al. Causes and consequences of deviation from multidisciplinary care in thoracic oncology. J Thorac Oncol 2011;6:510–6.

Screening, Early Detection, and Diagnosis

Current Status of Lung Cancer Screening

Ugo Pastorino, MD

KEYWORDS

- Lung cancer screening • Early detection • Low-dose computed tomography • Overdiagnosis
- Biomarkers

KEY POINTS

- Lung cancer risk: Risk is related to age and extent of tobacco smoking. It is less than 1% per year in typical screening populations of heavy smokers above the age of 50.
- Low-dose CT: Multi-slice spiral CT has dramatically improved the detection rate of small pulmonary lesions, in a few seconds, with lower radiation exposure and no intravenous contrast.
- Screening efficacy: This can be assessed by mortality reduction in the whole population under screening but not by the improvement of survival in CT-detected lung cancers.
- Overdiagnosis: Detection and treatment of indolent or slow-growing lung cancer, which would not affect patient's life expectancy without screening, can include resection of benign nodules.
- Biomarkers: There are promising developments of new blood biomarkers that combine safety and better accuracy for individual risk assessment, lung cancer detection, and prediction of outcome.

INTRODUCTION OR BACKGROUND

Lung cancer kills 1.3 million people every year[1] (more than breast, colon, and prostate cancer together)[2] and mortality is constantly rising in countries such as China.[3] In developed countries, smoking regulation has achieved a significant reduction in the prevalence of active smokers and lung cancer mortality in men but not in women.[4] As a consequence of smoking cessation, millions of former smokers remain at high risk of cancer for many years.

Improvements in clinical management of lung cancer have been modest over the last 20 years, with an overall 5-year survival rate just above 10% in Europe and 16% in the United States.[5,6] Presence of metastatic disease at diagnosis, occurring in 70% of all patients, is the main reason for treatment failure,[6] whereas the 5-year survival of patients resected in stage IA is higher than 70%.[7]

HISTORICAL NOTES: EARLY SCREENING TRIALS

Early detection trials with chest radiography (CR) and sputum cytology, funded by the US National Cancer Institute in 1970s, did not reduce lung cancer mortality, despite the higher proportion of early stage cancer identified through screening.[8–12] Active screening with 4-monthly CR doubled the number of early stage lung cancer in the interventional arm compared with annual CR arm, and survival rate of lung cancer patients diagnosed at an early stage in the screening arm was significantly higher (69% vs 54% at 5 years, median 16 years vs 5 years, respectively). Nonetheless, the 25 year follow-up of the Mayo trial showed that overall mortality was higher in the 4-monthly CR arm compared with the annual CR arm, even though the difference did not reach statistical significance ($P = .09$).[13] The reasons for such a detrimental

Division of Thoracic Surgery, Istituto Nazionale Tumori, Via Venezian 1, 20133 Milan, Italy
E-mail address: Ugo.Pastorino@istitutotumori.mi.it

Thorac Surg Clin 23 (2013) 129–140
http://dx.doi.org/10.1016/j.thorsurg.2013.01.018
1547-4127/13/$ – see front matter © 2013 Elsevier Inc. All rights reserved.

effect of screening have never been explored. Altogether, long-term results of the Mayo trial proved the inefficacy and potential danger of CR screening, as well as the occurrence of overdiagnosis in the intervention arm.

OBSERVATIONAL STUDIES WITH LDCT

The introduction of spiral chest LDCT in clinical practice opened a new perspective for early detection, and initial studies conducted in Japan in the 1990s demonstrated the potential value of LDCT for lung cancer screening.[14] The continuous technological development of multi-slice machines improved both sensitivity and reliability of spiral CT, providing a new chance for detecting pulmonary lesions of 3 to 4 mm in size in a few seconds, without the use of intravenous contrast.

In 1999, Cornell University of New York published the first results of Early Lung Cancer Action Project (ELCAP), showing that spiral CT scans had accuracy and sensitivity rates sixfold higher than CR, in identifying very small lung tumors (56% <1 cm) with a 96% resectability rate and an 85% frequency of stage I tumors. This study generated new guidelines for the management of CT-detected pulmonary lesions and needle aspiration biopsy of small nodules.[15]

Table 1 summarizes the results of LDCT screening in observational studies that include more than 70,000 subjects. Median age was 59 (range 53–67), with minimum age ranging from 40 to 60. Five studies included nonsmokers, representing 14% to 54% of participants in each trial, and an overall proportion of 18%. In the remaining 11 studies, the median pack-years (p-y) was 41 (range 30–47).

At baseline, the overall frequency of participants with noncalcified solid lesions was 21% (range 7–53), lung cancer detection rate 1% (range 0.2–2.7), and proportion of stage I lung cancer 78% (range 50%–100%). The two larger Japanese studies,[16,17] including a significant proportion of nonsmokers (38%–54%), also showed the lowest

Table 1
Lung cancer screening: Results of LDCT in observational studies

	Subjects	Age[a]	Nsm[b]	P-Y[c]	CT Lesions[d]	Lung Cancers Baseline[e]	Stage I[f]	First Repeat[g]
Henschke et al,[15] 1999	1,000	67	0	45	233 (23)	27 (2.7)	85	—
Sone et al,[16] 2001	5,483	64	54	—	588 (11)	23 (.4)	100	27 (.5)
Nawa et al,[17] 2002	7,956	56	38	—	541 (7)	36 (.5)	78	4 (.1)
Sobue et al,[18] 2002	1,611	59	14	—	186 (12)	14 (.9)	71	22 (1.4)
Swensen et al,[19] 2003	1,520	59	0	45	780 (51)	27 (1.7)	74	13 (.9)
Pastorino et al,[20] 2003	1,035	58	0	40	199 (19)	11 (1.1)	55	11 (1.1)
Diederich et al,[21] 2004	817	53	0	45	350 (43)	12 (1.5)	64	—
Bastarrika et al,[22] 2005	911	55	0	30	291 (32)	12 (1.3)	83	2 (.2)
Chong et al,[23] 2005	6,406	55	23	—	2,255 (35)	23 (.4)	56	—
Novello et al,[24] 2005	519	59	0	—	241 (47)	5 (1.0)	67	3 (.6)
MacRedmond et al,[25] 2006	449	55	0	45	111 (25)	2 (.4)	50	4 (.9)
I-ELCAP,[26] 2006	31,567	61	17	30	4,186 (13)	410 (1.3)	85	74 (.2)
Callol et al,[27] 2007	466	61	0	36	98 (21)	1 (.2)	100	4 (.9)
Veronesi et al,[28] 2008	5,201	58	0	44	2,754 (53)	55 (1.1)	66	37 (.7)
Wilson et al,[29] 2008	3642	59	0	47	1,477 (41)	53 (1.5)	58	24 (.7)
Menezes et al,[30] 2010	3352	60	0	30	600 (18)	44 (1.3)	65	10 (.3)
Overall	71,935	59	18	41	14,890 (21)	755 (1.0)	78	235 (.4)

[a] Median age of participants.
[b] Proportion of nonsmokers.
[c] Median pack-years.
[d] Subjects with noncalcified solid lesions (percent of participants).
[e] Lung cancers detected at baseline (percent of participants).
[f] Percent of lung cancers detected in stage I at baseline.
[g] Lung cancers detected at first annual CT repeat.

frequency of baseline lesions (7%–11%) and lung cancer detection rates (0.4–0.5%). On the other hand, the highest baseline detection rate (2.7%), reported by Henschke and colleagues,[15] can be explained by the accrual of heavier smokers above the age of 60 (median 67 years, 45 p-y), but also to the prolonged diagnostic workup of lesions detected at baseline (up to 2 years). In fact, in the more recent Korean study,[23] in which nearly half of the 6,406 participants were low risk and 23% were nonsmokers, the lung cancer detection rate at baseline was only 0.4%. Interestingly, the use of the latest generation spiral CTs (8–16-slice) has increased the proportion of subjects with noncalcified solid nodules above 50%, but the lung cancer detection rate has remained relatively stable.[28]

In most studies, lung cancer detection rate declined after baseline CT. Thirteen studies reported the number of lung cancers detected at first annual CT repeat (see **Table 1**): a total of 235 cases from 63,712 subjects, corresponding to 0.4% rate (range 0.1–1.4) and a cumulative frequency at two years of 1.4% (range 0.6–2.6).

The difference observed in baseline detection rate are mainly due to the heterogeneity of cancer risk among the various study populations, but also to the diagnostic algorithm, the methodology of analysis of CT images and the definition of a positive screen applied by each center. If one excludes the two Japanese studies with a high proportion of nonsmokers,[16,17] cumulative lung cancer detection rate of baseline and second year of screening is 1.6% (range 1.1–2.6).

RANDOMIZED TRIALS WITH LOW-DOSE SPIRAL CT
Differences in Study Design

Several randomized lung cancer screening trials are currently ongoing worldwide, with more than 90,000 recruited subjects (**Table 2**). A major difference between the American and European trials design is the nature of control arm, which is annual CR in the United States and observational in Europe. In the United States, CR was chosen for the control group to facilitate accrual, improve compliance, and avoid potential interference with the results of the larger ongoing Prostate, Lung, Colorectal, and Ovarian Cancer (PLCO) screening study.[10,39]

The methodology of accrual also differed among the various studies. The two US studies recruited smoking volunteers (or former smokers) through direct mailings from hospital lists and use of mass media. The NELSON trial extracted potentially eligible subjects from population registries: 335,441 individuals born between 1928 and 1953 received a questionnaire about general health, life style, and smoking habits; 32% replied and 5% were then selected based on their individual cancer risk.[34] The ITALUNG trial contacted 71,232 candidates identified through 269 general practitioner's lists, and randomized 5% of them.[35] The LUSI trial adopted a population-based recruitment from three cities in the Rhine-Neckar region (Mannheim, Ludwigshafen, Heidelberg), sending more than 300,000 questionnaires to randomize 1.4% of the population.[38,40,41]

Table 2
Lung cancer screening: Design of randomized LDCT trials

Study	Country	Study Design	Year Started	Subjects Enrolled	Age Range	Number of CTs	Years Screen
LSS[31]	USA	CT vs CR	2000	3,318	55–74	2	2
DANTE[32]	Italy	CT vs observation	2001	2,811	60–74	5	5
NLST[33]	USA	CT vs CR	2002	53,454	55–74	3	3
NELSON[34]	Netherlands	CT vs observation	2003	15,822	50–74	3	4
ITALUNG[35]	Italy	CT vs observation	2004	3,206	55–69	4	4
DLCST[36]	Denmark	CT vs observation	2004	4,104	50–70	5	5
MILD[37]	Italy	CT vs observation	2005	4,099	49–75	5–10	10
LUSI[38]	Germany	CT vs observation	2007	4,052	50–69	5	5
Total	—	—	—	90,866	—	—	—

The Lung Screening Study (LSS) was a pilot trial performed in six centers of the United States in 2000 that randomized 3,318 smokers (age 55–74, ≥30 p-y, median 54 p-y) to LDCT or CR, performed at baseline and first year repeat.[31,42]

Based on the success of LSS, in 2002, the National Cancer Institute, in collaboration with the American College of Radiology Imaging Network, launched the National Lung Screening Trial (NLST), which was the largest randomized clinical trial (RCT) worldwide comparing LDCT versus CR, with lung cancer mortality as the endpoint.[33] A total of 53,454 participants (age 55–74, ≥30 p-y) have been enrolled from 33 centers across the United States. The NLST has 90% statistical power to detect a 20% reduction in lung cancer mortality in the LDCT arm. The three planned annual screening examinations were completed in 2006.

The European screening program currently includes six randomized studies: the NELSON trial in the Netherlands, the Danish Lung Cancer Screening Trial (DLCST) trial in Denmark, the LUSI trial in Germany, and three Italian studies: DANTE-Milan, ITALUNG-Florence, and Multicentric Italian Lung Detection (MILD)-Milan, all comparing annual CT versus observation without CR screening.

The NELSON trial was designed to detect a 25% reduction of lung cancer mortality in subjects aged 50 to 74 having smoked more than 15 cigarettes per day for more than 25 years, or more than 10 cigarettes per day for more than 30 years, with a planned population of 20,000 subjects and three 16-slice LDCT examinations at year 1, 2, and 4 in the screening arm.[34] The NELSON trial accrued 15,822 individuals in the Netherlands and Belgium.

The DLCST trial has recruited 4,104 individuals with a similar risk population (50–70 years, ≥20 p-y) but includes annual LDCT screening for 5 years, with results regularly uploaded to the NELSON database. The LUSI trial had a similar design, with annual LDCT for 5 years and 4,052 randomized subjects.[38,40]

The DANTE study in Milan was the first European randomized trial to be launched in 2001, enrolling 2,811 male subjects (60–74 years, ≥20 p-y) in annual LDCT screenings or observation for 5 years.[32] At baseline, participants in both arms had to undergo one single CR and sputum cytology examination, which led to lung cancer detection in eight patients in the control arm. The ITALUNG-Florence trial randomized 3,206 subjects (55–69 years, ≥20 p-y) to annual CT versus observation for 4 years.

The MILD trial started in Milan in 2005 and enrolled 4,099 participants at the Istituto Nazionale Tumori of Milan.[37] Volunteers were assigned to LDCT or control and, in the LDCT arm, further randomized to annual LDCT versus biennial LDCT, for a period of 10 years. All participants had to undergo an anti-tobacco counseling program, pulmonary function test evaluation, and tissue sampling for extensive biomarker assessment.

A pilot trial, Depiscan, was launched in France in 2002 to assess the feasibility of a screening program with the accrual based on 232 general practitioners and occupational physicians. This trial entered only 621 subjects in 2 years and was closed due to insufficient accrual (41% active investigators) and poor compliance.[42]

A new randomized trial, the United Kingdom Lung Screening (UKLS) trial started in 2011 with a pilot phase of 4,000 subjects selected according to the Liverpool Lung Project risk model, to achieve a higher lung cancer incidence (1% per year).[43] This trial will test the efficacy of one-shot screening. Participants will be randomized to only one screening CT or observation. After the pilot phase, the trial will proceed to the total accrual of 32,000 subjects.

Accrual Status and Detection Rates

The population features and nodule detection rate of the LDCT arm is illustrated in **Table 3**. Overall, median age was 60 years (range among trials 57–65), male proportion 65% (55%–100%), and median p-y 51 (36–56).

LSS confirmed the higher lung cancer detection rate of LDCT as compared with CR: 1.8% versus 0.5% at baseline, and 2.4 versus 1.3% cumulative after the first year repeat.

In the NLST trial, participants showed the highest smoking intensity (median 56 p-y) but also the highest proportion of former smokers (52%). The frequency of noncalcified solid nodules in the LDCT arm was 25% at baseline, 28% at first LDCT repeat, and 17% at second repeat; lung cancer detection rate was 1% at baseline, 0.6% at first LDCT repeat, and 0.9% at second repeat.

Initial results of NELSON have shown a 0.9% lung cancer detection rate at baseline and 0.7% at first LDCT repeat.[44] Lung cancer detection rate of DLCST was similar to that of NELSON: 0.8% at baseline and 0.6% at first LDCT repeat.[47] Baseline LDCT of ITALUNG detected 21 lung cancers in 20 subjects (1.5%).[35] Detection rates of the MILD trial were 0.7% at baseline and 0.8% (17 and 18 cases, respectively).[48] The Depiscan trial detected at baseline 8 lung cancers (2.4%) in the CT arm and 1 (0.4%) in the CR arm.[42]

Lung Cancer Incidence and Mortality

In October 2010, an National Cancer Institute press release announced that the NLST trial was

Table 3
Lung cancer screening: Results of LDCT arm in randomized studies

						Lung Cancers		
	Subjects	Age	Male	P-Y	CT Lesions	Baseline	Stage I	First Repeat
LSS,[31] 2005	1,629	62	58	54	316 (17)	30 (1.8)	48	8 (.6)
NELSON,[44] 2009	7,557	59	84	42	1,570 (21)	70 (.9)	64	54 (.7)
DANTE,[45] 2009	1,276	65	100	47	226 (18)	47 (3.7)	66	13 (1)
ITALUNG,[35] 2009	1,406	61	65	39	426 (30)	20 (1.5)	48	—
NLST,[46] 2011	26,309	60	59	56	6561 (25)	270 (1)	63	168 (.6)
DLCST,[47] 2012	2,047	58	55	36	179 (9)	17 (.8)	53	11 (.6)
MILD,[48] 2012	2,376	57	68	39	335 (14)	17 (.7)	57	18 (.8)
LUSI,[38] 2012	2,029	57	65	—	540 (27)	22 (1.1)	—	—
Overall	44,629	60	65	51	10,153 (23)	493 (1.1)	62	272 (.7)

prematurely stopped due to the different mortality rates observed in the two arms, which reached the anticipated goal of 20% reduction in lung cancer mortality rate, corresponding to a 6.9% reduction in total mortality. In the full paper, published the following year[46] with a median follow-up of 6.5 years, there was an absolute difference of 87 lung cancer deaths (356 in the LDCT arm vs 443 in the CR arm, −20%) and of 123 deaths for all causes (1877 in the CT arm vs 2000 in the CR arm, −6.7%), and an excess of 119 detected lung cancers (1060 in the LDCT arm vs 941 in the CR arm).

At present, three European trials have published lung cancer incidence and mortality data. In the DANTE study, after a median follow-up of only 3 years, lung cancer was detected in 60 (4.7%) subjects receiving LDCT and 34 (2.8%) controls (P = .016), with a higher percentage of stage I (54% vs 34%, respectively; not significantly different: P = .06), corresponding to a threefold excess in the total number of stage I (33 vs 12; P = .004).[45] However, the number of stage III to IV lung cancers was not reduced in the LDCT arm

(24 vs 21 cases) and lung cancer mortality was identical in the two arms (20 deaths each), as well as mortality for other causes (26 vs 25). The DLCST trial also showed more lung cancers in the screening arm (69 vs 24, P<.001) and more patients with stage I to IIB (48 vs 21, P = .002) at 5 years follow-up.[47] However, the number of lung cancer deaths was higher in the screening arm (15 vs 11, P = .428) as well as the total number of deaths (61 vs 42, P = .059). In the MILD trial, at 5 years follow-up, a total of 34 lung cancers were observed in the annual LDCT arm, 25 in the biennial LDCT arm, and 20 in the control arm (P = .036).[48] Lung cancer deaths were 12, 6, and 7 (P = .21), and the total number of deaths in the three arms was 31, 20, and 20, respectively (P = .13).

Given the relevant differences in sample size and follow-up among the various trials, one way to compare the results is to look at observed numbers over person-years. The observed lung cancer incidence and mortality rates are illustrated in **Table 4** as percentage per year. The lung cancer mortality reduction in the NLST, although statistically

Table 4
Lung cancer incidence and mortality in randomized screening trials (percent per year)

Study	Trial Arm	Person-years (%)	Lung Cancer Incidence (%)	Lung Cancer Mortality (%)	Total Mortality (%)
NLST[46]	LDCT	144,103	0.65	0.25	1.30
	CR	143,368	0.57	0.31	1.40
PLCO[a,39]	CR	85,428	0.61	0.36	—
	Observation	85,474	0.61	0.38	—
DLCST[47]	LDCT	9,769	0.66	0.15	0.62
	Observation	9,794	0.25	0.11	0.43
MILD[48]	LDCT annual	5,482	0.62	0.22	0.56
	LDCT biennial	5,471	0.46	0.11	0.36
	Observation	6,433	0.31	0.11	0.31

[a] Subset of 30,321 PLCO participants eligible for NLST trial.

significant owing to the large number of randomized subjects, was only 0.06% per year (or 6 out of 10,000 individuals). Such a difference is very similar to the one observed between the control arm of the NLST and the intervention arm of the PLCO, both receiving annual CR.[39] A fourfold bigger difference between lung cancer incidence and mortality was observed in the control arm of the NLST and the PLCO (0.26% and 0.25%, respectively), which is difficult to explain in a disease that kills 85% of diagnosed patients. The difference in lung cancer incidence rates between the annual LDCT arm and the control arm was only 0.08% in the NLST, much lower than 0.41% observed in the DLCST, and 0.31% in the MILD trials.

CRITICAL ISSUES IN LDCT SCREENING TRIALS
False-Positive Findings

The frequency of noncalcified pulmonary lesions in heavy smokers aged 50 or older receiving LDCT examination varies according to population characteristics, but the probability of detecting benign lesions at first LDCT is 20 times higher than the lung cancer detection rate (see **Tables 1** and **3**).

The overall screening performance depends on the diagnostic algorithm chosen in the research protocol, and the threshold applied to define suspicious lesions. As an example, in the Mayo CT trial, the cumulative frequency of subjects with suspicious lesions was 74% at 5 years, but only 6% of them proved to have cancer, with a 70% rate of false-positive findings among all participants to the study.[49] In the Milan pilot study, using single-slice CT and a cut-off diameter above 5 mm, the cumulative frequency of subjects with suspicious lesions that were recalled for LDCT or positron emission tomography (PET) was only 19% at 5 years (193 out of 1035), 20% of whom (38 out of 193) proved to have cancer, with only 15% false-positive CTs.[37] Of interest, the cumulative lung cancer detection rate at 5 years was 4% in both trials (average 0.8% per year), with the same resectability rate (94%) and a very similar proportion of stage I disease (68% vs 63%).

Diagnostic Evaluation of Positive CT Screens

Diagnostic assessment of small indeterminate pulmonary nodules requires serial CT scanning for the detection of morphology and volume changes and the availability of reliable software for fully automated three-dimensional segmentation and highly consistent volume measurement of lung nodules havebecome helpful in evaluating even limited growth as a marker of potential malignancy.[50,51]

Long-term follow-up of lesions less than or equal to 5 mm has proven that these nodules do not require additional workup. For lesions between 5 and 10 mm, surveillance of growth should be performed by three-dimensional volumetry because volume doubling is equivalent to only 26% increase of diameter, a difference that may be difficult to detect with manually-guided diameter measurements. Changes in size indicating a doubling time ranging from 30 to 360 days are consistent with cancer and require further investigation.[52]

The diagnostic algorithm of the NELSON trial, based on the automated assessment of volume and doubling time, without the help of computer aided detection or PET, obtained a 99.9% negative predictive value, but the frequency of invasive procedures for benign disease was very high (27%).[44]

Pure nonsolid lesions, or ground-glass opacities, have a low risk of malignancy (10%–15%), usually represented by well differentiated bronchioloalveolar carcinomas (BAC) or in situ adenocarcinoma, but their volume and growth are more difficult to evaluate. Part-solid lesions have a higher risk of malignancy (up to 50%), which is directly related to the size and growth of the solid component.[53]

Large meta-analyses have demonstrated the clinical value of PET in the differential diagnosis of undetermined pulmonary nodules detected by spiral CT, with a sensitivity rate of 96% to 97%, a specificity of 78% to 82%,[54] and an accuracy rate reaching 92% with the CT/PET fusion machine.[55] Moreover, a randomized trial demonstrated that preoperative PET is an essential component of lung cancer staging.[56] The Milan trial was the first screening protocol to include selective use of PET in the diagnostic algorithm, thus showing that PET may be helpful in the management of CT detected lesions greater than or equal to 7 mm. In the first 5 years of screening, PET was applied to only 1.4% of spiral CTs, with an overall sensitivity rate of 94%, specificity of 82%, and an accuracy rate of 88%.[37,57,58]

Overdiagnosis of Indolent Tumors

Overdiagnosis refers to LDCT-detected lung cancers that would not affect patient lifetime because of competing causes of death or because the lesion would never progress to symptomatic cancer without screening. Detection and treatment of "indolent" or "slow-growing" disease are the most likely explanations for the lack of mortality reduction observed in CR screening trials, despite a significant increase in the resectability rate and proportion of early stage cancers in the intervention arm.[13] The occurrence of slow growing lung cancer has been often rejected on the grounds that screening-detected and symptomatic tumors show similar histopathologic and, sometimes, molecular features, particularly when comparison is restricted to stage I patients.[59] However, the significant rise in the frequency of adenocarcinoma from 32% of all cases in the SEER database from the years 1983 to 1987[60] to over 70% (range 55%–95%) in CT screening trials[8–21] indicates overdiagnosis. An international panel has reviewed the histopathological features of 279 stage IA adenocarcinomas belonging to the I-ELCAP database to determine whether survival differed from the proportion of the BAC component.[61] The revision confirmed that 81% of CT-detected adenocarcinomas show a substantial BAC component, and that 5-year survival was 100% for pure BAC and 95% for mixed BAC. Such a sudden shift toward adenocarcinoma and BAC cannot be explained by well-known changes in the epidemiology of tobacco consumption, and is indicative overdiagnosis by CT screening.

Analysis of metabolic activity by PET has shown that a standardized uptake value less than or equal to 2.5 can identify patients with 100% 5-year survival among all screening-detected lung cancers.[58] In addition, long-term follow-up of 76 ground-glass nodules in the MILD trial demonstrated that only a minimal fraction of these lesions evolve to adenocarcinoma without progression-advanced stage, so that active surveillance of these lesions is justified.[62] If confirmed by prospective studies, these results might improve the clinical management of LDCT-detected tumors, reducing the risk of unnecessary treatment of indolent disease.

The awareness of overdiagnosis as a consequence of screening programs for each and every solid tumor is increasing and the magnitude of the problem requires adequate approaches to keep the human and economic costs of anticipated treatments for healthy or asymptomatic population under control.[63,64]

Survival of LDCT-detected Lung Cancers and Mortality in the Screening Cohort

In 2005, Swensen and colleagues,[49] comparing the lung cancer mortality rates in the Mayo CT study with those observed in the previous CR trial, found no differences in lung cancer mortality rates between the two studies in the subset of men aged 50 years or older (2.8 vs 2.0 per 1000 person-years). On the other hand, in 2006, the International ELCAP study group published a report on the efficacy of CT screening in which the overall survival of 484 screening-detected lung cancer patients was 80% at 10 years, regardless of stage and treatment, and reached 92% in the subset of clinical stage I resected within 1 month of diagnosis.[26] The investigators, therefore, concluded that CT screening could prevent 80% of all lung cancer deaths in high-risk individuals. However, the analysis was focused only on cancer detected at baseline and first CT repeat, without long-term follow-up of the entire cohort. Moreover, patients' outcome at 10 years was projected from a median follow-up of only 3 years, using lung cancer specifically instead of overall survival.

A concurrent meta-analysis of three single-arm studies (Mayo Clinic, Milan, and Lee Moffitt Cancer Center) including 3,246 subjects and 10,942 person-years, showed that CT screening resulted in a 3.5-fold increase of lung cancer diagnoses, a 10-fold increase of surgical resections; however, the number of advanced lung cancers and lung cancer deaths did not differ from those expected from a simulation model.[65] Interestingly, the results were consistent among all three centers, despite the potential differences in epidemiologic risk and screening methodology.

It is clear from these data that an excellent survival of patients with LDCT-detected lung cancer cannot predict a positive outcome in the entire cohort under screening.

Morbidity of CT Screening

The side-effects and morbidity of LDCT screening are difficult to assess in a comprehensive way. **Table 5** reports the frequency of surgical procedures for benign disease, not including bronchoscopy and fine-needle aspiration biopsy. Invasive biopsies for benign lesions represent 22% (range 0%–34%) of all surgical procedures and 0.5% of individuals undergoing CT screening. In particular, the frequency of invasive surgical procedures for benign disease was 24% in the NLST and 27% in the NELSON trial.[44,46]

Mortality and morbidity is not reported in most screening studies. In the NLST trial, the frequency of death within 2 months of diagnostic evaluation of a detected finding in the LDCT arm was 0.08%, the frequency of major complications 0.33%, and 60-day perioperative mortality after surgical procedures 1%.

The damage attributable to prolonged exposure of current smokers to ionizing radiations is probably underestimated on the grounds that average dose for yearly LDCT (1.5 mSv) is below the recommended safety dose for the general population. However, a significant proportion of screened individuals have to undergo further and more complex

Table 5
Lung cancer screening: Surgical procedures for benign disease

	Subjects	Number of Surgical Procedures			
		Total	Cancer	Benign	% Benign
Henschke et al,[15] 1999	1,000	28	27	1	4
Sone et al,[16] 2001	5,483	72	56	16	22
Nawa et al,[17] 2002	7,956	58	40	18	31
Sobue et al,[18] 2002	1,611	36	31	5	14
Diederich et al,[21] 2004	817	14	11	3	21
Swensen et al,[19] 2003	1,520	83	68	15	18
Pastorino et al,[20] 2003	1,035	43	36	7	16
Bastarrika et al,[22] 2005	911	14	14	0	0
Novello et al,[24] 2005	519	14	12	2	14
MacRedmond et al,[25] 2006	449	9	6	3	33
Caillol et al,[27] 2007	466	7	5	2	29
Veronesi et al,[28] 2008	5,201	107	92	15	14
Wilson et al,[29] 2008	3642	82	54	28	34
Menezes et al,[30] 2010	3352	57	44	13	23
NELSON,[44] 2009	7,557	91	67	24	27
DANTE,[45] 2009	1,276	72	55	17	24
ITALUNG[35]	1,406	17	16	1	6
NLST,[46] 2011	26,309	673	509	164	24
DLCST,[47] 2012	2,047	25	17	8	32
MILD,[48] 2012	2,376	51	47	4	8
LUSI,[38] 2012	2,029	31	22	9	29
Overall	76,962	1,584	1,229	355	22

diagnostic examinations to rule out false-positive lesions, with radiation doses largely exceeding the one of single LDCT. It has been estimated that NLST participants received an average of 8 mSv over three years, and that one cancer death per 2,500 persons screened may be caused by radiation.[66] The interaction between diagnostic radiations and persisting exposure to smoking carcinogens, particularly in young individuals, is substantially unknown[67] and needs to be better investigated within current randomized trials.

ROLE OF BIOMARKERS IN LUNG CANCER SCREENING

In the last decade, clinical research on CT screening has determined a profound and valuable mutation in our understanding of lung cancer biology, a change that might carry important advances in the management of such a dreadful disease, the outcome of which has not improved for a very long time.

Recent publications have launched biomarker tests for early lung cancer detection. MicroRNAs are small noncoding RNAs that modulate gene activity and are aberrantly expressed in most types of cancer.[68] Because of their small size and stability, they can be also tracked in biologic fluids such as plasma and serum and serve as circulating biomarkers.[69] A recent study from the author's group showed that a combination of 24 microRNAs circulating in plasma detects lung cancer up to 2 years earlier than LDCT and also identifies tumor aggressiveness.[10,70] These findings were confirmed by another group with 34 serum circulating microRNA, in patients detected by LDCT screening.[71] Overall, these studies highlight the potential of circulating microRNAs as screening biomarkers for lung cancer, which seem to be superior to autoantibodies assay[72] and serum proteomic signatures.[73]

These results indicate that microRNA assay could overcome some of the problems encountered with the use of LDCT in lung cancer screening by exploiting the synergy between the molecular and imaging tests to reduce individual radiation exposure, harmful diagnostic procedures, unnecessary surgery, overload of highly specialized medical centers, and costs for the health care system.[66]

If these data are confirmed in the future, the use of plasma assay as the first line examination could avoid unnecessary LDCT in a large proportion of subjects or substantially increase the sensitivity of imaging tools by the integrated use of microRNA and LDCT.

COMMENTS AND CONTROVERSIES

Why is earlier detection by LDCT screening not able to prevent the occurrence of metastatic lung cancer, nor to substantially reduce mortality in the long term? One possible explanation is that spiral CT is unable to intercept the fast-growing or most aggressive lung cancers before the onset of metastases.

Implementing annual LDCT screening for millions of current or former smokers would require the investment of enormous resources, particularly in European countries where the national health services are guaranteed and free for the whole population. Several critical factors need to be taken into account. The study population of the NLST was quite different from that of European studies: 52% were former smokers and 41% were women.[74] The control arm did not represent current practice (observation) but was indeed a screening arm with annual CR.

Moreover, premature interruption of RCTs for ethical reasons is a dangerous decision. In fact, a recent review and meta-regression analysis by Cochrane Institute showed that, in most instances, truncated trials are associated with greater effect sizes, which are not confirmed by nontruncated RCTs.[75] With the specific limitations of smaller size, when compared with NLST, and 3 to 5 years follow-up, the midterm results of European trials have not confirmed that LDCT screening has a measurable effect in diminishing lung cancer mortality.

Even assuming that the NLST policy and quality of management can be reproduced in general hospitals, it will take 900 CTs, 18 PETs, 3 bronchoscopies or needle aspiration biopsies, and 2 pulmonary resections for benign disease to avoid one lung cancer death.

In the end, the cost-benefit balance of screening for a preventable disease must carefully compared with the one of alternative policies such as systematic use of effective anti-tobacco drugs (varenicline).

SUMMARY

Randomized trials are the most appropriate instrument to test the efficacy of CT screening in heavy smokers. The ongoing randomized studies around the world have the adequate size and appropriate design to provide unequivocal evidence of even modest reductions in lung cancer mortality. In the meantime, CT screening for lung cancer should be considered an experimental procedure, not to be offered or promoted outside controlled clinical trials. Innovative strategies, based on lung cancer biology and tissue biomarkers, should be implemented to improve or replace radiological screening, boost primary prevention through pharmacologic smoking cessation, and identify specific inhibitors of lethal cancers that still elude imaging techniques.

ACKNOWLEDGMENTS

The Milan Early Detection Research program is supported by a Research Grant from the Italian Ministry of Health (Ricerca Finalizzata), the Italian Association for Cancer Research (AIRC), and the Cariplo Foundation.

REFERENCES

1. Peto R, Lopez AD, Boreham J, et al. Mortality from smoking worldwide. Br Med Bull 1996;52:12–21.
2. Jemal A, Siegel R, Xu J, et al. Cancer statistics, 2010. CA Cancer J Clin 2010;60(5):277–300.
3. Yang L, Parkin DM, Li LD, et al. Estimation and projection of the national profile of cancer mortality in China: 1991–2005. Br J Cancer 2004;90:2157–66.
4. Levi F, Lucchini F, Negri E, et al. Mortality from major cancer sites in the European Union, 1955-1998. Ann Oncol 2003;14:490–5.
5. Verdecchia A, Franceschi S, Brenner H, et al. Recent cancer survival in Europe: a 2000–02 period analysis of EUROCARE 4 data. Lancet Oncol 2007; 8:784–96.
6. Howlander N, Noone AM, Krapcho M, et al, editors. SEER Cancer statistics review, 1975–2008. Bethesda (MD): National Cancer Institute.
7. Goldstraw P, Crowley J, Chansky K, et al. The IASLC lung cancer staging project: proposals for the revision of the TNM stage groupings in the forthcoming (seventh) edition of the TNM classification of malignant tumours. J Thorac Oncol 2007;2:706–14.
8. Melamed MR, Flehinger BJ, Zaman MB, et al. Screening for lung cancer: results of the Memorial Sloan-Kettering study in New York. Chest 1984;86: 44–53.
9. Tockman MS. Survival and mortality from lung cancer in a screened population. Chest 1986; 89(Suppl 4):324S–5S.
10. Prorok PC, Andriole GL, Bresalier RS, et al, Prostate, Lung, Colorectal and Ovarian Cancer Screening Trial Project Team. Design of the

Prostate, Lung, Colorectal and Ovarian (PLCO) Cancer Screening trial. Control Clin Trials 2000; 21(Suppl 6):273S–309S.

11. Melamed MR. Lung cancer screening results in the National Cancer Institute New York study. Cancer 2000;89(Suppl 11):2356–62.

12. Kubík A, Polak J. Lung cancer detection: results of a randomized prospective study in Czechoslovakia. Cancer 1986;57(12):2427–37.

13. Marcus PM, Bergstralh EJ, Zweig MH, et al. Extended lung cancer incidence follow-up in the Mayo lung project and overdiagnosis. J Natl Cancer Inst 2006;98:748–56.

14. Kaneko M, Eguchi K, Ohmatsu H, et al. Peripheral lung cancer: screening and detection with low-dose spiral CT versus radiography. Radiology 1996;201:798–802.

15. Henschke CI, McCauley DI, Yankelevitz DF, et al. Early lung cancer action project: overall design and findings from baseline screening. Lancet 1999;354:99–105.

16. Sone S, Li F, Yang ZG, et al. Results of three-year mass screening programme for lung cancer using mobile low-dose spiral computed tomography scanner. Br J Cancer 2001;84:25–32.

17. Nawa T, Nakagawa T, Kusano S, et al. Lung cancer screening using low-dose spiral CT: results of baseline and 1-year follow-up studies. Chest 2002;122: 15–20.

18. Sobue T, Moriyama N, Kaneko M, et al. Screening for lung cancer with low-dose helical computed tomography: anti-lung cancer association project. J Clin Oncol 2002;20:911–20.

19. Swensen SJ, Jett JR, Hartman TE, et al. Lung cancer screening with CT: Mayo Clinic experience. Radiology 2003;226:756–61.

20. Pastorino U, Bellomi M, Landoni C, et al. Early lung-cancer detection with spiral CT and positron emission tomography in heavy smokers: 2-year results. Lancet 2003;362:593–7.

21. Diederich S, Thomas M, Semik M, et al. Screening for early lung cancer with low-dose spiral computed tomography: results of annual follow-up examinations in asymptomatic smokers. Eur Radiol 2004; 14:691–702.

22. Bastarrika G, García-Velloso MJ, Lozano MD, et al. Early lung cancer detection using spiral computed tomography and positron emission tomography. Am J Respir Crit Care Med 2005;171:1378–83.

23. Chong S, Lee KS, Chung MJ, et al. Lung cancer screening with low-dose helical CT in Korea: experiences at the Samsung Medical Center. J Korean Med Sci 2005;20:402–8.

24. Novello S, Fava C, Borasio P, et al. Three-year findings of an early lung cancer detection feasibility study with low-dose spiral computed tomography in heavy smokers. Ann Oncol 2005;16:1662–6.

25. MacRedmond R, McVey G, Lee M, et al. Screening for lung cancer using low dose CT scanning: results of 2 year follow up. Thorax 2006;61:54–6.

26. The International Early Lung Cancer Action Program Investigators (I-ELCAP). Survival of patients with stage I lung cancer detected on CT screening. N Engl J Med 2006;355:1763–71.

27. Callol L, Roig F, Cuevas A, et al. Low-dose CT: a useful and accessible tool for the early diagnosis of lung cancer in selected populations. Lung Cancer 2007;56(2):217–21.

28. Veronesi G, Bellomi M, Mulshine JL, et al. Lung cancer screening with low-dose computed tomography: a non-invasive diagnostic protocol for baseline lung nodules. Lung Cancer 2008;61:340–9.

29. Wilson DO, Weissfeld JL, Fuhrman CR, et al. The Pittsburgh Lung Screening Study (PLuSS): outcomes within 3 years of a first computed tomography scan. Am J Respir Crit Care Med 2008;178(9): 956–61.

30. Menezes RJ, Roberts HC, Paul NS, et al. Lung cancer screening using low-dose computed tomography in at-risk individuals: the Toronto experience. Lung Cancer 2010;67(2):177–83.

31. Gohagan JK, Marcus PM, Fagerstrom RM, et al, The Lung Screening Study Research Group. Final results of the Lung Screening Study, a randomized feasibility study of spiral CT versus chest X-ray screening for lung cancer. Lung Cancer 2005;47:9–15.

32. Infante M, Lutman FR, Cavuto S, et al, DANTE Study Group. Lung cancer screening with spiral CT: baseline results of the randomized DANTE trial. Lung Cancer 2008;59:355–63.

33. Clark KW, Gierada DS, Marquez D, et al. Collecting 48,000 CT exams for the Lung Screening Study of the National Lung Screening Trial. J Digit Imaging 2008;22(6):667–80.

34. van den Bergh KA, Essink-Bot ML, Bunge EM, et al. Impact of computed tomography screening for lung cancer on participants in a randomized controlled trial (NELSON trial). Cancer 2008;113:396–404.

35. Lopes Pegna A, Picozzi G, Mascalchi M, et al, ITALUNG Study Research Group. Design, recruitment and baseline results of the ITALUNG trial for lung cancer screening with low-dose CT. Design, recruitment and baseline results of the ITALUNG trial for lung cancer screening with low-dose CT. Lung Cancer 2009;64(1):34–40.

36. Pedersen JH, Ashraf H, Dirksen A, et al. The Danish randomized lung cancer CT screening trial–overall design and results of the prevalence round. J Thorac Oncol 2009;4:608–14.

37. Pastorino U. Early detection of lung cancer. Respiration 2006;73:5–13.

38. Becker N, Motsch E, Gross ML, et al. Randomized study on early detection of lung cancer with MSCT in Germany: study design and results of the first

screening round. J Cancer Res Clin Oncol 2012; 138(9):1475–86.

39. Oken MM, Hocking WG, Kvale PA, et al, PLCO Project Team. Screening by chest radiograph and lung cancer mortality: the Prostate, Lung, Colorectal, and Ovarian (PLCO) randomized trial. JAMA 2011; 306(17):1865–73.

40. Becker N, Delorme S, Kauczor HU. LUSI: the German component of the European trial on the efficacy of multislice-CT for the early detection of lung cancer. Onkologie 2008;31:PO320.

41. Gohagan JK, Marcus PM, Fagerstrom RM, et al. The Lung Screening Study: the National Cancer Institute's randomized feasibility study of spiral CT versus chest X-ray in lung cancer screening. Chest 2004;126:114–21.

42. Blanchon T, Bréchot JM, Grenier PA, et al, "Dépiscan" Group. Baseline results of the Depiscan study: a French randomized pilot trial of lung cancer screening comparing low dose CT scan (LDCT) and chest X-ray (CXR). Lung Cancer 2007;58:50–8.

43. Field JK, Baldwin D, Brain K, et al, UKLS Team. CT screening for lung cancer in the UK: position statement by UKLS investigators following the NLST report. Thorax 2011;66(8):736–7.

44. van Klaveren RJ, Oudkerk M, Prokop M, et al. Management of lung nodules detected by volume CT scanning. N Engl J Med 2009;361:2221–9.

45. Infante M, Cavuto S, Lutman FR, et al, DANTE StudyGroup*. A randomized study of lung cancer screening with spiral computed tomography (The DANTE Trial) three-year results. Am J Respir Crit Care Med 2009;180:445–53.

46. Kramer BS, Berg CD, Aberle DR, et al. Lung cancer screening with low-dose helical CT: results from the National Lung Screening Trial (NLST). J Med Screen 2011;18:109–11.

47. Saghir Z, Dirksen A, Ashraf H, et al. CT screening for lung cancer brings forward early disease. The randomised Danish Lung Cancer Screening Trial: status after five annual screening rounds with low-dose CT. Thorax 2012;67:296–301.

48. Pastorino U, Rossi M, Rosato V, et al. Annual or biennial CT screening versus observation in heavy smokers: 5-year results of the MILD trial. Eur J Cancer Prev 2012;21:308–15.

49. Swensen SJ, Jett JR, Hartman TE, et al. CT screening for lung cancer: five-year prospective experience. Radiology 2005;235:259–65.

50. Wiemker R, Rogalla P, Blaffert T, et al. Aspects of computer-aided detection (CAD) and volumetry of pulmonary nodules using multislice CT. Br J Radiol 2005;78:S46–56.

51. Marchianò A, Calabrò E, Civelli E, et al. Pulmonary nodules: volume repeatability at multidetector CT lung cancer screening. Radiology 2009;251: 919–25.

52. Libby DM, Smith JP, Altorki NK, et al. Managing the small pulmonary nodule discovered by CT [review]. Chest 2004;125:1522–9.

53. Henschke CI, Yankelevitz DF, Mirtcheva R, et al, ELCAP Group. CT screening for lung cancer: frequency and significance of part-solid and non-solid nodules. AJR Am J Roentgenol 2002;178: 1053–7.

54. Gould MK, Maclean CC, Kuschner WG, et al. Accuracy of positron emission tomography for diagnosis of pulmonary nodules and mass lesions: a meta-analysis. JAMA 2001;285:914–24.

55. Kim SK, Allen-Auerbach M, Goldin J, et al. Accuracy of PET/CT in characterization of solitary pulmonary lesions. J Nucl Med 2007;48:214–20.

56. van Tinteren H, Hoekstra OS, Smit EF, et al, PLUS study group*. Effectiveness of positron emission tomography in the preoperative assessment of patients with suspected non-small-cell lung cancer: the PLUS multicentre randomised trial. Lancet 2002; 359:1388–92.

57. Veronesi G, Bellomi M, Veronesi U, et al. Role of positron emission tomography scanning in the management of lung nodules detected at baseline computed tomography screening. Ann Thorac Surg 2007;84:959–66.

58. Pastorino U, Landoni C, Marchianò A, et al. Fluoro-deoxyglucose (FDG) uptake measured by positron emission tomography (PET) and standardised uptake value (SUV) predicts long-term survival of CT screening-detected lung cancer in heavy smokers. J Thorac Oncol 2009;11:1352–6.

59. Bianchi F, Hu J, Pelosi G, et al. Lung cancers detected by screening with spiral computed tomography have a malignant phenotype when analyzed by cDNA microarray. Clin Cancer Res 2004;10:6023–8.

60. Travis DL, Travis LB, Devesa SS. Lung cancer. Cancer 1995;75:191–202.

61. Vazquez M, Carter D, Brambilla E, et al, The International Early Lung Cancer Action Program Investigators. Solitary and multiple resected adenocarcinomas after CT screening for lung cancer: histopathologic features and their prognostic implications. Lung Cancer 2009;64(2):148–54.

62. Silva M, Sverzellati N, Manna C, et al. Long-term surveillance of ground glass nodules. Evidence from the MILD Trial. J Thorac Oncol 2012;7(10):1541–6.

63. Welch HG, Black WC. Overdiagnosis in cancer. J Natl Cancer Inst 2010;102:605–13.

64. Esserman L, Thompson I. Solving the overdiagnosis dilemma. J Natl Cancer Inst 2010;102:582–3.

65. Bach PB, Jett JR, Pastorino U, et al. Computed tomography screening and lung cancer outcomes. JAMA 2007;297:953–61.

66. Bach PB, Mirkin JN, Oliver TK, et al. Benefits and harms of CT screening for lung cancer: a systematic review. JAMA 2012;307:2418–29.

67. Stiles BM, Stowe CW, Mirza FM, et al. Cumulative radiation dose from medical imaging procedures in patients undergoing resection for lung cancer. Proceedings of the 47th Annual Meeting of the Society of Thoracic Surgeons, San Diego, February 1, 2011.

68. Iorio MV, Croce CM. MicroRNA dysregulation in cancer: diagnostics, monitoring and therapeutics. A comprehensive review. EMBO Mol Med 2012;4: 143–59.

69. Mitchell PS, Parkin RK, Kroh EM, et al. Circulating microRNAs as stable blood-based markers for cancer detection. Proc Natl Acad Sci U S A 2008; 105:10513–8.

70. Boeri M, Verri C, Conte D, et al. MicroRNA signatures in tissues and plasma predict development and prognosis of computed tomography detected lung cancer. Proc Natl Acad Sci U S A 2011;108: 3713–8.

71. Bianchi F, Nicassio F, Marzi M, et al. A serum circulating miRNA diagnostic test to identify asymptomatic high-risk individuals with early stage lung cancer. EMBO Mol Med 2011;3:495–503.

72. Lam S, Boyle P, Healey GF, et al. Early CDT-Lung: an immunobiomarker test as an aid to early detection of lung cancer. Cancer Prev Res (Phila) 2011; 4:1126–34.

73. Pecot CV, Li M, Zhang XJ, et al. Added value of a serum proteomic signature in the diagnostic evaluation of lung nodules. Cancer Epidemiol Biomarkers Prev 2012;21:786–92.

74. Aberle DR, Adams AM, Berg CD, et al, The National Lung Screening Trial Research Team. Baseline characteristics of participants in the randomized national lung screening trial. J Natl Cancer Inst 2010; 102(23):1771–9.

75. Bassler D, Briel M, Montori VM, et al, STOPIT-2 Study Group. Stopping randomized trials early for benefit and estimation of treatment effect. Systematic review and meta-regression analysis. JAMA 2010;303:1180–7.

Systematic Approach to the Management of the Newly Found Nodule on Screening Computed Tomography
Role of Dedicated Pulmonary Nodule Clinics

Robert J. Korst, MD

KEYWORDS

- Pulmonary nodule clinic • Lung cancer screening • Volumetric analysis • Computed tomography

KEY POINTS

- With the adoption of lung cancer screening programs and the increasing use of computed tomography for nonscreening purposes, the detection of indeterminate pulmonary nodules is increasing.
- Indeterminate pulmonary nodules are inconsistently managed by a variety of caregivers.
- A dedicated clinic affords an opportunity to provide evidence-based, standardized care for patients with indeterminate pulmonary nodules.
- A dedicated indeterminate pulmonary nodule clinic should be multidisciplinary and offer state-of-the-art technology and expertise, as well as a navigator service for patient convenience and smooth operation.

INTRODUCTION

One of the central controversies concerning the performance of low-dose computed tomography (LDCT) for lung cancer screening has been the high frequency of screening scans that show 1 or more indeterminate pulmonary nodules (IPNs), and the potential for subsequent, potentially unnecessary testing regarding these nodules.[1] With the publication of the results of the National Lung Screening trial (NLST) in 2011, which showed a significant decrease in lung cancer–specific mortality as a result of LDCT screening,[2] it can be expected that screening using LDCT will become more commonplace, as will the detection of IPNs. This article examines the concept of a clinic or service dedicated to the management of patients with newly diagnosed IPNs.

HISTORICAL NOTES

A solitary pulmonary nodule was traditionally defined as a round opacity less than 3 cm in size and surrounded by lung parenchyma, detected on chest radiograph.[3] With the advent of computed tomography (CT) of the chest, pulmonary nodules became detectable at smaller sizes, and at higher frequencies. The modern era of lung cancer screening began in 1993, when investigators began evaluating LDCT as a screening tool.[4,5] Using this modality, it became apparent that many asymptomatic individuals possessed small IPNs, most of which were benign. This finding prompted the development of the first algorithms aimed at managing small indeterminate lung nodules.[5]

Conflict of interest/Financial relationships: None.
Division of Thoracic Surgery, Department of Surgery, The Daniel and Gloria Blumenthal Cancer Center, The Valley Hospital, Ridgewood, New Jersey, 1 Valley Health Plaza, Paramus, NJ 07652, USA
E-mail address: korsro@valleyhealth.com

Thorac Surg Clin 23 (2013) 141–152
http://dx.doi.org/10.1016/j.thorsurg.2013.01.007

PULMONARY NODULES

Nodular pulmonary parenchymal opacities detected using chest CT are common. In contrast with the initial definition of a solitary pulmonary nodule, nodules detected using screening LDCT are smaller and more likely to be multiple,[6,7] with many abutting other structures including the chest wall and blood vessels. Although it is generally agreed that nodules with a benign calcification pattern or small size (<5 mm) have negligible malignant potential,[8] a significant number of nodules do not possess these features, making management strategies an essential part of the clinical armamentarium.

Lung Cancer Screening and Pulmonary Nodules

In 2011, the NLST showed that screening using LDCT resulted in a 20% relative reduction in lung cancer–specific mortality in high-risk patients (aged 55–74 years; >30 pack years of cigarette smoking; quit smoking <15 years earlier if a former smoker) compared with the use of plain chest radiography.[2] This study also revealed that IPNs greater than 4 mm in size were detected in 7191 (27%) of the 26,309 individuals screened in the LDCT arm at the initial (prevalence) screen, with more than 90% of these patients undergoing further work-up or surveillance as a result. In this regard, the frequency of a positive prevalence screen is 24% (range 3%–51%) in published randomized and cohort studies evaluating screening LDCT.[1] Adding to these numbers is the observation that many other IPNs are detected using screening LDCT, but do not meet size or morphologic criteria for a positive screen,[7] which indicates that the number of total nodules detected using LDCT screening is higher than is reported in some studies. As an example, in the prevalence screen from the Danish Lung Cancer Screening Trial, 75% of the participants in whom IPNs were detected had lesions that were either less than 5 mm or possessed a benign calcification pattern.[7] The NLST did not report total nodules. As lung cancer screening using LDCT becomes more commonplace as a result of the NLST results, it can be anticipated that many more pulmonary nodules will be discovered, even if only the individuals with the highest risk are screened.

Pulmonary Nodules and Nonscreening CT

It has been estimated that the use of CT scans in the United States tripled between 1993 and 2006.[9] Given the anatomic detail provided using this imaging modality, CT has become the test of choice for the evaluation of patients in acute care settings, including trauma and acute pain syndromes, as well as surveillance and follow-up of nonmalignant, chronic processes. In 2007, an estimated 72 million CT scans were performed in the United States, 11 million of which included the chest, and 20 million of the abdomen.[10]

Although the frequency at which IPNs are detected on nonscreening chest CT cannot directly be extrapolated from LDCT screening studies, evidence exists that IPNs are commonly detected in patients undergoing chest CT for nonpulmonary indications, including atherosclerotic heart disease and thoracic aortic surveillance (**Table 1**).[11–13] Further, CT scans of the abdomen include limited cuts through the lower pulmonary parenchyma. Patients undergoing abdominal CT scanning also have a significant likelihood of being diagnosed with an IPN (see **Table 1**).[14,15] In addition, there is evidence to suggest that the presence of IPNs on abdominal scans may be overlooked by radiologists in a significant proportion of scans.[16]

Factors Affecting the Prevalence of Malignancy in IPNs

The overall prevalence of malignancy in screen-detected IPNs is low, ranging from 0.3% to 3.7%

Table 1
Prevalence and cancer risk of IPNs detected using abdominal CT and nonscreening chest CT

Author/Year	Type of Scan	Indication	# Patients	# IPNs (%)	# Cancers (%)
Iribarren et al,[11] 2008	Cardiac CT	ASHD	459	81 (18)	0 (0)
Kasirajan & Dayama,[12] 2012	Chest CT angiography	Aortic surveillance	242	83 (34)	8 (3)
Alpert et al,[14] 2012	Abdominal	All scans[a]	12,287	364 (3)	NS
Harthun & Lau,[15] 2011	Abdominal	AAA stent surveillance	138	25 (18)	6 (4)
Hall et al,[13] 2009	Chest CT angiography	Pulmonary embolism	589	127 (22)	NS

Abbreviations: ASHD, atherosclerotic heart disease; NS, not stated.
[a] All abdominal CT scans at a single institution over a 1-year period.

of positive screens.[1] This percentage is even lower when IPNs of all sizes and densities are included. When a patient or lung cancer screening participant is found to have an IPN, several factors affect the likelihood that the nodule represents lung cancer. These include:

- Clinical parameters (independent of CT images)
- CT parameters
  ○ Size
  ○ Shape
  ○ Density
  ○ Growth

Clinical parameters

The major risk factors for lung cancer that are independent of CT imaging (referred to as pretest risk) include increasing age and a history of cigarette smoking.[17,18] Other factors that may be important are the presence of chronic obstructive pulmonary disease (COPD), the exposure to secondhand smoke, toxic exposures (radon, asbestos), as well as a family history of the disease.[19] Important factors with regard to smoking are the number of cigarettes smoked, and the time since quitting (if a former smoker).[17,18] Many patients with IPNs that are detected as a result of newly adopted screening programs are high risk in terms of age and smoking history, simply because many such programs are being modeled after the NLST. However, patients with IPNs detected using CT independently of screening need to be assigned a pretest risk, which factors into the decision making.[8] Assigning pretest risk is a subjective process and clinician dependent, but objective attempts at quantification of this risk have been made using mathematical models.[18,20]

CT parameters

The most important CT criteria that are used to assess the risk of malignancy in an IPN include size, shape, density, and growth rate. The multiplicity of nodules is not easily interpreted, however. Although it is generally accepted that abundant (>10) small (<5 mm) nodules are almost universally benign, many lung cancers are detected as a larger lesion existing in the presence of satellite lesions, many of which are benign.[5] Further, abundant (>10) nodules of a larger size may represent metastatic disease to the lungs.

Size The size of an IPN is strongly correlated with the risk of malignancy.[5,21–24] Data from an early LDCT observational study showed that the prevalence of malignancy in IPNs less than 5 mm in diameter was 0%.[5] Further, a review of the LDCT screening literature reported in 2007 showed that the risk of malignancy increased with increasing

size: 0% to 1% for less than 5 mm, 6% to 28% for 5 to 10 mm, 33% to 64% for 11 to 20 mm, and 64% to 82% for greater than 20 mm.[25]

Shape IPNs that are round are more likely to represent malignancy, compared with flat, tubular, or polygonal lesions.[6,26,27] Edge characteristics are also important, with lobulated or spiculated edges more likely to represent cancer than a smooth surface.[6,25,27] Intraparenchymal lymph nodes tend to be small (3–8 mm), smooth bordered, coffee bean–shaped or polygonal nodules in a subpleural location in the lower lung fields.[6,28]

Density The density on CT is an important factor to be considered when evaluating an IPN. Lesions with specific calcification patterns (popcorn, central, or laminated) are almost always benign; however, nonspecific (stippled or eccentric) calcification may be a feature of lung cancer.[25,29] Fat density may indicate a hamartoma.[30] Noncalcified IPNs can be further characterized as solid, nonsolid (pure ground-glass opacity), or part solid based on CT density. Although highly variable, data obtained from LDCT screening studies suggest that the prevalence of malignancy tends to be lower in solid lesions compared with nonsolid and part-solid IPNs.[25,31] Of particular concern are nonsolid lesions that begin to solidify over time (**Fig. 1**), a process that may indicate the development of an invasive malignant component.[31]

Growth The mainstay of IPN evaluation is the assessment of nodule growth, as measured using serial CT scans. This is based on malignant tumors being mitotically active, and growing over time. Multiple retrospective studies have evaluated malignant lung tumor growth over successive CT scans, with a wide range of tumor growth rates reported.[32] However, additional literature confirms that individual cancers may exhibit wide variation in growth rates over time, with some cancers shrinking at some point.[33,34] Many inflammatory lesions also grow in size to varying degrees, which further confounds the use of growth rates to determine malignancy. Acute inflammatory lesions may display rapid growth over a short time, whereas chronic inflammatory or otherwise benign nodules may grow extremely slowly.[35]

RATIONALE FOR THE IMPLEMENTATION OF DEDICATED IPN CLINICS

A program, or clinic, dedicated to IPNs implies that an institution has invested in the necessary infrastructure, personnel, and expertise aimed at streamlining and optimizing the management of patients with IPNs. There are several reasons

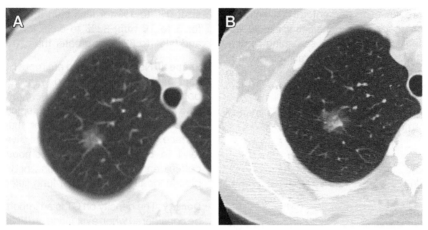

Fig. 1. Solidification of a nonsolid nodule over time. (*A*) Initial CT image of a nonsolid right upper lobe nodule. Note that the blood vessels that pass through the lesion are readily visible. (*B*) Corresponding CT image 3 years later showing the development of a solid, central component. The patient underwent a transthoracic needle aspiration, which revealed adenocarcinoma.

why such a program may be beneficial for these patients.

Adoption of Lung Cancer Screening and False-Positive Screens

The results of the NLST have prompted major medical societies and organizations, including the American Society of Clinical Oncology, The American Thoracic Society, The American College of Chest Physicians (ACCP), and The National Comprehensive Cancer Network, to endorse lung cancer screening using LDCT.[36,37] These events have led to the implementation of dozens of lung cancer screening programs throughout the United States over the past year. Given the prevalence of IPNs detected on screening LDCT previously mentioned, combined with the finding that more than 90% of positive screens represent a benign process,[1] a dedicated IPN clinic aimed at minimizing harm to screening subjects is logical, especially at an institution that has implemented a screening program.

Limitations and Inconsistencies of Currently Published Recommendations Regarding IPNs

Algorithms for the management of CT-detected IPNs were first proposed by organizations initially involved with LDCT screening for lung cancer.[5] Following these initial cohort studies, several organizations published guidelines and position papers on this topic, including the Fleischner Society,[38] the ACCP,[8] The American Association for Thoracic Surgery (AATS),[39] and the American College of Radiology (ACR).[40] The Fleischner guidelines, published in 2005, give specific recommendations for

the radiographic follow-up of IPNs less than 8 mm in diameter, but do not specifically comment on the work-up of lesions greater than 8 mm.[38] The ACCP guidelines accept the follow-up algorithms proposed by the Fleischner Society for small IPNs (less than 8 mm), but go further and emphasize the importance of the pretest probability of malignancy to dictate management of larger nodules.[8] According to the ACCP, the pretest probability of malignancy can be determined either by clinical judgment or by mathematical modeling. The AATS guidelines are also similar to the Fleischner recommendations for small nodules, but are not specific for the work-up of IPNs greater than 8 mm, instead deferring to specialists in lung cancer to dictate further management.[39] This latter approach was used in the NLST, in which work-up of a positive screen was left to each institution's own discretion.[2] The implementation of a dedicated IPN clinic allows for the standardization of institutional guidelines for the management of pulmonary nodules.

Lack of Use and Adherence to Guidelines

Despite the availability of guidelines for the management of IPNs, published evidence suggests that many institutions and physician practices either do not have a policy for guideline use or, in those that do have such policies, adherence to the guidelines is limited.[41–43] In a survey of 834 radiologists throughout the United States, 37% of respondents worked in practices that used no written policy outlining recommendations for the management of IPNs. Of those with an established policy, 79% used the Fleischner guidelines, 14% the ACCP guidelines, and the remaining 7% used an internally developed written policy.[41] However, even when such a policy exists, adherence is limited, ranging from 27% to 60%.[41–43] Nonadherence usually tends toward overmanagement of IPNs.[43] The implementation of a dedicated IPN clinic may be helpful in this regard, because it mandates adherence to management algorithms. As a result, it gives the host institution the opportunity to standardize the management of patients with IPNs according to evidence-based guidelines.

Varying Expertise of Physicians Managing IPNs

Many physicians are involved in the management of IPNs detected on CT. Although specialists including pulmonologists and thoracic surgeons have the most clinical expertise in addressing lung cancer, and are responsible for writing many of the guidelines for management of lung cancer and IPNs, it is likely that most IPNs are, at least initially, managed by primary care physicians. By the nature of their practice, primary care physicians most likely see only a small number of patients with lung cancer and may not have experience interpreting CT examinations of the chest. As a result, the radiologist's report and recommendations are central to the management of IPNs in these circumstances, which may increase liability from a medicolegal standpoint.[44] However, diagnostic radiologists lack the clinical exposure to patients with lung cancer, as well as the outcomes of management of lung cancer and IPNs. The development of a dedicated IPN clinic fosters a multidisciplinary approach to patients with an IPN, which may help reduce potential liability for involved caregivers, including primary care physicians, who are initially presented with a patient who has an IPN.

PRACTICAL ASPECTS OF A PULMONARY NODULE CLINIC

Instituting a program dedicated to the management of IPNs requires a multidisciplinary effort, coordination of services, as well as institutional investment in infrastructure, which includes investment in personnel, technology, and community outreach.

Imaging

Since the introduction of helical CT scanning in the 1990s,[45] the technology has improved to the point at which high-resolution scans of the chest can be performed during a single breath hold. It is generally agreed that intravenous contrast is not necessary for the detection and growth assessment of pulmonary nodules.[8] Institutional CT protocols should be standardized as much as possible to limit variability caused by scanning technique.[46]

In this regard, many outside patients are referred to a dedicated pulmonary nodule clinic with CT images obtained using a variety of scanning protocols and image qualities. This source of variability needs to be considered when assessing nodule growth on successive scans. The institution should store images in a picture archive and communication system (PACS) to facilitate future scan comparisons.

Section thickness

A scanning variable that deserves particular attention is the section thickness used during measurements of size. Many IPNs that are detected during screening are small (<8 mm) and may require thinner sections for accurate size measurement. Further, small IPNs may be missed if the section thickness is too large.[8,47] The use of advanced technology such as navigational bronchoscopy requires thin sections to achieve accurate image-to-body registration. In addition, established LDCT screening programs have adopted thin sections in their protocols.[27,48] For all of these reasons, thin-section imaging seems to be the most attractive for monitoring IPNs in a dedicated clinic. Section thickness becomes even more important when volumetric analysis is performed. Error rates in volumetric measurement of IPNs ranging from 10% to 40% have been reported to be caused by differences in section thickness.[46] This large source of error must be considered when comparing sequential scans acquired with different section thicknesses from the same patient to evaluate growth.

Radiation exposure

Follow-up scans for evaluation of nodule growth are best performed using a low-dose protocol, especially because an individual patient may require several scans to monitor for nodule growth.[8,27,48,49] In situations in which other disorders are suggested on an initial screening LDCT (eg, mediastinal mass, adenopathy), follow-up scans can be performed at a full dose (potentially with intravenous contrast) to enhance resolution. CT scan manufacturers have incorporated automatic dose modulation for diagnostic CT imaging, in which the radiation dose is automatically adjusted and potentially reduced on an individual basis according to the size and attenuation characteristics of the body part being scanned, while keeping CT image quality constant. This advance has the potential advantage of eliminating arbitrary selection by radiologists and technologists.[50]

Adoption of Algorithms

One of the greatest benefits of a dedicated IPN clinic is the ability to provide patients and caregivers a unified, evidence-based approach to the management of IPNs. To achieve this goal, stakeholders at the participating institution must agree on, adopt, and adhere to management guidelines. In addition, a physician leader should be identified to facilitate the adoption of guidelines. The management of small nodules (<8 mm) is probably best modeled after the Fleischner Society guidelines, which have also been generally endorsed by the ACCP and the AATS. For lesions greater than 8 mm, individual programs need to establish their own protocols for management, which can be loosely based on previously published guidelines. Management strategies, especially those for obtaining a tissue diagnosis, may vary between institutions, given that the available expertise may differ.

Assessment of Nodule Size and Determination of Growth

At the center of any management strategy for patients with IPNs is the assessment of nodule growth. An institution desiring to construct a dedicated IPN clinic should adopt standards for measuring nodule growth from the outset. Nodule growth is most commonly assessed by comparing sequential scans, and the diameter of the IPN in question measured in 2 dimensions using electronic calipers. Nodule diameter was used in both the NLST and ITALUNG trials to assess growth.[2,51] Limitations of measuring IPN size using this technique are well described:

- High degree of interobserver and intraobserver variability in the measurement of IPN size.[52,53]
- An increase in diameter may grossly underestimate an increase in tumor volume. For example, a lesion 5 mm in diameter that grows to 6.3 mm has doubled in volume, assuming spherical growth.

- Tumors do not grow symmetrically, and two-dimensional measurements may miss such asymmetric growth.
- Volumetric tumor doubling time cannot be calculated using two-dimensional measurements, unless a spherical shape is assumed.

Despite these potential shortcomings, the current standard of care involves two-dimensional assessments of IPN growth.

Given these limitations of two-dimensional measurement, assessment of nodule growth in 3 dimensions (volumetric analysis) is an area of active investigation.[46] Volumetric analysis can be conducted using manually derived measurements from individual CT sections or, more commonly, by the use of semiautomated software (**Fig. 2**).[46] Initial evaluation of volumetric analysis used phantom studies to show reproducibility.[54] The use of semiautomated software may possess real benefits compared with standard, two-dimensional measurements in multiple regards:

- Reproducibility of IPN size measurements is enhanced.[55,56]
- Volume doubling time (VDT), or the number of days required for a specific lesion to double in volume, is calculated. VDT incorporates the time interval between scans in the growth measurement.
- Asymmetric growth is accounted for using some semiautomated volumetric software packages.[46]

Despite these potential benefits of volumetric analysis of nodule growth, limitations of the technology exist, and include:

- Volumetric analysis of IPNs abutting the pleura or vascular structures results in higher error rates, because nodules may have the same attenuation as these structures. The

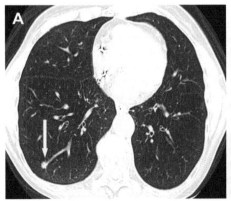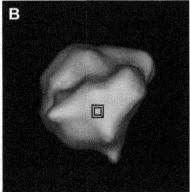

Fig. 2. Volumetric image of a small lung cancer. (*A*) CT image of a 9-mm right lower lobe lung cancer (*arrow*). (*B*) Three-dimensional image of the same lesion created by semiautomated volumetric software.

user may have to correct the software in such instances.[57,58]

- The evaluation of nonsolid and part-solid lesions is problematic.[59]
- The definition of a malignant doubling time of an IPN remains controversial and arbitrary. In the NELSON LDCT screening trial, high-risk IPNs were those with a VDT of less than 400 days, whereas IPNs with a VDT greater than 600 days were considered low risk.[27] Despite these thresholds, multiple studies have shown that the VDT of malignant lung tumors is variable, and dependent on factors such as patient gender (tumors in women have longer mean doubling times), radiographic appearance (tumors presenting as nonsolid nodules have longer doubling times than solid tumors), histology (adenocarcinomas have longer mean doubling times than squamous lesions), and, perhaps most importantly, the context in which the tumor was detected (LDCT screen–detected cancers have longer doubling times than those detected by chest radiograph or by routine medical care).[32] Further complicating the use of VDT is the finding that individual cancers may have wide variation in VDT over time, with some cancers shrinking at some point when growth is measured using volumetric software.[33,34]
- The performance of volumetric analysis adds time to the scan interpretation process and adds cost in that it is a billable service to the patient.[34]

In summary, although the decision to perform volumetric analysis of all IPNs has theoretic advantages, it has not definitively been shown to be of benefit in the clinical arena compared with thin-section two-dimensional measurements of growth.

Work-up of Suspicious Nodules

When an IPN is deemed suspicious by assessment of pretest risk of malignancy and CT criteria, further work-up is mandated.[8] Selection of further studies or maneuvers depends on characteristics of the nodule itself (size, shape, location, growth rate, increasing solid component), as well as the technology and expertise available at a given institution. It needs to be reiterated that most nodules managed in a dedicated IPN clinic are benign, with cancer being detected in only 3% to 29% of participants.[34,60]

Fluorodeoxyglucose positron emission tomography

Fluorodeoxyglucose positron emission tomography (FDG-PET) is a noninvasive functional imaging modality that is widely used in lung cancer staging. The sensitivity of FDG-PET in detecting malignant IPNs is high (>80%), but it is generally accepted that this sensitivity decreases for subcentimeter lesions as well as certain subtypes of adenocarcinoma.[25] The specificity of FDG-PET is highly variable because of the detection of inflammatory lesions as well. Given these shortcomings, combined with most screen-detected IPNs being less than 1 cm in size and screen-detected cancers having longer doubling times, FDG-PET plays a limited role in a dedicated IPN clinic.[1,32]

Antimicrobials

Certain IPNs may possess features more consistent with an inflammatory process than malignancy. As an example, a rapidly growing lesion, or one with a thin-walled cavity, can be treated with a limited course of broad-spectrum antimicrobials as a diagnostic maneuver. This course is followed by repeat LDCT in 1 to 2 months to determine whether the lesion decreases in size (**Fig. 3**).[48]

Biopsy techniques

When biopsy of an IPN is warranted, several techniques are available, including CT-guided transthoracic needle aspiration, endobronchial ultrasound (**Fig. 4**), and transbronchial biopsy with or without electromagnetic navigation (**Fig. 5**). The choice of approach depends on nodule size and location as well as other factors, including the need to potentially stage the mediastinum. For peripherally located IPNs in patients thought to have a high likelihood of malignancy, minimally invasive (eg, thoracoscopic or robotic) surgical wedge resection may be the best option. If pathologic assessment of the nodule on frozen section reveals malignancy, definitive lobectomy and mediastinal lymph node dissection can be performed at the same setting.

The Multidisciplinary Team

The implementation of a dedicated IPN clinic requires a multidisciplinary team working in coordination to provide a user-friendly service to patients with nodules, as well as referring physicians. The physician component includes diagnostic imaging (preferable a chest radiologist), interventional radiology, and a pulmonologist and/or thoracic surgeon. Any pulmonologists who are involved should have a special interest in lung cancer and interventional skills. A thoracic surgeon should ideally be involved, and should be a fellowship-trained general thoracic surgeon with experience in minimally invasive biopsy and surgical techniques. A physician champion should be identified (usually a clinician) to serve as a facilitator to bring all of the components together and act as a supervisor.

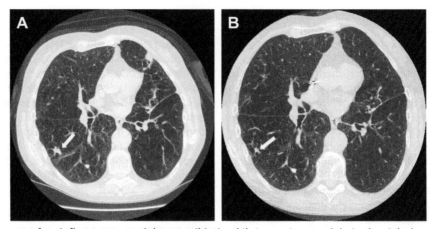

Fig. 3. Response of an inflammatory nodule to antibiotics. (*A*) A new 1-cm nodule in the right lower lobe with spiculated edges (*arrow*) in a heavy smoker with a history of stage 1 lung cancer. The nodule was not present on CT obtained 6 months earlier, suggesting an inflammatory lesion. (*B*) CT image of the same lesion (*arrow*) 4 weeks later after a short course of broad-spectrum antibiotics.

An essential part of any dedicated, highly specialized clinical program is a nurse navigator.[61] The navigator is the backbone of the program and is responsible for moving patients through the program, providing counseling for patients, organizing clinical results, and mediating the physician/patient interaction. Data entry personnel are also beneficial to record data pertaining to defining the success of the program. In addition, a multidisciplinary lung cancer team (medical and radiation oncology, support services) should be available to address any malignant diagnoses that are made.

Patient Flow

Referrals
A dedicated IPN clinic has the potential to receive patient referrals from a variety of sources.

Physician referral Physicians who may receive benefit from referral of their patients into a dedicated IPN clinic mainly comprise primary care physicians and pulmonologists, although any caregiver who orders a CT scan of the chest and/or abdomen is a potential source of referrals. This type of clinic may be inherently attractive to primary care physicians for several reasons:

- They can obtain a second, standardized opinion about nodule management.
- Organization and follow-up of subsequent imaging may be burdensome in a busy primary care practice.
- Given that a pulmonary nodule usually represents only a small component of an individual patient's active medical history, it is unlikely

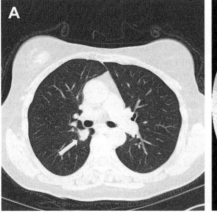
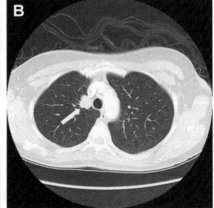

Fig. 4. Stage 1 lung cancer biopsied using endobronchial ultrasound. (*A*) A right lower lobe lesion (*arrow*) adjacent to the distal bronchus intermedius. (*B*) A right upper lobe cancer (*arrow*) adjacent to the trachea.

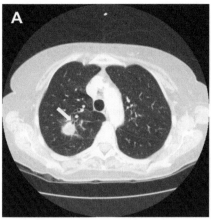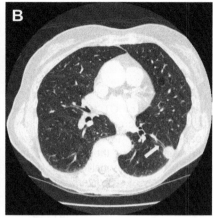

Fig. 5. Stage 1 lung cancer biopsied using electromagnetic navigational bronchoscopy showing the bronchus sign (*arrows*). (*A*) A right upper lobe lesion adjacent to the major fissure. (*B*) A peripheral left lower lobe cancer.

that a primary care physician will view the IPN clinic as competitive.

- Missed lung cancer is a major source of malpractice litigation, which commonly involves primary care physicians.[62]

However, community pulmonologists are consulted routinely for IPN management and may be more likely to view an institutional program as competitive. A helpful strategy in this regard would be for the physician leader of the IPN clinic to meet with individual pulmonologists to reinforce that the purpose of the clinic is to provide a second opinion, and to inform them regarding nodule management algorithms.

Self-referral Patients diagnosed with IPNs may self-refer into the clinic. Community outreach programs may be helpful in raising awareness of lung cancer and pulmonary nodules, especially if a screening program is instituted.

Lung cancer screening program A lung cancer screening program is likely to be the largest source of referrals for a dedicated IPN clinic.[60] Given the large number of IPNs detected using LDCT for lung cancer screening, implementation of an IPN clinic is most logical and practical if an institution elects to begin lung cancer screening.

Initial consultation

An initial consultation with a new patient should involve the nurse navigator as well as one of the clinicians (pulmonologist/thoracic surgeon) who are part of the program. CT scans from outside the institution should then be reviewed and subsequently scanned into the institutional PACS system for future comparisons. Patients are counseled, informed of the next step in their management, and, if indicated, follow-up studies are ordered.

Follow-up

A follow-up strategy that fits for a given institution needs to be implemented to provide convenient and effective care, but not waste resources. As an example, not all patients need to be seen by a physician for every follow-up event. One strategy is to divide patients into groups based on nodule size. Patients with IPNs less than 8 mm in diameter may be followed by the nurse navigator according to the Fleischner Society guidelines, using the radiologists' reports for scan comparisons. Physician visits are reserved for larger nodules, those that have shown growth or other concerning characteristics, and those that require additional testing. In the cases that require additional testing, a multidisciplinary conference may be useful in deciding on further action.

Communication with patients and referring physicians

In addition to discussing the plan of action with the patient at each follow-up event, letters are sent via certified mail to each patient outlining the impression and plan of action. A letter is also sent in a similar fashion to each referring physician and to the patient's primary care physician if they are self-referred. Referring and primary care physicians are also contacted by the clinician (pulmonologist/thoracic surgeon) by telephone for all lesions that require further diagnostic studies other than a follow-up LDCT.

Discharge from the clinic

ACCP guidelines state that solid IPNs that have been stable for more than 2 years do not require specific follow-up; however, nonsolid and part-solid lesions may require longer follow-up imaging.[8] If it is decided that a patient does not require further follow-up, discharge from the IPN clinic is reasonable. However, because many patients are referred from an LDCT screening program, they continue to be screened as per the screening regimen.

SUMMARY

With the increasing use of CT for lung cancer screening as well as nonscreening purposes, the number of patients with IPNs will markedly increase. Given that most of these nodules are benign, combined with the potential for inconsistent management by a variety of caregivers, a program dedicated to dealing with IPNs should be considered, especially if a lung cancer screening program has already been implemented. A dedicated IPN clinic should be multidisciplinary and offer state-of-the-art technology and expertise, as well as a navigator service for patient convenience. The incidence of lung cancer detection is variable, and depends on the pattern of referrals into the clinic.

REFERENCES

1. Bach PB, Mirkin JN, Oliver TK, et al. Benefits and harms of CT screening for lung cancer. A systematic review. JAMA 2012;307:2418–29.
2. Aberle DR, Adams AM, Berg CD, et al. Reduced lung-cancer mortality with low-dose computed tomographic screening. N Engl J Med 2011;365:395–409.
3. Tuddenham WJ. Glossary of terms for thoracic radiology: recommendations of the Nomenclature Committee of the Fleischner Society. AJR Am J Roentgenol 1984;143:509–17.
4. Kaneko M, Eguchi K, Ohmatsu H, et al. Peripheral lung cancer: screening and detection with low-dose spiral CT versus radiography. Radiology 1996;201:798–802.
5. Henschke CI, McCauley DI, Yankelevitz DF, et al. Early Lung Cancer Action Project: overall design and findings from baseline screening. Lancet 1999; 354:99–105.
6. Edey AJ, Hansell DM. Incidentally detected small pulmonary nodules on CT. Clin Radiol 2009;64: 872–84.
7. Pederson JH, Ashraf H, Dirksen A, et al. The Danish Randomized Lung Cancer CT Screening Trial – overall design and results of the prevalence round. J Thorac Oncol 2009;4:608–14.
8. Gould MK, Fletcher J, Iannettoni MD, et al. Evaluation of patients with pulmonary nodules: when is it lung cancer? Chest 2007;132:108S–30S.
9. Mettler FA Jr, Thomadsen BR, Bhargavan M, et al. Medical radiation exposure in the U.S. in 2006: preliminary results. Health Phys 2008;95:502–7.
10. Berrington de Gonzalez A, Mahesh M, Kim KP, et al. Projected cancer risks from computed tomographic scans performed in the United States in 2007. Arch Intern Med 2009;169:2071–7.
11. Iribarren C, Hlatky MA, Chandra M, et al. Incidental pulmonary nodules on cardiac computed tomography: prognosis and use. Am J Med 2008;121: 989–96.
12. Kasirajan KI, Dayama A. Incidental findings in patients evaluated for thoracic aortic pathology using computed tomography angiography. Ann Vasc Surg 2012;26:306–11.
13. Hall WB, Truitt SG, Scheunemann LP, et al. The prevalence of clinically relevant incidental findings on chest computed tomographic angiograms ordered to diagnose pulmonary embolism. Arch Intern Med 2009;169:1961–5.
14. Alpert JB, Fantauzzi JP, Melamud K, et al. Clinical significance of lung nodules reported on abdominal CT. AJR Am J Roentgenol 2012;198:793–9.
15. Harthun NL, Lau CL. The incidence of pulmonary neoplasms discovered by serial computed tomography scanning after endovascular abdominal aortic aneurysm repair. J Vasc Surg 2011;53:738–41.
16. Rinaldi MF, Bartalena T, Giannelli G, et al. Incidental lung nodules on CT examinations of the abdomen: prevalence and reporting rates in the PACS era. Eur J Radiol 2010;74:e84–8.
17. Cassidy A, Duffy SW, Myles JP, et al. Lung cancer risk prediction: a tool for early detection. Int J Cancer 2006;120:1–6.
18. Gould MK, Anath L, Barnett PG. A clinical model to estimate the pretest probability of lung cancer in patients with solitary pulmonary nodules. Chest 2007;131:383–8.
19. Matakidou A, Eisen T, Houlston RS. Systematic review of the relationship between family history and lung cancer risk. Br J Cancer 2005;93:825–33.
20. Swensen SJ, Silverstein MD, Ilstrup DM, et al. The probability of malignancy in solitary pulmonary nodules: application to small radiographically indeterminate nodules. Arch Intern Med 1997;157:849–55.
21. Gohagan J, Marcus P, Fagerstrom R, et al. Baseline findings of a randomized feasibility trial of lung cancer screening with spiral CT scan vs. chest radiograph: the lung screening study of the national cancer institute. Chest 2004;126:114–21.
22. Henschke CI, Yankelevitz DF, Nadich DP, et al. CT screening for lung cancer: suspiciousness of nodules according to size on baseline scans. Radiology 2004;231:164–8.
23. Swenson SJ, Jett JR, Hartman TE, et al. CT screening for lung cancer: five-year prospective experience. Radiology 2005;235:259–65.
24. Blanchon T, Brechot JM, Grenier PA, et al. Baseline results of the Despiscan study: a French randomized pilot trial of lung cancer screening comparing low dose CT scan (LDCT) and chest X-ray (CXR). Lung Cancer 2007;58:50–8.

25. Wahidi MM, Govert JA, Goudar RK, et al. Evidence for the treatment of patients with pulmonary nodules: when is it cancer? Chest 2007;132:94S–107S.

26. Takashima S, Sone S, Li F, et al. Small solitary pulmonary nodules (< or = 1 cm) detected at population-based CT screening for lung cancer: reliable high resolution CT features of benign lesions. AJR Am J Roentgenol 2003;180:955–64.

27. Xu DM, Gietama H, de Koning H, et al. Nodule management protocol of the NELSON randomized lung cancer screening trial. Lung Cancer 2006;54:177–84.

28. Yankelevitz D, Vasquez M, Bogot NR, et al. CT features of intraparenchymal lymph nodes confirmed by cytology. Clin Imaging 2010;34:185–90.

29. Siegelman SS, Zerhouni EA, Leo FP, et al. CT of the solitary pulmonary nodule. AJR Am J Roentgenol 1980;135:1–13.

30. Siegelman SS, Khouri NF, Scott WW Jr, et al. Pulmonary hamartoma: CT findings. Radiology 1986;160:313–7.

31. Henschke CI, Yankelevitz DF, Mirtcheva R, et al. CT screening for lung cancer: frequency and significance of part-solid and nonsolid nodules. AJR Am J Roentgenol 2002;178:1053–7.

32. Detterbeck FC, Gibson CJ. Turning gray: the natural history of lung cancer over time. J Thorac Oncol 2008;3:781–92.

33. Lindell RM, Hartman TE, Swenson SJ, et al. Five-year lung cancer screening experience: CT appearance, growth rate, location, and histologic features of 61 lung cancers. Radiology 2007;242:555–62.

34. Korst RJ, Lee BE, Krinsky GA, et al. The utility of automated volumetric growth analysis in a dedicated pulmonary nodule clinic. J Thorac Cardiovasc Surg 2011;142:372–7.

35. Revel M-P, Merlin A, Peyrard S, et al. Software volumetric evaluation of doubling times for differentiating benign versus malignant pulmonary nodules. AJR Am J Roentgenol 2006;187:135–42.

36. Available at: http://www.asco.org/ASCOv2/Press+Center/Latest+News+Releases/General+News+Releases/Statement+from+the+American+Society+of+Clinical+Oncology+and+the+American+College+of+Chest+Physicians+on+the+Joint+Systematic+Review+and+Clinical+Practice+Guideline+on+the+Role+of+CT+Screening+for+Lung+Cancer+(Endorsed+by+the+American+Thoracic+Society). Accessed September 30, 2012.

37. Available at: http://www.tju.edu/jmc/medicine/pulmonary_critical_care/clinical_programs/documents/NCCN_Guidelines_%20Lung_Cancer_Screening.pdf. Accessed September 18, 2012.

38. McMahon H, Austin JH, Gamsu G, et al. Guidelines for the management of small pulmonary nodules detected on CT scans: a statement from the Fleischner Society. Radiology 2005;237:395–400.

39. Jacobson FL, Austin JH, Field JK, et al. Development of The American Association for Thoracic Surgery guidelines for low-dose computed tomography scans to screen for lung cancer in North America: recommendations of The American Association for Thoracic Surgery Task Force for Lung Cancer Screening and Surveillance. J Thorac Cardiovasc Surg 2012;144:25–32.

40. Khan A. ACR appropriateness criteria on solitary pulmonary nodule. J Am Coll Radiol 2007;4:152–5.

41. Eisenberg RL, Bankier AA, Boiselle PM. Compliance with Fleischner Society guidelines for management of small lung nodules: a survey of 834 radiologists. Radiology 2010;255:218–24.

42. Lacson R, Prevedello LM, Andriole KP, et al. Factors associated with radiologists' adherence to Fleischner Society guidelines for the management of pulmonary nodules. J Am Coll Radiol 2012;9:468–73.

43. Masciocchi M, Wagner B, Lloyd B. Quality review: Fleischner criteria adherence by radiologists in a large community hospital. J Am Coll Radiol 2012;9:336–9.

44. Berlin L. Failure to diagnose lung cancer: anatomy of a malpractice trial. AJR Am J Roentgenol 2003;180:37–45.

45. Kalender WA, Seissler W, Klotz E, et al. Spiral volumetric CT with single-breath-hold technique, continuous transport, and continuous scanner rotation. Radiology 1990;176:181–3.

46. Gavrielides MA, Kinnard LM, Myers KJ, et al. Noncalcified lung nodules: volumetric assessment with thoracic CT. Radiology 2009;251:26–37.

47. Fischbach F, Knollmann F, Greisshaber V, et al. Detection of pulmonary nodules by multislice computed tomography: improved detection rate with reduced slice thickness. Eur Radiol 2003;13:2378–83.

48. Available at: http://www.ielcap.org/professionals/docs/ielcap.pdf. Accessed September 22, 2012.

49. Christie A, Torrente JC, Lin M, et al. CT screening and follow-up of lung nodules: effects of tube current-time setting and nodule size and density on detectability and of tube current-time setting on apparent size. AJR Am J Roentgenol 2011;197:623–30.

50. Kalra MK, Maher MM, Rizzo S, et al. Radiation exposure and projected risks with multidetector-row computed tomography scanning: clinical strategies and technologic developments for dose reduction. J Comput Assist Tomogr 2004;28:S46–9.

51. Lopes Pegna A, Picozzi G, Mascalchi M, et al. Design, recruitment and baseline results of the ITALUNG trial of lung cancer screening with low-dose CT. Lung Cancer 2009;64:34–40.

52. Bogot NR, Kazerooni EA, Kelly AM, et al. Interobserver and intraobserver variability in the assessment of pulmonary nodule size on CT using film and computer display methods. Acad Radiol 2005;12:948–56.

53. Erasmus JJ, Gladish GW, Broemeling L, et al. Interobserver and intraobserver variability in measurement of no-small-cell lung carcinoma lesions: implications for assessment of tumor response. J Clin Oncol 2003;21:2574–82.

54. Yankelevitz DF, Reeves AP, Kostis WJ, et al. Small pulmonary nodules: volumetrically determined growth rates based on CT evaluation. Radiology 2000;217:251–6.

55. Revel MP, Lefort C, Bissery A, et al. Pulmonary nodules: preliminary experience with three-dimensional evaluation. Radiology 2004;231:459–66.

56. Goodman LR, Gulsun M, Washington L, et al. Inherent variability of CT lung nodule measurements in vivo using semiautomated volumetric measurements. AJR Am J Roentgenol 2006;186:989–94.

57. Ko JP, Marcus R, Bomsztyk E, et al. Effect of blood vessels on measurement of nodule volume in a chest phantom. Radiology 2006;239:79–85.

58. Gietema HA, Wang Y, Xu D, et al. Pulmonary nodules detected at lung cancer screening: interobserver variability of semiautomated volume measurements. Radiology 2006;241:251–7.

59. Ko JP, Rusinek H, Jacobs EL, et al. Small pulmonary nodules: volume measurement at chest CT-phantom study. Radiology 2003;228:864–70.

60. Veeramachaneni NK, Crabtree TD, Kreisel D, et al. A thoracic surgery clinic dedicated to indeterminate pulmonary nodules: too many scans and too little pathology? J Thorac Cardiovasc Surg 2009;137: 30–5.

61. Hunnibell LS, Rose MG, Connery DM, et al. Using nurse navigation to improve timeliness of lung cancer care at a veterans hospital. Clin J Oncol Nurs 2012; 16:29–36.

62. McLean TR. Why do physicians who treat lung cancer get sued? Chest 2004;126:1672–9.

Fluorescence and Navigational Bronchoscopy

Annette McWilliams, MB, FRCPC[a,b],
Tawimas Shaipanich, MD, FRCPC[c,d],
Stephen Lam, MD, FRCPC[e,f,*]

KEYWORDS

- Bronchoscopy • Lung cancer • Computed tomography

KEY POINTS

- Autofluorescence bronchoscopy and narrow band imaging provide a sensitive means to localize preinvasive bronchial cancers and preneoplastic lesions in the central airways.
- Choice of bronchoscopy versus computed tomography (CT)-guided biopsy of peripheral lung lesions is guided by the size and location of the lesion and other factors such as presence or absence of emphysema surrounding the lesion.
- Bronchoscopy has a lower diagnostic yield than CT-guided transthoracic lung biopsy for lesions no more than 20 mm but has a lower complication rate of pneumothorax and bleeding.

 Video of 'peripheral adenocarcinoma diagnosed by virtual bronchoscopy and R-EBUS' accompanies this article at http://www.thoracic.theclinics.com/

INTRODUCTION

In patients suspected to have lung cancer based on radiographic and clinical features, a tissue biopsy using the least invasive and safest method is needed not only to confirm the diagnosis but also for molecular analysis. Unless the patient presents with extrathoracic spread such as a palpable supraclavicular lymph node, pleural effusion, or skin metastasis that is readily accessible to biopsy, bronchoscopy or computed tomography (CT)-guided transthoracic needle/core biopsy is the method of choice. Bronchoscopy has the advantage that staging can be performed at the same time, providing a 1-stop approach for the patient to shorten the time between diagnosis, staging, and treatment. In this article, the bronchoscopic approaches for diagnosis of central and peripheral lung tumors are discussed.

PRINCIPLES OF BRONCHOSCOPIC IMAGING

White light bronchoscopy (WLB), the simplest and most commonly used bronchoscopic imaging method, makes use of the specular reflection, back-scattering, and absorption properties of broadband visible light from approximately 400 nm to 700 nm to define the structural features of the bronchial surface to discriminate between normal and

[a] Department of Integrative Oncology, British Columbia Cancer Agency, 6-108, 675 West 10th Avenue, Vancouver, British Columbia V5Z 1L3, Canada; [b] Department of Medicine, University of British Columbia, 6-108, 675 West 10th Avenue, Vancouver, British Columbia V5Z 1L3, Canada; [c] Department of Integrative Oncology, British Columbia Cancer Agency, 6th Floor, 675 West 10th Avenue, Vancouver, British Columbia V6Z 1Y6, Canada; [d] Department of Medicine, University of British Columbia, 6th Floor, 675 West 10th Avenue, Vancouver, British Columbia V6Z 1Y6, Canada; [e] Department of Integrative Oncology, British Columbia Cancer Agency, 6-113, 675 West 10th Avenue, Vancouver, British Columbia V5Z 1L3, Canada; [f] Department of Medicine, University of British Columbia, 6-113, 675 West 10th Avenue, Vancouver, British Columbia V5Z 1L3, Canada
* Corresponding author. 675 West 10 Avenue, Vancouver, British Columbia V5Z 1L3, Canada.
E-mail address: slam@bccancer.bc.ca

Thorac Surg Clin 23 (2013) 153–161
http://dx.doi.org/10.1016/j.thorsurg.2013.01.008
1547-4127/13/$ – see front matter © 2013 Elsevier Inc. All rights reserved.

abnormal tissues. To highlight the vasculature, narrow band imaging (NBI),[1–3] using blue light centered at 415 nm (range 400–430 nm) and green light centered at 540 nm (range 530–550 nm) corresponding to the maximal hemoglobin absorption peaks is used. The blue light highlights the superficial capillaries, while the green light can penetrate deeper to highlight the larger blood vessels in the submucosa. The narrow bandwidths reduce the scattering of light from other wavelengths that are present in a broad-spectrum white light and enable enhanced visualization of blood vessels. Preneoplastic lesions and invasive cancers can be highlighted by their increase in angiogenesis. Autofluorescence bronchoscopy (AFB) makes use of fluorescence and absorption properties to provide information about the biochemical composition and metabolic state of endogenous fluorophores in bronchial tissues.[4] Most endogenous fluorophores are associated with the tissue matrix or are involved in cellular metabolic processes. The most important fluorophores are structural proteins, such as collagen and elastin, and those involved in cellular metabolism, such as nicotinamide adenine dinucleotide (NADH) and flavins.[5] Upon illumination by violet or blue light (380–460 nm), normal bronchial tissues fluoresce strongly in the green light (480–520 nm). In bronchogenic carcinoma, as the bronchial epithelium changes from normal to dysplasia, and then to carcinoma in situ and invasive cancer, there is a progressive decrease in green autofluorescence but proportionately less decrease in the red fluorescence intensity. These differences can be exploited to detect preinvasive and invasive bronchial cancers.[4] Commercially available AFB devices make use of a combination of autofluorescence and reflectance imaging to optimize the image quality.[6,7] Small amounts of reflected light (blue, green, or near infrared) are employed to form a reflectance image that is used to enhance the chromatic contrast and to normalize the green autofluorescence image to correct for nonuniformity caused by optical and geometric factors such as variable distances and angles between the endoscope tip and the bronchial surface. Depending on the type of reflected light used to combine with the fluorescence image for display, abnormal areas appear brownish red, red, purple, or magenta, while normal areas appear green or light blue.[6,8–11] Some devices allow simultaneous display of the white light and fluorescence images.[7,12] An example of a carcinoma in situ detected by autofluorescence bronchoscopy is shown in **Fig. 1**.

WHITE LIGHT AND AFB

Flexible bronchoscopy is a valuable tool for lung cancer diagnosis. It has a high diagnostic yield for tumors proximal to a subsegmental bronchus. For central tumors that present as polypoid or nodular lesions, the diagnostic sensitivity of forceps biopsy is over 90%.[13,14] False-negative biopsies are usually from necrotic tumors. Bronchial brushing and washing that are frequently done along with forceps biopsy can increase the sensitivity further, although by themselves, the sensitivity is lower.[15,16] For submucosal and peribronchial tumors, multiple biopsies in the same site are needed or transbronchial needle aspiration.[17]

In contrast to invasive carcinoma, carcinoma in situ (CIS) and high-grade dysplasia are difficult to visualize by WLB. AFB allows rapid scanning of large areas of the bronchial surface for subtle abnormalities that are not visible to white light examination. In addition to multiple single-center studies,[4] there are 2 randomized trials[18,19] and 3 large multicenter trials,[9,20,21] comparing WLB and AFB. The studies showed an improvement in the detection rate of high-grade dysplasia, CIS, and microinvasive cancer with AFB compared with WLB. In general, there is a twofold improvement in the relative sensitivity with AFB. However, the specificity of AFB is lower (~60% vs ~90% for WLB) due to false-positive fluorescence with inflammation, mucous gland hyperplasia, and interobserver error. A recent meta-analysis reported a pooled sensitivity on a per lesion basis to detect preinvasive lesions of 85% for WLB combined with AFB. The overall relative sensitivity

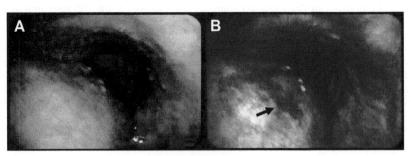

Fig. 1. White light (*A*) and autofluorescence (*B*) image of an area with CIC (*arrow*).

compared with WLB alone was 2.04 (95% confidence interval [CI]: 1.56–11.55).[22] However, the pooled sensitivity of WLB combined with AFB versus WLB alone for invasive squamous cell carcinoma was only marginally improved (95% vs 89%, respectively; relative sensitivity 1.15, 95% CI: 1.05–1.26). The specificity of WLB combined with AFB was lower than for WLB alone, with a pooled specificity of 61% and 80%, respectively.[22] The specificity of AFB can be improved to 80% by quantifying the red-to-green fluorescence ratio (R/G) of the target lesion during the bronchoscopic procedure.[23] Combining the R/G ratios with the visual score improved the specificity further to 88%. A higher false-positive rate was also found in a multicenter trial where the R/G ratios were hidden from the bronchoscopists when making the visual classification of the bronchial mucosal changes.[9] Quantitative imaging decreases intra- and interobserver variation.

NARROW BAND IMAGING

Narrow band imaging (NBI) is now classified as an image-enhanced endoscopy (IEE) technology.[24,25] It is widely used in gastrointestinal endoscopy for classification of lesions.[26,27] Its place in routine bronchoscopic examination has not been established. The advantage of NBI over other techniques is its ability to enhance fine superficial microvessel patterns. Angiogenesis is a relatively early event during lung cancer pathogenesis.[28] NBI can target the angiogenic features of neoplasia to improve the detection of preinvasive lesions and to differentiate these lesions from invasive carcinoma. There is a progressive pattern of neovascularization correlating with the progression of invasiveness. Dotted vessels, increased vessel growth, and complex networks of tortuous vessels of various sizes are observed with angiogenic squamous dysplasia. With CIS, dotted vessels and small spiral or corkscrew-type tumor vessels are observed. Prominent spiral or corkscrew-type tumor vessels of various sizes and grades are visible in microinvasive or invasive lung cancer.[29] A prospective study compares the performance of WLB followed by either autofluorescence imaging or NBI as determined by a randomized code in the diagnosis of intraepithelial neoplasia.[30] The sensitivity of WLB to detect high-grade dysplasia or CIS was 0.18 and the specificity was 0.88. The relative sensitivity of WLB + AFB versus WLB alone was 3.7 compared with 3.0 with WLB plus NBI, but the difference was not statistically significant. The relative specificities of WLB plus AFB and WLB plus NBI were 0.5 and 1.0 respectively. WLB plus NBI showed a significantly higher specificity compared with WLB plus AFB (P<.001).

Currently it is not known how NBI compares to high-definition white light endoscopy that makes use of charge coupled device with markedly higher pixel densities and high-definition images. The issue of training to recognize vascular patterns versus abnormal autofluorescence has not been investigated. Application of AFB and NBI technologies is also limited by the size of the bronchoscopes. With the shift in lung cancer cell types from predominant squamous and small cell carcinomas in the central airways to adenocarcinomas that are located in smaller airways, reduction in the size of the bronchoscope from 5 to 6 mm to no more than 3 mm outer diameter with an adequate biopsy channel is needed.

OPTICAL COHERENCE TOMOGRAPHY

Optical coherence tomography (OCT) is an optical imaging method that can offer near histologic resolution for visualizing cellular and extracellular structures at and below the tissue surface.[31–34] OCT is similar to ultrasound, but properties of light waves instead of sound waves are used for imaging. Optical interferometry is used to detect the light that is scattered or reflected by the tissue to generate a 1-dimensional tissue profile along the light direction. By scanning the light beam over the tissue, 2-dimensional images or 3-dimensional volumetric images can be recorded. The imaging procedure is performed using fiberoptic probes that can be miniaturized to enable imaging of airways down to the terminal bronchiole. These probes can be inserted down the instrument channel during standard bronchoscopic examination under conscious sedation. The axial and lateral resolutions of OCT range from approximately 5 to 30 μm depending on imaging conditions, and the imaging depth is 2 to 3 mm. This combination of resolution and imaging depth is ideal for examining preneoplastic changes originating in epithelial tissues or tumors involving smaller airways. Additionally, unlike ultrasound, light does not require a liquid coupling medium, and thus is more compatible with airway imaging. There are no associated risks from the weak near-infrared light sources that are used for OCT.

OCT images of normal bronchus, primary tumors, and alveoli from 7 human lung cancer lobectomy specimens have been compared with the histopathology.[33] OCT images were also collected in vivo from 5 patients. OCT imaging revealed a layered bronchial wall structure in normal bronchus that is lost in lung cancer. In peripheral lung, air-containing alveoli are imaged by OCT as a honeycomb structure beyond the bronchial wall. Lam and colleagues[34] investigated the ability of OCT to discern invasive cancer versus CIS or dysplasia. Normal or hyperplasia is characterized by 1 or 2 cell layers above a highly scattering basement membrane and upper submucosa. As the epithelium changes from normal/hyperplasia to metaplasia, various grades of dysplasia, and CIS, the thickness of the epithelial layer increases. Quantitative measurement of the epithelial thickness showed that invasive carcinoma was significantly thicker than carcinoma in situ ($P = .004$), and dysplasia was significantly thicker than metaplasia or hyperplasia ($P = .002$). The nuclei became more readily visible in high-grade dysplasia or CIS. The basement membrane was still intact in CIS but became discontinuous or no longer visible with invasive cancer (**Fig. 2**). Squamous cell carcinoma has different volumetric features than adenocarcinoma.[35] OCT may be useful for confirming the nature of the lesion before taking a biopsy.

BRONCHOSCOPIC DIAGNOSIS OF PERIPHERAL LUNG LESIONS

With the positive finding by the National Lung Screening Trial (NLST) that low-dose thoracic CT (LDCT) in high-risk smokers can reduce lung cancer mortality by 20%[36] and increasing use of CT for cardiac and abdominal imaging that includes parts of the lungs, growing numbers of patients are found to have small lung nodules. Over 50% of the nonsmall cell lung cancers found by screening LDCT are 2 cm or less.[36,37] The distribution of the lung cancer cell types has also changed. **Table 1** shows the cell type distribution in the usual care (unscreened) group of the Prostate, Lung, Colorectal, and Ovarian (PLCO) study,[38] conducted between 1993 and 2001, and the low-dose CT-detected lung cancers in NLST[36] conducted from 2002 to 2010. The former reflects the cell type distribution in the community setting and the latter the lung cancer screening setting. Only 20% of the lung cancers are now squamous cell carcinoma, while most are peripherally located adencarcinomas. On the average, 25% of the surgically resected lung lesions found on a screening LDCT turn out to be a benign diagnosis.[36,37,39] Imaging methods such as positron emission tomography (PET) scan do not have sufficient sensitivity and specificity to replace a tissue diagnosis. In a meta-analysis, the pooled sensitivity and specificity of FDG-PET for identifying malignancy were 85% (95% CI 82%–89%) and 77% (95% CI 72%–81%), respectively.[40] The addition of a biopsy result to the clinical history and chest CT findings reduced the frequency of unnecessary surgery for a benign lesion from 39% to 15% and the frequency of missed surgical cure from 10% to 7%.[41] Confirmation of the diagnosis using the least invasive and safest method before making a decision regarding management is preferred.

The general approach to bronchoscopic diagnosis of peripheral lung lesions is summarized in **Box 1**. Up until recently, the bronchoscopist would review the CT imaging data. Based on the anatomic knowledge, the bronchoscope is steered to the segment where the lung lesion is located. If the lesion is not visible with a standard 5 to 6 mm flexible bronchoscope, an ultrathin bronchoscope (2.8 mm) can be used to extend the range of the examination. If the lesion is visible, a biopsy is taken under direct

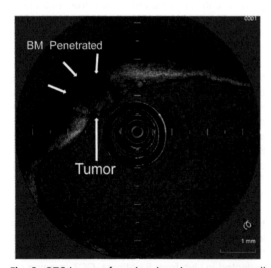

Fig. 2. OTC image of a micro-invasive squamous cell carcinoma. Basement membrane (BM) has high scattering and appears as a brighter line. The basement membrane is disrupted by tumor invasion (*arrows*).

Table 1		
Distribution of lung cancer cell types		
Cell Types	**PLCO[a]**	**NLST[b]**
Squamous	20%	21%
Small cell	15%	8%
Adenocarcinoma	41%	55%
NSCLC-NOS[c]	21%	12%
Other	3%	4%

[a] PLCO, Prostate, Lung, Colorectal, and Ovarian randomized trial usual care group from 1993 to 2001.
[b] National Lung Screening Trial low-dose CT group from 2002 to 2010.
[c] NSCLC-NOS, Non-small cell lung cancer-not otherwise specified.

vision. If the lesion is invisible, a biopsy forceps, brush, and curette are introduced blindly or under fluoroscopy to the target lesion to take a sample.[42,43] However, bronchial path selection based on 2-dimensional CT data is inaccurate even at the third-to fourth generation bronchial level.[44] Since the number of bronchial branches increases as the bronchoscope advances further into the periphery, and the path leading to the lesion is unknown at each branching point, the trial-and-error approach can be difficult within the limited examination time. Some lesions may not have a bronchus leading

into them. Nonsolid or part solid lesions are not visible or poorly visible on fluoroscopy. For these reasons, the diagnostic yield is poor, with an average sensitivity of only 34% for lesions that are no more than 20 mm and 63% for those that are greater than 20 mm.[45,46] Fluoroscopy also carries a radiation risk to the staff and the patient.

With the development of thin-slice CT and better image reconstruction technology, a three-dimensional virtual road map can be constructed, with the path leading to the lung lesion displayed as virtual bronchoscopy images. At each branching point, the bronchoscopist can match the actual videobronchoscopy image with the virtual image to steer the bronchoscope to the right direction.[47] An example is shown in Video 1. A randomized trial by Ishida and colleagues[48] showed that the diagnostic yield was significantly higher with virtual bronchoscopy navigation (VBN) compared with no VBN assistance (75.9% vs 59.3 mm for lesions <20 mm). The duration of the bronchoscopic examination was also significantly shorter with VBN.[48] Another recent advance is the development of real-time coregistration of the videobronchoscopy image with the virtual bronchoscopy image. An overlay on the real-time videobronchoscopy image indicates which airway to follow as well as the location and distance of the lesion behind the bronchial wall if there is no airway leading to the lesion directly. In a pilot study using this approach, the diagnostic yield was found to be 80% for lesions less than 42 mm.[49]

Virtual bronchoscopy can also be used for real-time steering by coregistering a steerable catheter, a bronchoscope, or biopsy forceps with a sensor at the tip that can be tracked by an external electromagnetic device similar in concept to a global positioning system. The procedure is known as electromagnetic navigation (EMN). Once the target lesion is reached on the virtual image, the location may be further confirmed by radial endoscopic ultrasound or fluoroscopy before taking a biopsy to minimize registration error, especially for lesions in the lower lobes, where the difference between a single breath hold CT that is used for planning the virtual path and the actual location of the bronchoscope or catheter is the greatest due to respiratory movement.[50] A recent multicenter experience with EMN showed a sensitivity of 50% for lesions no larger than 2 cm and 76% for lesions greater than 2 cm.[51] A meta-analysis of EMN showed an average diagnostic yield of 67% (95% CI 62.6%–71.4%).[52] A disadvantage of EMN is the significant cost implication of the single-use catheters compared with reusable instruments.

Radial ultrasound (R-EBUS) with a 1.4 mm probe with or without a guide sheath is used to localize peripheral lung lesions or to confirm arrival at the target lesion before taking a biopsy.[53] R-EBUS can localize lesions that are invisible or poorly visible on fluoroscopy.[54] R-EBUS by itself does not provide the road map to the lesion. The path is decided by the bronchoscopist by trial and error, with the use of VBN or used in conjunction with EMN, fluoroscopy, or CT. A meta-analysis of the performance of R-EBUS showed an average sensitivity of 56% for lesions no bigger than 20 mm and 78% for lesions greater than 20 mm.[55] When used in conjunction with VBN, the sensitivity is higher at 76% and 88% respectively.[48] Randomized trials of a combination of technologies showed improved sensitivity of 90% for lesions no bigger than 20 mm with VBN plus EMN plus R-EBUS compared to 78% with R-EBUS alone and 75% for EMN alone.[56] A recent meta-analysis of guided bronchoscopy showed similar results.[52] The presence of a bronchus sign (airway leading to the lesion) is associated with a higher diagnostic yield.[57,58] The diagnostic yield of R-EBUS is also determined by whether the probe can be placed at the center of the lesion. If only part of the lesion is visualized, or if the lesion is outside the airway, the diagnostic yield is reduced.[53,58] Newer technologies such as OCT,[34,35] which allows visualization with micron resolution, or SpyGlass (Boston Scientific, Natick, MA),[59] which allows direct visualization of the airways as small as 1 mm using fiberoptic probe, has the potential to improve the diagnostic yield and real time sampling.

The role of a guide sheath to allow insertion and removal of R-EBUS probe, biopsy forceps, or brushes is not clear, although it is widely used.[53,60] A recent randomized trial showed that the diagnostic yield is similar with or without a guide sheath when a thin (3.4 mm) bronchoscope is used.[61]

BRONCHOSCOPY VERSUS CT-GUIDED TRANSTHORACIC NEEDLE/CORE BIOPSY

CT-guided transthoracic needle/core biopsy has an average diagnostic yield of 90%.[62] For lesions not more than 15 mm, the sensitivity is lower, at 70% to 82%.[63,64] Transthoracic needle biopsy has an average pneumothorax rate of 15%. Chest tube drainage is required in approximately 6.6% of patients.[62] Hemoptysis occurs in about 1% of the procedures. The risk of pneumothorax is higher for smaller-sized lesions, deeper location, emphysema surrounding the lesion, and the need to traverse fissures.[64] Two small randomized trials comparing transthoracic needle biopsy and R-EBUS bronchoscopy have shown a similar

overall diagnostic yield.[65,66] Bronchoscopy has a lower diagnostic yield for lesions less than 20 mm, but the incidence of pneumothorax and other complications is significantly lower.[52,65,66] In a meta-analysis, the incidence of pneumothorax was 1% (range 0%–5%) with R-EBUS.[55]

The safest and most accurate method to diagnose peripheral lung lesions depends on the location and size of the lesion as well as the status of the surrounding lung parenchyma. For lesions that touch the pleura, without emphysema surrounding the lesion or the need for the needle to traverse fissures and for lesions less than 10 mm,[67] transthoracic needle biopsy is the method of choice. Image-guided bronchoscopy results in similar diagnostic yields to CT-guided transthoracic biopsy, with a significant reduction in adverse events, particularly for lesions with a bronchus sign on the CT and lesions surrounded by emphysema. When lung cancer is suspected based on clinical and radiographic findings, bronchoscopy has the advantage in that it can provide diagnostic and staging information by combining guided bronchoscopy with linear EBUS to sample mediastinal and hilar lymph nodes in a single procedure. Further advances in optical and image guidance technologies will likely further improve the diagnostic yield of bronchoscopy.

SUPPLEMENTARY DATA

Supplementary data related to this article can be found online at http://dx.doi.org/10.1016/j.thorsurg.2013.01.008.

REFERENCES

1. Shibuya K, Hoshino H, Chiyo M, et al. High magnification bronchovideoscopy combined with narrow band imaging could detect capillary loops of angiogenic squamous dysplasia in heavy smokers at high risk for lung cancer. Thorax 2003;58:989–95.
2. Vincent B, Fraig M, Silvestri G. A pilot study of narrow-band imaging compared to white light bronchoscopy for evaluation of normal airways and premalignant and malignant airways disease. Chest 2007;131:1794–9.
3. Gono K, Obi T, Yamaguchi M, et al. Appearance of enhanced tissue features in narrow-band endoscopic imaging. J Biomed Opt 2004;9:568–78.
4. Lam S. The role of autofluorescence bronchoscopy in diagnosis of early lung cancer. In: Hirsch FR, Bunn PA Jr, Kato H, et al, editors. IASLC textbook for prevention and detection of early lung cancer. London: Taylor & Francis; 2006. p. 149–58.
5. Wagnieres G, McWilliams A, Lam S. Lung cancer imaging with fluorescence endoscopy. In: Mycek M,

Pogue B, editors. Handbook of biomedical fluorescence. New York: Marcel Dekker; 2003. p. 361–96.

6. Chiyo M, Shibuya K, Hoshino H, et al. Effective detection of bronchial preinvasive lesions by a new autofluorescence imaging bronchovideoscope system. Lung Cancer 2005;48:307–13.

7. Ikeda N, Honda H, Hayashi A, et al. Early detection of bronchial lesions using newly developed videoendoscopy-based autofluorescence bronchoscopy. Lung Cancer 2006;52:21–7.

8. Lam S, MacAulay C, Hung J, et al. Detection of dysplasia and carcinoma in situ with a lung imaging fluorescence endoscope device. J Thorac Cardiovasc Surg 1993;105:1035–40.

9. Edell E, Lam S, Pass H, et al. Detection and localization of intraepithelial neoplasia and invasive carcinoma using fluorescence-reflectance bronchoscopy: an international, multicenter clinical trial. J Thorac Oncol 2009;4:49–54.

10. Häussinger K, Stanzel F, Huber RM, et al. Autofluorescence detection of bronchial tumors with the D-Light/AF. Diagn Ther Endosc 1999;5:105–12.

11. Tercelj M, Zeng H, Petek M, et al. Acquisition of fluorescence and reflectance spectra during routine bronchoscopy examinations using the ClearVu Elite device: pilot study. Lung Cancer 2005;50:35–42.

12. Lee P, Brokx HAP, Postmus PE, et al. Dual digital video-autofluorescence imaging for detection of preneoplastic lesions. Lung Cancer 2007;58:44–9.

13. Popp W, Rauscher H, Ritschka L, et al. Diagnostic sensitivity of different techniques in the diagnosis of lung tumors with the flexible fiberoptic bronchoscope. Comparison of brush biopsy, imprint cytology of forceps biopsy, and histology of forceps biopsy. Cancer 1991;67:72–5.

14. Zavala DC. Diagnostic fiberoptic bronchoscopy: techniques and results of biopsy in 600 patients. Chest 1975;68:12–9.

15. Kvale PA, Bode FR, Kini S. Diagnostic accuracy in lung cancer; comparison of techniques used in association with flexible fiberoptic bronchoscopy. Chest 1976;69:752–7.

16. Lam WK, So SY, Hsu C, et al. Fibreoptic bronchoscopy in the diagnosis of bronchial cancer: comparison of washings, brushings and biopsies in central and peripheral tumours. Clin Oncol (R Coll Radiol) 1983;9:35–42.

17. Shure D, Fedullo PF. Transbronchial needle aspiration in the diagnosis of submucosal and peribronchial bronchogenic carcinoma. Chest 1985;88:49–51.

18. Hirsch FR, Prindiville SA, Miller YE, et al. Fluorescence versus white-light bronchoscopy for detection of preneoplastic lesions: a randomized study. J Natl Cancer Inst 2001;93:1385–91.

19. Häussinger K, Becker H, Stanzel F, et al. Autofluorescence bronchoscopy with white light bronchoscopy compared with white light bronchoscopy alone for the detection of precancerous lesions: a European randomized controlled multicentre trial. Thorax 2005;60:496–503.

20. Lam S, Kennedy T, Unger M, et al. Localization of bronchial intraepithelial neoplastic lesions by fluorescence bronchoscopy. Chest 1998;113:696–702.

21. Ernst A, Simoff P, Mathur P, et al. D-Light autofluorescence in the detection of premalignant airway changes; A Multicenter Trial. J Bronchol 2005;12:133–8.

22. Sun J, Garfield DH, Lam B, et al. The value of autofluorescence bronchoscopy combined with white light bronchoscopy compared with white light alone in the diagnosis of intraepithelial neoplasia and invasive lung cancer: a meta-analysis. J Thorac Oncol 2011;6(8):1336–44.

23. Lee P, van den Berg RM, Lam S, et al. Color fluorescence ratio for detection of bronchial dysplasia and carcinoma in situ. Clin Cancer Res 2009;15:4700–5.

24. Tajiri H, Niwa H. Proposal for a consensus terminology in endoscopy: how should different endoscopic imaging techniques be grouped and defined? Endoscopy 2008;40:775–8.

25. Kaltenbach T, Sano Y, Friedland S, et al. American Gastroenterological Association (AGA) institute technology assessment on image-enhanced endoscopy. Gastroenterology 2008;134:327–40.

26. Curvers WL, Singh R, Song LM, et al. Endoscopic trimodal imaging for detection of early neoplasia in Barrett's oesophagus: a multi-centre feasibility study using high-resolution endoscopy, autofluorescence imaging and narrow band imaging incorporated in one endoscopy system. Gut 2008;57:167–72.

27. Van den Broek FJ, Fockens P, van Eeden S, et al. Endoscopic tri-modal imaging for surveillance in ulcerative colitis: randomized comparison of high-resolution endoscopy and autofluorescence imaging for neoplasia detection; and evaluation of narrowband imaging for classification of lesions. Gut 2008;57:1083–9.

28. Gazdar AF, Minna JD. Angiogenesis and the multistage development of lung cancers. Clin Cancer Res 2000;6:1611–2.

29. Shibuya K, Nakajima T, Fujiwara T, et al. Narrow band imaging with high-resolution bronchovideoscopy: a new approach for visualizing angiogenesis in squamous cell carcinoma of the lung. Lung Cancer 2010;69:194–202.

30. Herth FJ, Eberhardt R, Anantham D, et al. Narrowband imaging bronchoscopy increases the specificity of bronchoscopic early lung cancer detection. J Thorac Oncol 2009;4:1060–5.

31. Fujimoto JG, Brezinski ME, Tearney GJ, et al. Biomedical imaging and optical biopsy using optical coherence tomography. Nat Med 1995;1:970–2.

32. Tearney GJ, Brezinski ME, Bouma BE, et al. In vivo endoscopic optical biopsy with optical coherence tomography. Science 1997;276:2037–9.

33. Tsuboi M, Hayashi A, Ikeda N, et al. Optical coherence tomography in the diagnosis of bronchial lesions. Lung Cancer 2005;49:387–94.

34. Lam S, Standish B, Baldwin C, et al. In vivo optical coherence tomography imaging of preinvasive bronchial lesions. Clin Cancer Res 2008;14:2006–11.

35. Hariri LP, Applegate MB, Mino-Kenudson M, et al. Volumetric optical frequency domain imaging of pulmonary pathology with precise correlation to histopathology. Chest 2012 Mar 29. [Epub ahead of print].

36. National Lung Screening Trial Research Team. Reduced lung-cancer mortality with low-dose computed tomographic screening. N Engl J Med 2011;365:395–409.

37. Swensen SJ, Jett JR, Hartman TE, et al. CT screening for lung cancer: five-year prospective experience. Radiology 2005;235:259–65.

38. Oken MM, Hocking WG, Kvale PA, et al. Screening by chest radiograph and lung cancer mortality. The Prostate, Lung, Colorectal, and Ovarian (PLCO) randomized trial. JAMA 2011;306(17):1865–73. http://dx.doi.org/10.1001/jama.2011.1591.

39. Bach PB, Mirkin JN, Oliver TK, et al. Benefits and Harms of CT Screening for Lung Cancer. A Systematic Review. JAMA 2012;307(22):2418–29.

40. Barger RL Jr, Nandalur KR. Diagnostic performance of dual-time 18F-FDG PET in the diagnosis of pulmonary nodules: a meta-analysis. Acad Radiol 2012; 19:153–8.

41. Baldwin DR, Eaton T, Kolbe J, et al. Management of solitary pulmonary nodules: how do thoracic computed tomography and guided fine needle biopsy influence clinical decisions? Thorax 2002;57:817–22.

42. Yamamoto S, Ueno K, Imamura F, et al. Usefulness of ultrathin bronchoscopy in diagnosis of lung cancer. Lung Cancer 2004;46:43–8.

43. Oki M, Saka H, Kitagawa C, et al. Novel thin bronchoscope with a 1.7 mm working channel for peripheral pulmonary lesions. Eur Respir J 2008;32:465–71.

44. Dolina MY, Cornish DC, Merritt SA, et al. Interbronchoscopist variability in endobronchial path selection: a simulation study. Chest 2008;133(4):897–905.

45. Schreiber G, McCory DC. Performance characteristics of different modalities for diagnosis of suspected lung cancer: summary of published evidence. Chest 2003;123(Suppl 1):115S–28S.

46. Rivera MP, Mehta AC. Initial diagnosis of lung cancer: ACCP evidence-based clinical practice guidelines (2nd edition). Chest 2007;132(Suppl 3): 131S–48S.

47. Asano F. Virtual bronchoscopic navigation. Clin Chest Med 2010;31:75–85.

48. Ishida T, Asano F, Yamazaki K, et al. Virtual bronchoscopic navigation combined with endobronchial ultrasound to diagnose small peripheral pulmonary lesions: a randomised trial. Thorax 2011;66:1072–7.

49. Eberhardt R, Kahn N, Gompelmann D, et al. Lung-Point—a new approach to peripheral lesions. J Thorac Oncol 2010;5:1559–63.

50. Becker HD, Herth F, Ernst A, et al. Bronchoscopic biopsy of peripheral lung I lesions under electromagnetic guidance: a pilot study. J Bronchol 2005; 12:9–13.

51. Jensen KW, Hsia DW, Seijo LM, et al. Multi-center experience with electromagnetic navigation bronchoscopy for the diagnosis of pulmonary nodules. J Bronchology Interv Pulmonol 2012;19:195–9.

52. Wang Memoli JS, Nietert PJ, Silvestri GA. Meta-analysis of guided bronchoscopy for the evaluation of the pulmonary nodule. Chest 2012;143:385–93.

53. Kurimoto N, Miyazawa T, Okimasa S, et al. Endobronchial ultrasonography using a guide sheath increases the ability to diagnose peripheral pulmonary lesions endoscopically. Chest 2004;126:959–65.

54. Herth FJ, Eberhardt R, Becker HD, et al. Endobronchial ultrasound guided transbronchial lung biopsy in fluoroscopically invisible pulmonary nodules: a prospective trial. Chest 2006;129:147–50.

55. Steinfort DP, Khor YH, Manser RL, et al. Radial probe endobronchial ultrasound for the diagnosis of peripheral lung cancer: systematic review and meta-analysis. Eur Respir J 2011;37:902–10.

56. Eberhardt R, Anantham D, Ernst A, et al. Multimodality bronchoscopic diagnosis of peripheral lung lesions: a randomized controlled trial. Am J Respir Crit Care Med 2007;176:36–41.

57. Seijo LM, de Torres JP, Lozano MD, et al. Diagnostic yield of electromagnetic navigation bronchoscopy is highly dependent on the presence of a bronchus sign on CT imaging. Results from a prospective study. Chest 2010;138(6):1316–21.

58. Shinagawa N, Yamazaki K, Onodera Y, et al. Factors related to diagnostic sensitivity using an ultrathin bronchoscope under CT guidance. Chest 2007; 131:549–53.

59. Delage A, Godbout K, Martel S, et al. Evaluation of pulmonary nodules using the spyglass direct visualization system combined with radial endobronchial ultrasound: a feasibility study. Am J Respir Crit Care Med 2012;185;012:A1103.

60. Yoshikawa M, Sukoh N, Yamazaki K, et al. Diagnostic value of endobronchial ultrasonography with a guide sheath for peripheral pulmonary lesions without X-ray fluoroscopy. Chest 2007;131:1788–93.

61. Oki M, Saka H, Kitagawa C, et al. Randomized study of endobronchial ultrasound-guided transbronchial biopsy. Thin bronchoscope versus guide sheath method. J Thorac Oncol 2012;7:535–41.

62. Wiener RS, Schwartz LM, Woloshin S, et al. Population-based risk for complications after transthoracic needle lung biopsy of a pulmonary nodule: an analysis of discharge records. Ann Intern Med 2011;155: 137–44.

63. Kothary N, Lock L, Sze DY, et al. Computed tomography-guided percutaneous needle biopsy of pulmonary nodules: impact of nodule size on diagnostic accuracy. Clin Lung Cancer 2009;10:360–3.

64. Heyer CM, Reichelt S, Peters SA, et al. Computed tomography-navigated transthoracic core biopsy of pulmonary lesions: which factors affect diagnostic yield and complication rates? Acad Radiol 2008; 15:1017–26.

65. Steinfort DP, Vincent J, Heinze S, et al. Comparative effectiveness of radial probe endobronchial ultrasound versus CT-guided needle biopsy for evaluation of peripheral pulmonary lesions: a randomized pragmatic trial. Respir Med 2011;105:1704–11.

66. Fielding DI, Chia C, Nguyen P, et al. Prospective randomized trial of endobronchial ultrasound-guide sheath versus computed tomography-guided percutaneous core biopsies for peripheral lung lesions. Intern Med J 2012;42(8):894–900. http://dx.doi.org/10.1111/j.1445–5994. 2011.0707.x.

67. Ng YL, Patsios D, Roberts H, et al. CT-guided percutaneous fine-needle aspiration biopsy of pulmonary nodules measuring 10 mm or less. Clin Radiol 2008;63:272–7.

Advances in Cytopathology for Lung Cancer
The Impact and Challenges of New Technologies

Harmanjatinder S. Sekhon, MD, PhD[a],
Carolina A. Souza, MD, PhD[b], Marcio M. Gomes, MD, PhD[a],*

KEYWORDS

- Lung cancer • Cytology • Fine-needle aspiration biopsy • Immunohistochemistry

KEY POINTS

- The impact of new imaging technologies and sampling procedures.
- How multidisciplinary care and subspecialization are changing the face of cytopathology.
- The new techniques and ancillary tests for the diagnosis and management of lung cancer.
- Current cytologic diagnostic algorithm, techniques, and diagnostic values.

INTRODUCTION

Lung cancer remains one of the most prevalent cancers in both men and women. Despite new and improved therapies the outcome remains very poor in both genders. Along with progress in treatment modalities, the improved imaging techniques, new sampling procedures, pathologic ancillary tests, and identification of molecular targets have also evolved. With the development of new technologies and changes in the epidemiology and treatment of lung cancer, significant advances have been made in cytopathology. Among them, this article highlights fine-needle aspiration (FNA), which has emerged as a safe, cost-effective, and less invasive procedure without compromising the sensitivity, specificity, and accuracy of the diagnosis compared with histology specimens.[1] This article focuses on the impact of such new technologies, and the role of cytology in diagnosing lung cancer and facilitating multidisciplinary patient care. In addition, the current diagnostic cytologic techniques and their diagnostic values are briefly reviewed. A thorough review of cytologic techniques and diagnosis is beyond the scope of this article.

New Imaging Technologies and Sampling Procedures

Multidetector computed tomography and computed tomography–guided lung biopsy

The advances in cytopathology in the last 2 decades were made possible by advances in medical imaging technology. In particular, the advent of multidetector computed tomography (MDCT) has revolutionized thoracic imaging, allowing faster acquisition and multiplanar reconstruction (MPR), thus providing high-quality images. MDCT allows more accurate evaluation of lung lesions, hence assisting biopsy planning and the decision of biopsy approach and needle path, which influences both diagnostic yield and

[a] Department of Pathology and Laboratory Medicine, The Ottawa Hospital, University of Ottawa, 501 Smyth Road, Ottawa, Ontario, Canada K1H 8L6; [b] Department of Diagnostic Imaging, The Ottawa Hospital, University of Ottawa, 501 Smyth Road, Ottawa, Ontario, Canada K1H 8L6
* Corresponding author.
E-mail address: mgomes@toh.on.ca

Thorac Surg Clin 23 (2013) 163–178
http://dx.doi.org/10.1016/j.thorsurg.2013.01.011
1547-4127/13/$ – see front matter © 2013 Elsevier Inc. All rights reserved.

risk for complications.[2–5] Computed tomography (CT) is currently the modality of choice for imaging-guided biopsy in most centers and has largely replaced fluoroscopy alone or ultrasonography to guide percutaneous biopsies of parenchymal lung lesions.[1] CT has made transthoracic biopsy more accurate and safer, and has expanded the scope of lesions amenable to percutaneous biopsy (**Figs. 1** and **2**). CT is widely available, cost-effective, and allows radiologists to target smaller and deep-seated lesions with a better yield compared with transbronchial biopsy (**Figs. 3** and **4**).[6] The role of CT-guided biopsy has recently been established in the diagnosis of early adenocarcinoma (ADC) presenting as part-solid lesions (ie, lesions containing both ground-glass and solid components). The solid component in these lesions often correlates with the presence of tumor invasion on pathology.[7,8] Under CT guidance, the biopsy needle can be placed accurately within the solid component, thus increasing diagnostic accuracy (**Fig. 5**).

CT-guided biopsy is usually performed with coaxial technique, which involves imaging-guided placement of an introducer needle directed to the edge of the target lesion. Once adequate location of the introducer needle is confirmed with CT scan, tissue sampling is obtained with a biopsy needle through the introducer. With coaxial technique, several samples may be obtained through the same introducer, precluding

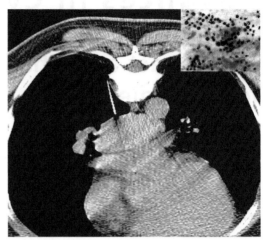

Fig. 2. CT-guided transthoracic biopsy in a 63-year-old man. Despite the challenging location for percutaneous biopsy, the subcarinal mass was targeted with precision using coaxial technique. The smear shows small cells with scanty cytoplasm and inconspicuous nucleoli in a necrotic background, typical of small cell lung carcinoma (SCLC - inset). Because SCLC are usually central, they were not frequently diagnosed by transthoracic FNA before CT-guided technique became widely available.

the need for repositioning the biopsy needle for each sample and avoiding several punctures of the pleura surface, thus decreasing procedure time and risk of complications.[2,3]

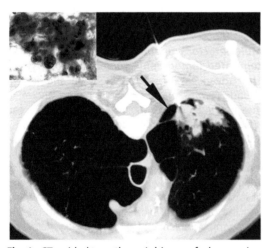

Fig. 1. CT-guided transthoracic biopsy of a large spiculated lesion in the left upper lobe. Using coaxial technique, the needle is accurately placed within the lesion, avoiding the large emphysematous bullae (*arrow*) adjacent to it, thus considerably decreasing the risk of pneumothorax. The smear shows markedly atypical tumor cells with large nuclei and high nuclear/cytoplasmic ratio, consistent with a poorly differentiated adenocarcinoma (inset).

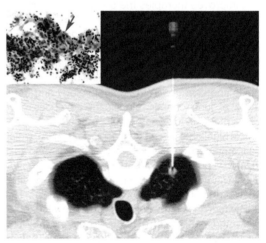

Fig. 3. CT-guided transthoracic FNA of a solid nodule in the left upper lobe of a 51-year-old man. Thin-slice CT scan allows accurate placement of the biopsy needle in the center of a subcentimeter (8 mm) nodule. The smear shows aggregates of histiocytes (*arrow*) and lymphocytes, indicating a granulomatous infection (inset). These lesions were not amenable to transthoracic FNA before the advent of CT-guided biopsies and the diagnosis depended on either wedge resection or radiological follow-up.

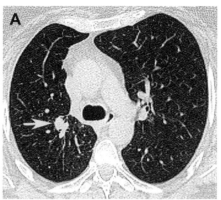
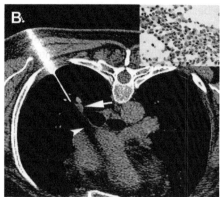

Fig. 4. CT scan of the chest with lung window settings showed a small central lesion in the right upper lobe (*arrow*) adjacent to a segmental bronchus (*A*). CT with mediastinal window settings obtained during biopsy shows the needle accurately placed in the center of the deep-seated lesion (*arrow*). Note the dark line beyond the lesion (*arrowhead*) consistent with metallic artifact from the biopsy needle (*B*). The FNA smear shows uniform neoplastic cells with rounded to oval nuclei and salt and pepper chromatin consistent with a typical carcinoid (inset). CT-guided biopsies can reach these deep-seated lesions with a higher yield than endoscopic transbronchial biopsies.

Impact of MDCT and CT-Guided Lung Biopsies:

- Increased accuracy and safety of transthoracic biopsies
- Expanded scope of lesions amenable to percutaneous biopsy
- Targeted biopsies of specific areas within lung lesions
- Increased detection of lesions and volume of cytopathology samples

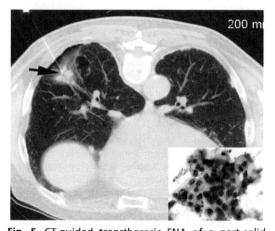

Fig. 5. CT-guided transthoracic FNA of a part-solid lesion in the right lower lobe in a 75-year-old woman. Using coaxial technique, the needle is accurately placed in the solid portion of the lesion (*arrow*). The smear shows atypical cells with prominent nucleoli and vacuolated cytoplasm in keeping with an adenocarcinoma (inset). CT-guided biopsies allow targeting of the solid area of a part-solid nodule, which is most likely to yield cells for cytologic diagnosis.

- Largely replaced fluoroscopy alone or ultrasonography for percutaneous lung biopsies

Endoscopic and endobronchial ultrasound-guided biopsies

Another major advance in the cytologic diagnosis and staging of lung cancer is biopsy guided by endoscopic ultrasound (EUS) and endobronchial ultrasound (EBUS). Both are minimally invasive techniques in which a small ultrasound (US) probe fitted to a special endoscope allows needle aspiration biopsy through the wall of hollow organs, using real-time US imaging to guide the biopsy. In EUS, the endoscope is introduced in the esophagus and the biopsy done through the esophageal wall, whereas, in EBUS, the probe is adapted to a bronchoscope and the biopsy is done through the tracheal and/or bronchial wall. EUS/EBUS had a great impact on the staging of lung cancer because it can sample peritracheal and periesophageal mediastinal node stations, and help to determine the resectability of a tumor.[9,10] This less invasive technique has shown high sensitivity and might replace mediastinoscopy to a great extent in the near future. In addition to staging of lung cancer, EUS/EBUS have become additional tools in the diagnosis of mediastinal lesions.[11,12] These techniques allow sampling of central lung lesions not involving the bronchial mucosa and otherwise not amenable to traditional bronchoscopic forceps biopsy, as well as biopsy of central/mediastinal lesions not amenable to transthoracic CT-guided biopsy. Although transbronchial needle aspiration (TBNA) has been done for a long time, the US probe has expanded its usefulness because of the improved detection of lesions, precision of needle placement, a decrease in complication rates, and an increase in the yield of cytology specimens. The EUS/EBUS will contribute to an increasing volume of cytopathology specimens as it becomes more widely available.

Impact of EUS and EBUS-Guided Biopsies:

- Expansion of the goal of cytopathology with sampling of mediastinal lymph node stations for lung cancer staging
- Expansion of the differential diagnosis in lung cytopathology with sampling of central and mediastinal lesions and lymph nodes
- Increase in the volume of cytopathology samples

Multidisciplinary care

The issue of subspecialization As in other fields of modern medicine, pathology practice is undergoing reform toward specialization. Histopathology has been subdivided into organ-specific subspecialties in most academic centers. Molecular pathology has emerged as a specific domain and cytopathology has become a well-established subspecialty, with board examinations in some jurisdictions and fellowship requirement in others.

As a subspecialty, cytopathology focuses on the cellular details and arrangements rather than the architectural features available in histologic sections. Because one of the morphologic parameters used for interpretation of biologic processes is absent, namely tissue architecture, cytopathologists have to be familiar with the cellular details to distinguish benign from malignant processes, or even make the diagnosis of specific cancer subtypes. If the lack of tissue architecture might render cytopathology less specific than histopathology, the ability to sample different areas of a lesion and the larger number of cells for morphologic assessment make it more sensitive in some instances.[1]

The role of a cytopathologist is broad because it covers diagnostic assessment of specimens from all body systems. One of the biggest challenges of the ever-increasing subspecialization is to be able to confidently integrate clinical, radiological, laboratory, and pathologic features, which tend to be highly organ specific. Personalized medicine is similarly showing many particularities in tumors from different organs. The response to the different therapies depends on the specific histologic subtype or genetic mutation, which vary greatly from organ to organ. Specific detailed guidelines are becoming the mainstream in the management of cancer by medical oncologists. A fast and clear communication between different disciplines is necessary to achieve specific diagnoses and identify pertinent molecular changes that would help to optimize therapy in a timely fashion.[7]

The pathologist plays a pivotal role in integrating clinical and radiological features when approaching the diagnosis of lung cancer. Knowledge of the clinical and radiological features of primary and metastatic thoracic malignancies, as well as integrating an epidemiologic approach into the diagnostic algorithm, allows more specific diagnoses and prevents unnecessary stains from being done, thus ensuring judicious use of limited health resources and preserving tissue for relevant molecular tests (**Fig. 6**).[7] Similar to other clinical specialties, the pathologist should incorporate concepts such as pretest probability and predictive values in routine clinical practice.

The current practice of lung cancer pathology requires the cytopathologist to master the technical skills for the morphologic interpretation of cytologic specimens and the use of ancillary techniques, and the organ-specific medical expertise to integrate the clinical context into daily diagnostic practice.

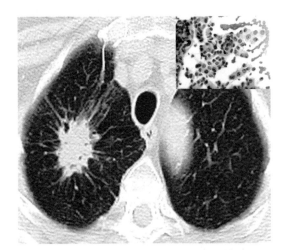

Fig. 6. CT scan of the chest in a 76-year-old woman shows a spiculated 3-cm lesion with pleural tags in the right upper lobe with features characteristic for a primary lung malignancy. The smear of the transthoracic FNA shows uniform cells with eccentric nuclei and conspicuous nucleoli, consistent with a well-differentiated lung adenocarcinoma. In a patient with no clinical or radiological features to suggest metastatic disease, and cytologic features consistent with a primary adenocarcinoma, the use of immunohistochemistry to confirm the primary site of the tumor is strongly discouraged. With the advent of targeted therapies, the pathologist should act as a gatekeeper, the guardian of the cell block, saving the available tissue for ancillary techniques whenever possible.

The impact of subspecialization:

- Cytopathology has become a well-established subspecialty
- Cytopathologists deal with lesions from all body systems
- Clinical practice and use of ancillary techniques has become organ specific
- Clinicopathologic correlation is necessary for optimal practice
- It is challenging to master the skills in both areas

Clinical-radiological-pathologic correlation The incidence of adenocarcinoma is steadily increasing in many countries, notably in Western societies. Different histologic subtypes and patterns of growth were shown to have different prognoses. For instance, adenocarcinoma in situ (formerly known as bronchioloalveolar carcinoma) has no metastatic potential, whereas micropapillary adenocarcinomas frequently metastasize to regional or distant sites.[13,14]

On radiology, lung adenocarcinomas also present with different patterns. Several recent studies with radiological-pathologic correlation have been able to better define the CT characteristics of different forms of lung adenocarcinoma and their prognostic implications. Concepts such as good prognosis and low metastatic potential for pure ground-glass lesions, high risk of malignancy in part-solid lesions, and consolidation as a common manifestation of mucin-producing adenocarcinoma are now well established and allow a better diagnostic approach and management of these lesions.[8,15] Although many centers prefer to remove any suspicious nodule to have a definite histologic diagnosis, others routinely perform FNA or core biopsies as the first diagnostic approach.

As a consequence, a more refined classification of lung adenocarcinoma is required. The International Association for the Study of Lung Cancer (IASLC)/American Thoracic Society /European Respiratory Society put together a multidisciplinary consensus classification in 2011.[7] A long existing, but poorly adhered to, category of adenocarcinoma in situ has been more precisely defined (formerly known as bronchioloalveolar carcinoma). The notion of minimally invasive adenocarcinoma was introduced, carrying with it the important prognostic implication of having virtually no metastatic potential. New morphologic subtypes were described and their validity is under scrutiny. Some of the new entities of the IASLC classification include size and tissue architecture in their definition, with important prognostic implications.

Therefore, the classification of the lesion based solely on cytologic features or on small tissue fragments is difficult or unfeasible. Diagnosing adenocarcinoma without knowledge of the radiological pattern and size of the lesion might lead to an incorrect interpretation and induce inadequate management (**Figs. 7** and **8**). In the current time of multidisciplinary care, it is an undeniable role of the pathologist to be able and make such integration of radiological and pathologic features, either alone or by discussing the case with the radiologist. Regardless the pathway, the final integrated interpretation should be part of a combined radiological-pathologic report.

The importance of clinical-radiological-pathologic correlation:

- Increased incidence and knowledge of lung adenocarcinoma
- New classification of lung adenocarcinoma including radiological and pathologic features
- Radiological features correlate with histologic subtypes of lung adenocarcinoma
- Integration of radiological and pathologic features may be necessary for a precise diagnosis

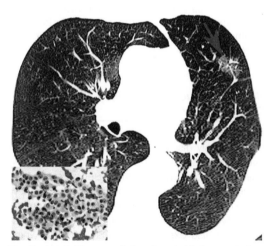

Fig. 7. Axial CT scan of the chest with lung window settings in a 54-year-old woman shows a well-circumscribed 2.7-cm pure ground-glass nodule in the left upper lobe (*red arrow*). The transthoracic FNA smear shows a monolayer of uniform cells with rounded nuclei and small nucleoli, consistent with a well-differentiated lung adenocarcinoma (inset). Although these features suggest a lepidic pattern of growth, the possibility of invasion cannot be ruled out. Therefore, the correlation with the radiological pattern is necessary. Adenocarcinoma in situ (noninvasive) has a better prognosis and usually presents as a pure ground-glass nodule in high-resolution CT.

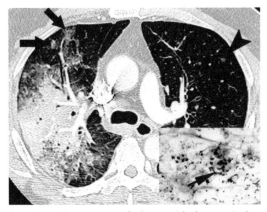

Fig. 8. Axial CT scan of chest with lung window settings in a 55-year-old man shows extensive airspace consolidation with air bronchograms in the right lung. Ground-glass opacities are also present including small ground-glass nodules in the right upper lobe (*arrows*) and left lung (*arrowhead*). The transthoracic FNA smear shows scattered atypical cells in a mucinous background (inset). The arrow highlights a neoplastic cell with a large cytoplasmic vacuole filled with mucin. Specific diagnosis of mucinous subtype in an FNA is important because it is considered an invasive neoplasm until proven otherwise, and it carries a worse prognosis for its aggressive behavior with frequent multicentricity and intrapulmonary metastatic spread. Furthermore, it is more frequently associated with the presence of EML4-ALK translocations. Because some radiological patterns are associated with mucinous phenotype, radiological-pathologic correlation is of paramount importance to achieve a more clinically relevant diagnosis.

New Techniques and Ancillary Tests on Cytopathology

Rapid on-site evaluation

As previously discussed, the incidence of adenocarcinoma, as well as the detection of early lung adenocarcinoma, is increasing. Because this type of tumor is more commonly located in the periphery of the lung, the most accurate cytologic diagnostic modality is FNA. The use of EUS and EBUS–guidance has also expanded the use of FNA, which has become the preferred technique for diagnosis and staging of lung cancer. The ease of performing the procedure, lower postprocedure complications, and cost-effectiveness have all contributed to this. However, rapid on-site evaluation (ROSE) is likely the main reason for its improved accuracy. Compared with core needle biopsy (CNB), FNA has traditionally had worse diagnostic values. However, the introduction of ROSE greatly increased the yield and sensitivity of FNA, to the point that no statistical differences exist between FNA and CNB when ROSE is done.[1]

ROSE is performed by an experienced cytotechnologist or cytopathologist. In most institutions in the United States, a preliminary diagnosis is rendered by the cytopathologist to initiate patient management. It not only assists in targeting the tissue of interest but also limits extra aspirates and reduces the number of unsatisfactory aspirates as well as guiding the operator to submit tissue for other studies including flow cytometric and cytogenetic analysis. These steps are critical to direct specific lesions for appropriate tests to attain accurate and specific diagnosis in a timely fashion and to direct patient management.

At our institution, after establishing adequacy by ROSE, at least 2 extra aspirates are added to the needle rinses in formalin for cell block. After instituting a protocol of 2 extra passes for cell block, our adequacy of cell block to perform ancillary studies has increased from 62% to 94% (>50 tumor cells). The formalin fixation and further processing are identical to the core needle biopsies or resection specimens. The cell block sections not only aid the interpretation of smears but also determine cellular differentiation and, in certain instances, are useful to subtype the pattern of adenocarcinoma. The formalin-fixed tissue is also optimal for immunohistochemical stains, molecular studies, and, if needed, for electron microscopy (**Fig. 9**).

New and expanded role of immunocytochemistry

The cytologic interpretation of malignant tumors in the past was primarily based on the morphologic (nuclear and cytoplasmic) features of the individual cells and/or their arrangement on limited material in the smears. Immunohistochemistry (IHC)/immunocytochemistry (ICC) started to be widely used in histologic specimens for clinical purposes in the 1990s. The technique is based on the identification of specific antigenic epitopes in tissues by designing specific antibodies. Its usefulness has been established and changes to the technical processing of cytologic specimens were made to allow the use of ICC. At first, ICC was used to determine the cellular lineage (eg, mesenchymal vs epithelial). With the advancement of the technique, organ and tissue specific antibodies were developed, which help in determining the primary site of a tumor (eg, breast vs lung carcinoma) and to distinguish among different subtypes of tumors (eg, adenocarcinoma vs squamous cell carcinoma (SqCCa)). This technique is part of the current routine cytologic assessment.

Primary lung carcinoma Although the cytomorphologic criteria for diagnosis of primary

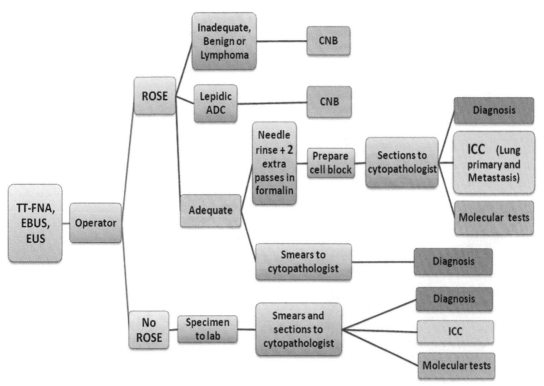

Fig. 9. Flow chart shows the steps of cytologic FNA specimen processing (with and without ROSE), integration of morphologic and ancillary studies to achieve specific diagnosis, and use of cell block for immunohistochemical stains and molecular tests to guide patient management.

squamous cell carcinoma and adenocarcinoma in cytologic samples are well defined more than a third of cases do not show clear squamous or glandular cellular differentiation in cytologic specimens or tissue biopsies.[16,17] ICC might help in that distinction and it requires a formalin-fixed cell block. In the past, a cell block was uncommonly prepared from the needle rinse to aid the interpretation of smears. With the new concepts of tumor-specific therapies, especially SqCCa versus ADC, the preparation of a cell block and the use of IHC have become important tools to subcategorize lung tumors.

Numerous ICC markers for SqCCa and ADC have been identified but none are absolutely sensitive or specific. Hence, the use of a panel of antibodies containing both SqCCa and ADC markers has been advocated at various consensus meetings. Among the different markers that are available, the use of TTF-1 and napsin for ADC, and p63 and CK5/6 for SqCCa, has been more widely tested and validated. Therefore, in the absence of clear cytomorphologic differentiation, the immunoprofile might help in determining the cellular differentiation and subtype.

Whithaus and colleagues[16] reported that a 4-stain panel can be successfully used to subtype SqCCa versus ADC. In adenocarcinoma cases, the sensitivity and specificity of napsin are 83% and 98% respectively, and of TTF-1 they are 60% and 98% respectively, whereas for SqCCa the p63 is 95% and 86%, respectively, and CK5/6 is 53% and 96%, respectively (**Figs. 10 and 11**).[16] There is only a 5% discrepancy between the immunoprofile of small tumor specimens and resected tumor.[18] In order to preserve tissue for molecular tests and other ancillary studies, the single most useful marker to distinguish ADC versus SqCCa is p63, with sensitivity of 84% and specificity of 85%,[19] whereas an addition of TTF-1 to p63 as a first step followed by CK5/6 aids in subclassifying most cases into SqCCa and ADC.[20] However, a 4-stain panel (TTF-1, napsin, p63, and CK5) is most commonly used (**Fig. 12**) and, to preserve tissue dual labeling, a combination of TTF-1 (nuclear) with napsin (cytoplasmic) and p63 (nuclear) with CK5/6 (cytoplasmic) is most informative by using only 2 sections (**Table 1**). Surfactant-A protein is less sensitive but more specific for lung adenocarcinoma. As presented

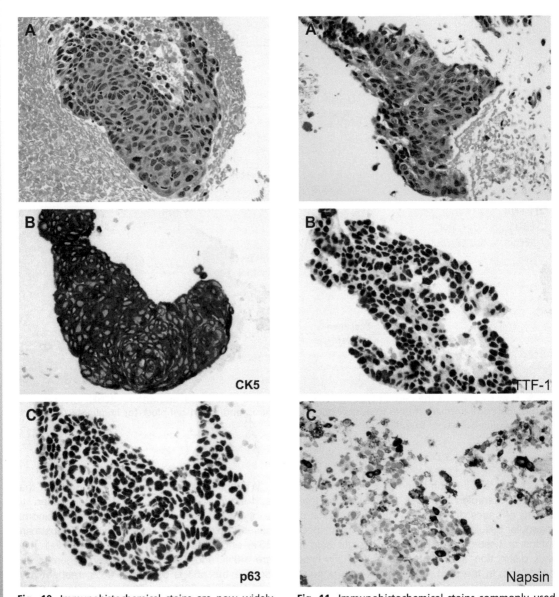

Fig. 10. Immunohistochemical stains are now widely used in FNA when cellular differentiation is not obvious. The photomicrographs show squamous cell carcinoma–specific immunostain profiles: (*A*) cell block section stained with hematoxylin-eosin (H&E), (*B*) CK5 (cytokeratin 5), a marker for squamous cell differentiation, shows diffuse and strong immunopositivity (dark brown color) in the cytoplasm, and (*C*) p63 is also a maker for squamous differentiation but stains nuclei. It is strongly and diffusely positive in nuclei of squamous cell carcinoma. These stains are particularly helpful in poorly differentiated squamous cell carcinoma cases because they lack typical squamous cytomorphologic features.

Fig. 11. Immunohistochemical stains commonly used for adenocarcinoma. (*A*) Cell block section stained with H&E show a large sheet of cells with a few slitlike glandular configurations; (*B*) TTF-1 stains the nuclei strongly and diffusely, whereas expression of the other adenocarcinoma immunomarker, napsin, is seen in cytoplasm (*C*). These markers are useful to distinguish poorly differentiated adenocarcinomas from poorly differentiated squamous cell carcinomas, which are negative for these immunostains.

in **Table 1**, there is significant overlapping in expression of cell markers in SqCCa and ADC. Most importantly, despite using immunohistochemical stains, a small proportion of poorly differentiated non–small cell lung carcinoma (NSCLC) cannot be subtyped.[21]

Metastatic tumors to the lung The lung is the most common site of systemic metastasis in the body. Several organ-specific and tissue-specific antibodies have been developed and a review of

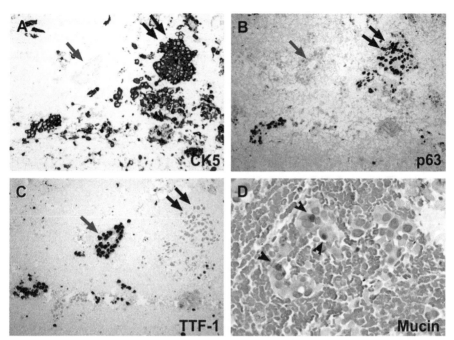

Fig. 12. Immunohistochemical stains showing differential immunoreactivity in adenosquamous carcinoma, showing mixed morphology of adenocarcinoma and squamous carcinoma. It can be challenging cytomorphologically to make definitive diagnosis. The FNA smear with Papanicolaou stain showed some cells arranged in a glandular configuration and others in sheets with hyperchromatic cells of squamous differentiation; similarly, the sections of cell block stained with H&E also showed glandular and squamous differentiation. The sections of cell block stained with CK5 (*A*) and p63 (*B*) are positive in the squamous cell carcinoma component (*double black arrows*), confirming a dual malignant cell population. (*C*) TTF-1 shows strong nuclear staining in adenocarcinoma (glands, *single red arrow*) and is negative in the squamous cell component (*double black arrow*). (*D*) In addition, the histochemical stain mucicarmine shows positive red color in mucin vacuoles in adenocarcinoma cells (*arrowheads*). These figures highlight the heterogeneity of lung tumors and show the value of immunohistochemical stains to determine cellular differentiation and make a challenging diagnosis even in rare lung tumors.

their indications is beyond the scope of this article. However, a few remarks about the general use of ICC in the distinction between primary and metastatic tumors are important. First, clinical history as well as imaging play a major role in designing an immunohistochemical staining panel to delineate whether or not the tumor is a lung primary. Again, ICC markers are not completely sensitive or specific and the choice of tests, as well as their interpretation, has to be done in association with the clinical findings. Second, ICC is usually performed to determine the primary site of an adenocarcinoma, because there are no tests so far for reliably determining the primary site of other tumor subtypes (eg, SqCCa). Third, TTF-1 and surfactant antibodies are most specific for primary lung adenocarcinomas and are used in conjunction with the markers for clinically expected/plausible metastatic cancers (**Fig. 13**). Immunohistochemical markers used to determine the ontogeny of most common carcinomas in the lung are shown in **Table 2**.

Detection of molecular targets in cytology specimens

NSCLC collectively represents 70% to 80% of all lung cancers and worldwide accounts for approximately 1.2 million cases out of 1.6 million lung cancers.[22] At the time of diagnosis, only about

Table 1
Frequency of positive immunocytochemical markers that are used to differentiate squamous cell carcinoma and adenocarcinoma in cases in which cytomorphologic features are ambiguous

IHC Marker	Squamous Cell Carcinoma (%)	Adenocarcinoma (%)
TTF-1	4	89
Napsin	21	84
Surfactant-A	2	54
p63	99	25
CK5/6	94	16

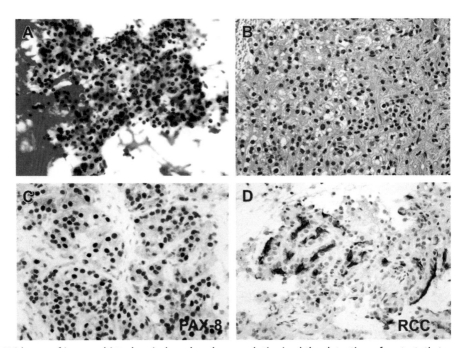

Fig. 13. Wide use of immunohistochemical markers has revolutionized the detection of metastatic tumors in the lung. A panel of figures shows immunohistochemical staining in metastatic clear cell renal cell carcinoma. (*A*) The smear of FNA and Papanicolaou stain show large cells with round, small nuclei and abundant clear or pale cytoplasm; and (*B*) section of cell block stained with H&E also shows similar features. (*C*) The cell block sections stained for PAX8 show strong and diffuse nuclear stains, and (*D*) renal cell carcinoma stain (RCC) shows strong luminal and apical staining. The TTF-1 (lung marker) and synaptophysin (neuroendocrine tumor) were negative (stains not shown). The 65-year-old man had a nephrectomy for renal cell carcinoma 5 years before and the immunoprofile and cytomorphologic features are consistent with metastatic clear cell renal cell carcinoma to the lung.

one-third of lung cancers are amenable to surgery, whereas the other two-thirds present with advanced and/or inoperable cancer because of comorbidities and either undergo radiation therapy, chemotherapy, or a combination thereof, with poor outcome. In the past decade, numerous molecular targets including EGFR, ELM4-ALK, KRAS, BRAF, PIK3CA, MEK, FGFR4, HER2,

Table 2
Some of the immunohistochemical markers used to delineate the origin of the tumor cells for common metastatic tumors in the lung

ICC Markers	Lung	Colon	Breast	Renal
CK7	+	−	+	−
CK20	−	+	−	−
TTF-1	+	−	−	−
CDX2	−	+	−	−
ER	−	−	+	−
Mammaglobin	−	−	+	−
RCC	−	−	−	+
PAX8	−	−	−	+

Abbreviation: RCC, renal cell carcinoma.

ROS1, ERCC1, MSH2, and RRM1 have been identified and new candidates are continuously added with the help of new-generation and high-throughput technologies.

As elucidated earlier, a distinction between ADC and SqCCa is important considering that certain agents such as the antiangiogenic bevacizumab (anti–vascular endothelial growth factor antibody) are contraindicated in SqCCa. Pemetrexed has shown increased overall survival in patients with nonsquamous histology, but not in SqCCa. Moreover, with the advent of tyrosine kinase inhibitors (TKIs), most of the attention has been shifted to adenocarcinoma, which might harbor several targetable genetic mutations. EML4-ALK translocation identified by IHC and confirmed by fluorescent in situ hybridization (FISH) (**Fig. 14**) and EGFR mutations by polymerase chain reaction (**Fig. 15**) are treated by TKIs including erlotinib (Tarceva), gefitinib (Iressa), and crizotinib (Xalkori) (see **Fig. 14**). EGFR and EML4-ALK are mutually exclusive, thus showing a better response to a single therapeutic agent, whereas the presence of KRAS is an indicator of poor prognosis, imparting refractoriness to TKI therapy. KRAS expression is also more

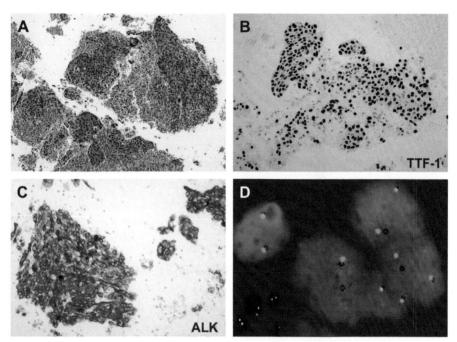

Fig. 14. Molecular test for ALK gene rearrangement using an FNA adenocarcinoma specimen in a 58-year-old nonsmoker. (*A*) H&E-stained section of cell block show features of adenocarcinoma, and (*B*) these cells are positive for TTF-1 nuclear expression, consistent with adenocarcinoma. (*C*) The same cells express diffuse and strong ALK immunoreactivity using 5A4 antibody (Dako); (*D*) the adenocarcinoma cells when tested with FISH using Vysis LSI dual color, break apart rearrangement probe (Abbott Molecular, Des Plaines, IL) show 2 separated red and green signals confirming the IHC test for ALK gene rearrangement (inset shows fused signals indicating normal ALK arrangement).

frequently present in patients with lung cancer who are heavy smokers.[23]

These targets also seem to be demographically driven because EGFR mutations are more frequent in young, Asian women and nonsmokers or light smokers.[24] Furthermore, most of the targetable identified molecular signatures are not only more frequently detected in adenocarcinoma but also certain subtypes of adenocarcinoma more commonly harbor particular genetic mutations.[25] EFGR mutation is more common in lepidic and micropapillary/papillary subtypes but the reverse is true for KRAS mutation, which is more common in solid subtypes.[23] In contrast, KRAS is frequently identified in mucinous adenocarcinoma but not EGFR mutation.[23] In addition, adenocarcinoma with signet ring or goblet cell cytomorphologic features expresses EML4-ALK gene rearrangement more frequently.[26] These findings highlight that histologic and cytomorphologic distinctions are important to guide the therapeutic approach in the future. More importantly, a large amount of tissue has to be harvested to allow the execution of ancillary techniques for research and clinical purposes, and the ancillary techniques have to be used judiciously to preserve tissue for the most important tests (see **Fig. 15**).

Current Cytologic Diagnostic Algorithm, Techniques, and Diagnostic Values

The impact of new technologies on the diagnostic algorithm of cytopathology

A distinction between small cell lung carcinoma (SCLC) or NSCLC was traditionally enough to guide therapeutic management. However, as discussed earlier, new treatment standards require more specific diagnoses to personalize patient care. IHC not only sometimes allows the specific subtype of NSCLC to be determined but also frequently distinguishes primary from metastatic tumors, which has a profound impact on management. After determining the subtype and/or the specific cell morphology as a screening for specific mutations, it is also important to establish the adequacy of material for the additional ancillary techniques needed (**Fig. 16**).

Over time, new and refined techniques have evolved to increase the adequacy of the specimens and interpretation of the material obtained. However, interinstitutional and intrainstitutional

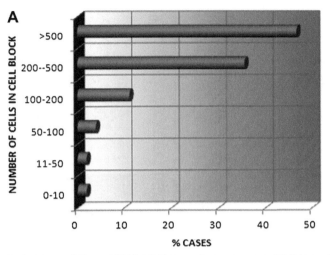

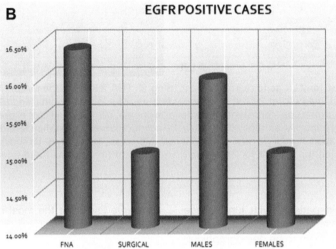

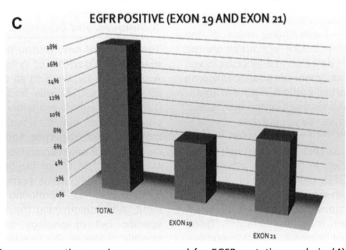

Fig. 15. FNA and biopsy or resection specimens were used for EGFR mutation analysis. (*A*) Bar plot shows that more than 90% of the cases had an adequate number of cells in the FNA cell blocks (>100 tumor cells) obtained by having 2 extra passes after establishing diagnostic adequacy with rapid on-site evaluation. (*B*) The percentage of EGFR mutation–positive FNA cases was similar to tissue biopsy and resection cases. (*C*) Bar graph shows that 46% of FNA cases harbored exon 19 deletion and 54% exon 21 point mutation (L858R). The data support that the FNA samples are optimal for molecular studies.

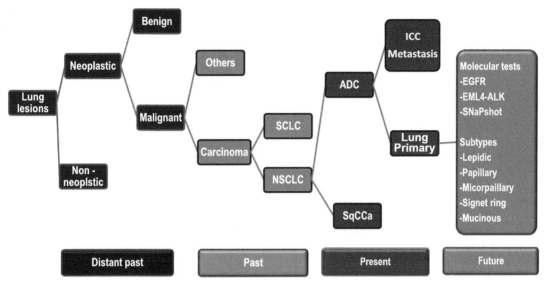

Fig. 16. The increased complexity of cytopathology diagnostic work-up. With time, the demand to provide specific diagnosis has progressed and molecular markers are becoming an important facet of patient care.

variations still remain because of practice guidelines regarding type of lesion, accessibility of lesion, techniques to obtain the specimen, preparation of material for cytologic assessment, resources, personal preferences, and expertise in cytopathology. The introduction of liquid-based cytology (LBC) has increased the efficiency by automation, better preservation of the cells, enrichment of the cell population, and use of single-specimen collection method. Despite the wide adoption of these new techniques for cervix pap smears, the use of LBC in respiratory cytology has not been widely adopted. The lung cancer diagnosis can be obtained from various types of samples. The diagnostic values of each of the samples currently used are briefly summarized.

CYTOLOGY SAMPLES

1. Exfoliative cytology:
   a. Sputum: once used as a screening tool for lung cancer in symptomatic smokers, sputum is at present less frequently used for diagnostic purposes.
      i. Induced sputum is high yield and the least invasive procedure with high specificity ranging from 96% to 99% with a positive predictive value (PPV) of 100% and negative predictive value (NPV) of 15%. Sensitivity is low for single samples (45%) but increases with multiple samples over multiple days (60% for 3 and 91% for 5 specimens).

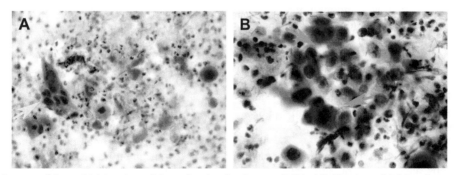

Fig. 17. Smears of bronchial brush and bronchoalveolar lavage (BAL). (*A*) The bronchial brush sample from a patient with 50-pack-year history and large cavitary central lesion shows malignant squamous cells characterized by dark hyperchromatic and angulated nuclei with moderate orangeophilic cytoplasm (*yellow arrow*). The background contains necrotic debris. (*B*) The BAL smear of a 55-year-old nonsmoking woman shows large polygonal cells containing large nuclei with pale blue or coarse chromatin, prominent cherry-red nucleoli and abundant vesicular cytoplasm. The green arrows point to gland formation. These features indicate an adenocarcinoma in the smears.

ii. Central tumors have high sensitivity (73%) compared with peripheral tumors (45%). However, accuracy of tumor classification is high (77%) for squamous cell carcinoma but low (40%) for adenocarcinoma.[27]

2. Minimally invasive cytology:

Bronchial cytology using rigid and/or flexible bronchoscope has improved over the past 5 decades with less than 0.5% major complications.[28]

  a. Bronchial brushing:

    i. Mainly performed for endobronchial or central lesions. Endobronchial lesions such as SqCCa (**Fig. 17**A) give higher cellular yield than subepithelial lesion (eg, metastasis).

    ii. Sensitivity is moderate (68.4%) but its combination with biopsy increases positive diagnosis from 82.7% of biopsy alone to 88.8%.[29] Accuracy of bronchial brushing is comparable with tissue biopsy and an addition of cell block to smears further increases the accuracy for lung cancer detection.[30,31] However, differentiation between in situ and invasive SqCCa or adenocarcinoma is not possible. Clinical-radiological-cytologic correlation is needed for such interpretation.

  b. Bronchial wash

    i. Commonly performed in conjunction with bronchial brushing and is cost-effective.

    ii. Sensitivity of bronchial wash varies from 36% to 72% in invisible and visible tumors.[32] However, bronchial wash sensitivity does not increase significantly whether bronchial wash is performed before or after endobronchial biopsy.[32,33]

  c. Bronchoalveolar lavage (BAL)

    i. BAL is usually performed for deeper/peripheral lesions (commonly adenocarcinoma, **Fig. 17**B) compared with bronchial brush and wash, which are used mainly for central or pericentral lesions (commonly SqCCa).

    ii. Sensitivity is moderate, ranging from 33% for lesions less than 2 cm and 62% for lesions greater than 2 cm.[34]

  d. Pleural fluid

    i. The thoracentesis is performed for infections and primary or metastatic pleural tumors.

    ii. The sensitivity for malignant pleural effusion is low (50%) and ranges from 4% to 77% depending on type on type of malignancy.[35] ICC further helps to refine the cytologic diagnosis.

3. FNA cytology:

Although the procedure is not new, FNA either under direct vision, US guidance, or CT guidance has become the preferred technique for primary diagnosis and staging of lung cancer. Using ROSE, the ease of performing the procedure, fewer postprocedure complications, and cost-effectiveness have all contributed to this.

  a. Mediastinal lymph nodes for lung cancer staging and central tumors:

    i. Procedures

      1. Transbronchial (Wang) needle aspiration

      2. EBUS-guided transbronchial FNA (EBUS-FNA)

      3. EUS-guided transesophageal FNA (EUS-FNA)

    ii. Frequently performed to target mediastinal lymph nodes for staging of lung cancer but also used for central or endobronchial lesion.

    iii. EBUS-FNA procedure has sensitivity of 95%, specificity 100%, NPV 94% and accuracy of 97%.[36] In another study, the sensitivity, accuracy, and NPV were comparable with mediastinoscopy (81%, 93%, and 91% vs 73%, 93%, and 90%).[37] No complications were observed in patients who underwent EBUS-FNA but 2.6% had minor complications when the same patients had mediastinoscopy.[37]

    iv. Some mediastinal lymph nodes that are inaccessible by EBUS are sampled using the transesophageal EUS approach. The EUS of mediastinal lymph nodes has a sensitivity of 82%, specificity 100%, accuracy 90%, NPV 80%, and PPV 100 in patients with known or suspected lung cancer.[38]

    v. On-site rapid evaluation helps in real time to guide the bronchoscopist if the specimen contains targeted tissue, and thus virtually eliminates false-negative sampling if elements of mediastinal lymph nodes are absent in the aspirates.

    vi. We found 100% correlation between smears and cell block of negative and malignant cases. Cell block prepared using additional aspirates also provide adequate material for immunophenotyping and molecular testing.

  b. Paracentral and peripheral lesions

    i. Procedures

      1. CT-guided percutaneous or transthoracic FNA: also used to sample central

tumors and lymph nodes, but less commonly

2. Fluoroscopic percutaneous or transthoracic FNA

ii. Diagnostic capabilities of FNA for malignant lesions are comparable with those of CNB. A recent systematic review of literature from 1991 to 2009 showed that the sensitivity range for FNA was 81.3% to 90.8%, specificity 75.4% to 100%, and accuracy 79.7% to 91.8%, compared with CNB with 85.7% to 97.4%, 88.6% to 100%, and 89% to 96.9%, respectively.[1]

iii. FNA is 350% less expensive than CNB but has a higher false-negative rate than CNB (19% vs 11%).[39] FNA is less useful for specific diagnoses of benign lung lesions (FNA 16.7% vs CNB 81.7%).[40]

SUMMARY

Cytopathology has evolved greatly over the last 3 decades. New technologies in imaging, ICC, and molecular biology have revolutionized the cytologic diagnosis of lung cancer. The current practice involves new and complex algorithms that require an integrated multidisciplinary approach to optimize tissue sampling, tissue processing, and the diagnostic approach. This process may take time, which most patients with lung cancer do not have because of the aggressive nature of the disease. The ongoing challenges are mainly related to the facilitation of this integration to improve and expedite patient care. Several initiatives are necessary and underway, including the development and adherence to an institutional multidisciplinary approach; fostering communication between team members, such as defining pertinent information in requisitions and providing access to clinical information and radiological images; establishing well-defined local standard operating procedures for the laboratory, which should incorporate clinical variables to standardize tissue processing; developing complete synoptic cytologic reports to avoid missing information; performing and updating quality assurance programs; and implementing continued interdisciplinary medical education programs and research projects. A combined action is more appropriate in this time of program-based clinical services. Cytopathology has become essential in defining lung cancer management and will remain so in the foreseeable future.

REFERENCES

1. Yao X, Gomes MM, Tsao MS, et al. Fine-needle aspiration biopsy versus core-needle biopsy in diagnosing lung cancer: a systematic review. Curr Oncol 2012;19:e16–27.

2. Li H, Boiselle PM, Shepard JO, et al. Diagnostic accuracy and safety of CT-guided percutaneous needle aspiration biopsy of the lung: comparison of small and large pulmonary nodules. AJR Am J Roentgenol 1996;167:105–9.

3. Oikonomou A, Matzinger FR, Seely JM, et al. Ultrathin needle (25 G) aspiration lung biopsy: diagnostic accuracy and complication rates. Eur Radiol 2004; 14:375–82.

4. Khouri NF, Stitik FP, Erozan YS, et al. Transthoracic needle aspiration biopsy of benign and malignant lung lesions. AJR Am J Roentgenol 1985;144:281–8.

5. Cox JE, Chiles C, McManus CM, et al. Transthoracic needle aspiration biopsy: variables that affect risk of pneumothorax. Radiology 1999;212:165–8.

6. Ohno Y, Hatabu H, Takenaka D, et al. CT-guided transthoracic needle aspiration biopsy of small (< or = 20 mm) solitary pulmonary nodules. AJR Am J Roentgenol 2003;180:1665–9.

7. Travis WD, Brambilla E, Noguchi M, et al. International Association for the Study of Lung Cancer/American Thoracic Society/European Respiratory Society international multidisciplinary classification of lung adenocarcinoma. J Thorac Oncol 2011;6: 244–85.

8. Naidich DP, Bankier AA, Macmahon H, et al. Recommendations for the management of subsolid pulmonary nodules detected at CT: a statement from the Fleischner Society. Radiology 2013;266:304–17.

9. Yasufuku K, Chiyo M, Koh E, et al. Endobronchial ultrasound guided transbronchial needle aspiration for staging of lung cancer. Lung Cancer 2005;50: 347–54.

10. ASGE Standards of Practice Committee, Jue TL, Sharaf RN, Appalaneni V, et al. Role of EUS for the evaluation of mediastinal adenopathy. Gastrointest Endosc 2011;74:239–45.

11. Devereaux BM, Leblanc JK, Yousif E, et al. Clinical utility of EUS-guided fine-needle aspiration of mediastinal masses in the absence of known pulmonary malignancy. Gastrointest Endosc 2002;56:397–401.

12. Yasufuku K, Nakajima T, Chiyo M, et al. Endobronchial ultrasonography: current status and future directions. J Thorac Oncol 2007;2:970–9.

13. Noguchi M, Morikawa A, Kawasaki M, et al. Small adenocarcinoma of the lung. Histologic characteristics and prognosis. Cancer 1995;75:2844–52.

14. Sanchez-Mora N, Presmanes MC, Monroy V, et al. Micropapillary lung adenocarcinoma: a distinctive histologic subtype with prognostic significance. Case series. Hum Pathol 2008;39:324–30.

15. Gaikwad A, Gupta A, Hare S, et al. Primary adeno-carcinoma of lung: a pictorial review of recent updates. Eur J Radiol 2012;81:4146–55.

16. Whithaus K, Fukuoka J, Prihoda TJ, et al. Evaluation of napsin A, cytokeratin 5/6, p63, and thyroid transcription factor 1 in adenocarcinoma versus squamous cell carcinoma of the lung. Arch Pathol Lab Med 2012;136:155–62.

17. Khayyata S, Yun S, Pasha T, et al. Value of P63 and CK5/6 in distinguishing squamous cell carcinoma from adenocarcinoma in lung fine-needle aspiration specimens. Diagn Cytopathol 2009;37:178–83.

18. Mukhopadhyay S, Katzenstein AL. Subclassification of non-small cell lung carcinomas lacking morphologic differentiation on biopsy specimens: utility of an immunohistochemical panel containing TTF-1, napsin A, p63, and CK5/6. Am J Surg Pathol 2011; 35:15–25.

19. Terry J, Leung S, Laskin J, et al. Optimal immunohistochemical markers for distinguishing lung adenocarcinomas from squamous cell carcinomas in small tumor samples. Am J Surg Pathol 2010;34: 1805–11.

20. Rekhtman N, Ang DC, Sima CS, et al. Immunohistochemical algorithm for differentiation of lung adenocarcinoma and squamous cell carcinoma based on large series of whole-tissue sections with validation in small specimens. Mod Pathol 2011;24:1348–59.

21. Noh S, Shim H. Optimal combination of immunohistochemical markers for subclassification of non-small cell lung carcinomas: a tissue microarray study of poorly differentiated areas. Lung Cancer 2012;76:51–5.

22. Ferlay J, Shin HR, Bray F, et al. Estimates of worldwide burden of cancer in 2008: GLOBOCAN 2008. Int J Cancer 2010;127:2893–917.

23. Li H, Pan Y, Li Y, et al. Frequency of well-identified oncogenic driver mutations in lung adenocarcinoma of smokers varies with histological subtypes and graduated smoking dose. Lung Cancer 2013;79: 8–13.

24. Rosell R, Moran T, Queralt C, et al. Spanish Lung Cancer G: screening for epidermal growth factor receptor mutations in lung cancer. N Engl J Med 2009;361:958–67.

25. An SJ, Chen ZH, Su J, et al. Identification of enriched driver gene alterations in subgroups of non-small cell lung cancer patients based on histology and smoking status. PloS One 2012;7:e40109.

26. Shaw AT, Yeap BY, Mino-Kenudson M, et al. Clinical features and outcome of patients with non-small-cell lung cancer who harbor EML4-ALK. J Clin Oncol 2009;27:4247–53.

27. Ammanagi AS, Dombale VD, Miskin AT, et al. Sputum cytology in suspected cases of carcinoma of lung (sputum cytology a poor man's bronchoscopy!). Lung India 2012;29:19–23.

28. Pue CA, Pacht ER. Complications of fiberoptic bronchoscopy at a university hospital. Chest 1995;107:430–2.

29. Karahalli E, Yilmaz A, Turker H, et al. Usefulness of various diagnostic techniques during fiberoptic bronchoscopy for endoscopically visible lung cancer: should cytologic examinations be performed routinely? Respiration 2001;68:611–4.

30. Popp W, Rauscher H, Ritschka L, et al. Diagnostic sensitivity of different techniques in the diagnosis of lung tumors with the flexible fiberoptic bronchoscope. Comparison of brush biopsy, imprint cytology of forceps biopsy, and histology of forceps biopsy. Cancer 1991;67:72–5.

31. Kawan E, Ulrich W, Redtenbacher S, et al. Kawan bronchial brush/cell block technique. Facilitation of the routine diagnosis of bronchial neoplasms. Acta Cytol 1998;42:1409–13.

32. van der Drift MA, van der Wilt GJ, Thunnissen FB, et al. A prospective study of the timing and cost-effectiveness of bronchial washing during bronchoscopy for pulmonary malignant tumors. Chest 2005; 128:394–400.

33. Sompradeekul S, Chinvetkitvanich U, Suthinon P, et al. Difference in the yields of bronchial washing cytology before and after forceps biopsy for lung cancer diagnosis. J Med Assoc Thai 2006; 89(Suppl 5):S37–45.

34. Schreiber G, McCrory DC. Performance characteristics of different modalities for diagnosis of suspected lung cancer: summary of published evidence. Chest 2003;123:115S–28S.

35. Bielsa S, Panades MJ, Egido R, et al. Accuracy of pleural fluid cytology in malignant effusions. An Med Interna 2008;25:173–7 [in Spanish].

36. Lee BE, Kletsman E, Rutledge JR, et al. Utility of endobronchial ultrasound-guided mediastinal lymph node biopsy in patients with non-small cell lung cancer. J Thorac Cardiovasc Surg 2012;143:585–90.

37. Yasufuku K, Pierre A, Darling G, et al. A prospective controlled trial of endobronchial ultrasound-guided transbronchial needle aspiration compared with mediastinoscopy for mediastinal lymph node staging of lung cancer. J Thorac Cardiovasc Surg 2011;142: 1393–1400.e1.

38. Srinivasan R, Bhutani MS, Thosani N, et al. Clinical impact of EUS-FNA of mediastinal lymph nodes in patients with known or suspected lung cancer or mediastinal lymph nodes of unknown etiology. J Gastrointestin Liver Dis 2012;21:145–52.

39. Vimpeli SM, Saarenmaa I, Huhtala H, et al. Large-core needle biopsy versus fine-needle aspiration biopsy in solid breast lesions: comparison of costs and diagnostic value. Acta Radiol 2008;49:863–9.

40. Greif J, Marmor S, Schwarz Y, et al. Percutaneous core needle biopsy vs. fine needle aspiration in diagnosing benign lung lesions. Acta Cytol 1999; 43:756–60.

Subtyping Lung Adenocarcinoma According to the Novel 2011 IASLC/ATS/ERS Classification
Correlation with Patient Prognosis

Morihito Okada, MD, PhD

KEYWORDS

- Subtype • Histology • Tumor grade • Therapy

KEY POINTS

- The term bronchioloalveolar carcinoma (BAC) is eliminated, adenocarcinoma in situ and minimally invasive adenocarcinoma are defined, and the term lepidic is resurrected in the 2011 International Association for the Study of Lung Cancer/American Thoracic Society/European Respiratory Society classification.
- The impact of subtyping according to the 2011 classification on patient survival is independent of known prognostic factors such as TNM stage.
- The role of clinical decision making for treating lung adenocarcinoma is predominantly based on subtyping similar to that of breast and prostate cancer.

INTRODUCTION

Primary lung cancer is the leading cause of cancer-related mortality worldwide, and non–small-cell lung cancer accounts for about 85% of all lung cancers, of which approximately 70% are adenocarcinomas. Lung adenocarcinoma is a radiologically, histomorphologically, molecularly, and clinically heterogeneous tumor with a broad range of malignant behavior that cannot be predicted by known prognostic factors such as the TNM staging system at diagnosis or surgery. Because a reliable and easily measured predictor of prognosis is tumor grade based on histomorphologic criteria for several cancer entities, different histopathologic features of adenocarcinoma subtypes might generate further survival evidence. The recent universally accepted criteria for adenocarcinoma subtypes, in particular tumors that were formerly classified as bronchioloalveolar carcinoma (BAC), are of considerable importance.

Cumulative data have shown that the nature of lung adenocarcinoma growth is associated with differences in survival.[1–11] In 1995, Noguchi and colleagues[1] examined the histologic characteristics of small lung adenocarcinoma, particularly those of BAC, and based an original classification system on tumor growth patterns that were closely related to prognosis. Type C in Noguchi's classification is a mixed subtype that comprises more than 60% of all small adenocarcinomas. The mixed BAC category was introduced in the 1999 World Health Organization (WHO) classification of lung adenocarcinoma,[2] and maintained in the 2004 WHO classification of lung tumors (**Box 1**).[3] The mixed subtype is the most frequent, accounting for more than 80% of all resected small adenocarcinomas[4]; this is a major limitation of these WHO

Department of Surgical Oncology, Hiroshima University, 1-2-3 Kasumi, Minami-ku, Hiroshima City, Hiroshima 734-0037, Japan
E-mail address: morihito@hiroshima-u.ac.jp

Thorac Surg Clin 23 (2013) 179–186
http://dx.doi.org/10.1016/j.thorsurg.2013.01.001
1547-4127/13/$ – see front matter © 2013 Elsevier Inc. All rights reserved.

Box 1
Summary of 1999 and 2004 classifications of lung adenocarcinoma

<1999 Classification>

Acinar

Papillary

BAC: Nonmucinous, Mucinous, Mixed mucinous/nonmucinous

Solid with mucin

Variants: Colloid, Fetal, Signet-ring, Clear-cell

<2004 Classification>

Mixed subtype

Acinar

Papillary

BAC: Nonmucinous, Mucinous

Solid with mucin production

Variants: Fetal, Mucinous (Colloid), Signet-ring, Clear-cell

Abbreviation: BAC, bronchioloalveolar carcinoma.

Box 2
IASLC/ATS/ERS classification of lung adenocarcinoma (2011)

Preinvasive lesions

   Atypical adenomatous hyperplasia

   Adenocarcinoma in situ ($\leq$3 cm, formerly BAC)

      Nonmucinous, Mucinous, Mixed mucinous/nonmucinous

Minimally invasive adenocarcinoma ($\leq$3 cm lepidic-predominant tumor with $\leq$5 mm invasion)

   Nonmucinous, Mucinous, Mixed mucinous/nonmucinous

Invasive adenocarcinoma

   Lepidic predominant (formerly nonmucinous BAC pattern)

   Acinar predominant

   Papillary predominant

   Micropapillary predominant

   Solid predominant with mucin production

Variants

   Invasive mucinous adenocarcinoma (formerly mucinous BAC)

   Colloid

   Fetal

   Enteric

Abbreviation: BAC, bronchioloalveolar carcinoma.

classifications. The histologic classification of lung adenocarcinoma must be improved, based on survival outcomes, to overcome this limitation. Thus the new International Multidisciplinary Lung Adenocarcinoma Classification (**Box 2, Figs. 1 and 2**) was established by the International Association for the Study of Lung Cancer, American Thoracic Society, and European Respiratory Society (IASLC/ATS/ERS),[12] containing several key modifications: (1) the term BAC is no longer applied and the type is described as lepidic; (2) adenocarcinoma in situ is suggested for small ($\leq$3 cm) tumors with completely lepidic growth and no invasion; (3) minimally invasive adenocarcinoma refers to small ($\leq$3 cm) predominantly lepidic tumors accompanied by slight invasion ($\leq$0.5 cm); and (4) invasive adenocarcinoma is grouped along with the predominant subtype.

EVIDENCE FROM THE LITERATURE

The correlation between adenocarcinoma classification based on the new definitions and prognosis has been reviewed. In 2011, Yoshizawa and colleagues[13] tested whether the new lung adenocarcinoma classification proposed by the IASLC/ATS/ERS defined the prognostic significance of this subgroup. These investigators retrospectively examined 514 patients who had undergone complete resection with nodal dissection for pathologic stage I adenocarcinoma classified according

to the Union for International Cancer Control/American Joint Committee on Cancer seventh edition. Most patients were female (63%), had stage IA disease (58%), and were a median of 69 years old (range 33–89 years). The median tumor size was 20 (range 3–50) mm and the median follow-up was 4 (range 0.02–13.3) years. Three prognostic groups were identified based on clinical behavior as follows: adenocarcinoma in situ (n = 1) and minimally invasive adenocarcinoma (n = 8), with 5-year disease-free survival rates of 100% for both (low grade); nonmucinous lepidic-predominant (n = 29), papillary-predominant (n = 143), and acinar-predominant (n = 232) adenocarcinoma, with 5-year disease-free survival rates of 90%, 83%, and 84%, respectively (intermediate grade); and invasive mucinous (n = 13), colloid-predominant (n = 9), solid-predominant (n = 67), and micropapillary-predominant (n = 12) adenocarcinoma, with 5-year disease-free survival rates of 75%, 71%, 70%, and 67%, respectively

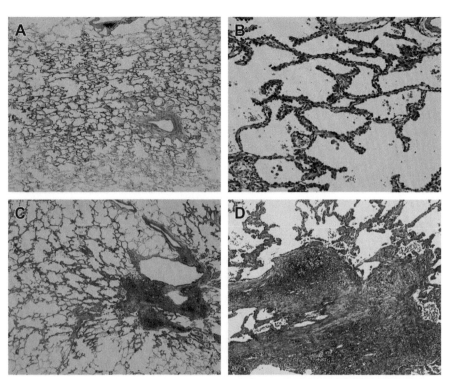

Fig. 1. Examples of early adenocarcinoma growth patterns. Representative hematoxylin and eosin–stained tumor slides of (*A, B*) adenocarcinoma in situ and (*C, D*) minimally invasive adenocarcinoma. *A* and *C* × 12.5; *B* × 100; *D* × 40.

(*P* = .001) (high grade). Univariate analysis demonstrated that male gender (*P* = .008), vascular invasion (*P* = .002), and higher stage, poor differentiation, and necrosis (all 3, *P*<.001) were significantly related to poor disease-free survival. Multivariate analysis indicated that the grade of the subtype classification (*P* = .038), male gender (*P* = .007), amount of tumor invasion adjusted for lepidic growth (*P* = .026), and necrosis (*P* = .002) were associated with a significantly worse prognosis. Thus, the new IASLC/ATS/ERS classification of lung adenocarcinoma identifies histologic subtyping with prognostic differences, which confers the potential to stratify patients with stage I disease for adjuvant therapy.

Soon after validating a North American series of 514 stage I lung adenocarcinomas,[13] Russell and colleagues[14] examined relationships between the new classification and survival in a series of Australian patients with stages I, II, and III lung adenocarcinoma. These investigators retrospectively analyzed data from 210 patients comprising 113 (54%) males and 97 (46%) females with a median age of 67 (range 30–91) years who underwent resection of lung adenocarcinoma with curative intent between 1996 and 2009. Tumor size ranged from 9 to 140 (median, 29) mm. Two pathologists, blinded to the background

and outcomes of the patients, independently reviewed the histologic classifications according to the new subtyping. All patients with adenocarcinoma in situ (n = 1), minimally invasive adenocarcinoma (n = 7), and lepidic-predominant invasive adenocarcinoma (n = 10) were stage I. The distribution of stages IA to IIIA was even with micropapillary-predominant (n = 14) and solid-predominant (n = 49) adenocarcinomas, whereas a greater proportion of papillary-predominant (n = 26) and acinar-predominant (n = 84) adenocarcinomas were classified as stage I while a substantial proportion was evident in stages II to IIIA. The median follow-up was 49 (range 3–176) months. The 5-year overall survival rate of the patients with adenocarcinoma in situ and minimally invasive adenocarcinoma was 100%, whereas that of patients with lepidic-predominant invasive adenocarcinoma was 86%, with only 1 death. Micropapillary-predominant and solid-predominant adenocarcinomas were associated with particularly poor 5-year overall survival rates of 38% and 39%, respectively, whereas papillary-predominant and acinar-predominant adenocarcinomas were associated with an intermediate prognosis (5-year overall survival rates of 71% and 68%, respectively). Both variants consisting of invasive mucinous (n = 10) and colloid

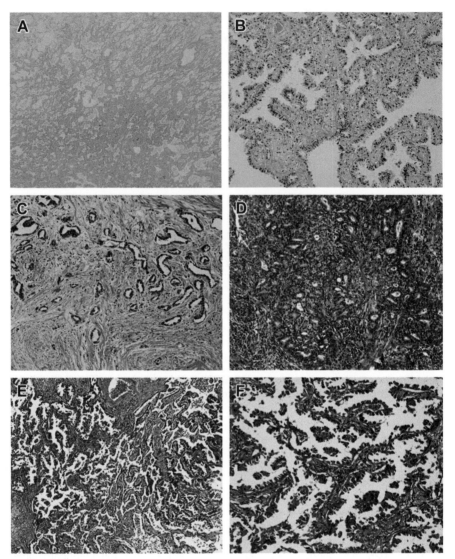

Fig. 2. Examples of invasive adenocarcinoma growth patterns. Representative hematoxylin and eosin–stained tumor slides of (*A, B*) lepidic-, (*C, D*) acinar-, (*E, F*) papillary-, (*G, H*) micropapillary-, and (*I, J*) solid-predominant adenocarcinomas. *A* × 12.5; *B, C, D, F, H* and *J* × 100; *E, G* and *I* × 40.

(n = 9) adenocarcinomas were associated with a 5-year overall survival rate of 51%. Subtyping lung adenocarcinoma according to the new IASLC/ATS/ERS classification correlated with 5-year overall survival rates, and the association persisted after controlling for known prognostic patient and tumor characteristics. This study suggested that the new classification has benefits not only for individual patient care but also for patient selection for clinical trials and molecular studies.

To further investigate the clinical relevance of the new classification, Warth and colleagues[15] examined the impact of tumor architecture defined according to the novel IASLC/ATS/ERS proposal on patient overall, disease-specific, and disease-free survival in 500 invasive pulmonary adenocarcinomas across all tumor stages under consideration of adjuvant therapy. These investigators retrospectively analyzed a cohort of 487 patients with resected invasive adenocarcinomas between 2002 and 2008. The reclassification of 487 specimens from these patients resulted in 207 (42.5%) acinar-predominant, 183 (37.6%) solid-predominant, 41 (8.4%) lepidic-predominant, 33 (6.8%) micropapillary-predominant, and 23 (4.7%) papillary-predominant adenocarcinomas. The lepidic-predominant adenocarcinomas were comparably smaller (mean diameter 3.37 cm), whereas the

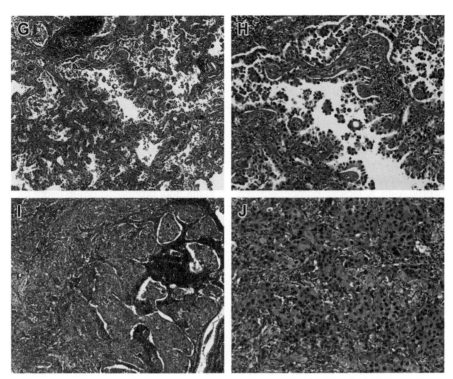

Fig. 2. (*continued*)

acinar-predominant subtypes were of intermediate size (mean diameter 3.89 cm), and the solid-predominant, papillary-predominant, and micropapillary-predominant subtypes had larger mean diameters of 4.54, 4.84, and 4.90 cm, respectively (*P*<.001). Although 93% of lepidic-predominant adenocarcinomas did not develop nodal metastases, 43%, 46%, 51%, and 76%, respectively, of papillary-predominant, acinar-predominant, solid-predominant, and micropapillary-predominant adenocarcinomas were node positive, indicating that the predominant growth pattern significantly differed with respect to nodal status. Mean overall survival significantly differed among lepidic-predominant, acinar-predominant, solid-predominant, papillary-predominant, and micropapillary-predominant adenocarcinomas, being 78.5, 67.3, 58.1, 48.9, and 44.9 months, respectively (*P* = .007). Survival differences became even more pronounced when the 3 latter subtypes were grouped according to growth patterns 1, 2, and 3, which were associated with survival durations of 78.5, 67.3, and 57.2 months, respectively (*P* = .001). Multivariate survival analyses indicated that both subtypes and pattern groups had a significant stage-independent, age-independent, sex-independent, and adjuvant treatment–independent impact on overall, disease-specific, and disease-free survival. Adjuvant therapy also influenced

survival differences based on subtypes. This study summarizes the grading of pulmonary adenocarcinomas according to the novel IASLC/ATS/ERS scheme as a rapid, straightforward, and efficient discriminator for patient prognosis that might support patient stratification for adjuvant therapy.

COMMENTS AND CONTROVERSIES

The management of BAC, which was originally defined as a well-differentiated tumor growing along the alveolar septae and as a combined invasive and noninvasive tumor, is of great consequence for evaluating the biological behavior of lung adenocarcinoma. Because several investigations mostly from Japan have indicated that pure BAC is noninvasive, small (≤20 or ≤30 mm) pure BACs were historically all essentially cured by resection.[1,16–19] Regarding noninvasive adenocarcinoma, BAC was reevaluated and eventually redefined, whereas invasive adenocarcinomas including BAC were grouped within the mixed subtype in the previous WHO classification. However, this classification did not provide useful prognostic information because more than 80% of total adenocarcinomas were classified as the mixed subtype. To overcome this limitation and to adapt to novel radiographic, pathologic, and molecular information, a series of IASLC workshops was designed to collect input from a panel of pathology experts about how to revise the classification in consideration of the radiologic/computed tomographic appearance of these tumors, widespread molecular alterations, and the prognosis of proposed histologic subtypes. As a result, one of the most significant changes in the latest classification was the exclusion of the term BAC. Adenocarcinoma that was formerly classified as BAC is now classified as adenocarcinoma in situ, minimally invasive adenocarcinoma, lepidic-predominant invasive adenocarcinoma, mucinous adenocarcinoma, and other invasive adenocarcinoma with a lepidic component. Of importance is that the term adenocarcinoma in situ refers to solitary, purely lepidic nodules of 3 cm or less in size, and a category of minimally invasive adenocarcinoma was launched because the prognoses of tumors with a small (<5 mm) invasive component and of adenocarcinoma in situ are similar. By contrast, invasive tumors are classified consistent with their predominant histologic subtype or the subtype that occupies the maximum cross-sectional area in histologic sections.

A significant correlation in lung adenocarcinoma between patient survival and histologic subtype along with the novel IASLC/ATS/ERS classification has been demonstrated in an American cohort of stage I diseases for disease-free survival,[13] in an Australian cohort of stage I, II, and III diseases for overall survival,[14] and most recently in a European cohort of stage I to IV diseases for overall and disease-free survival (**Table 1**).[15] The 3 categories of adenocarcinoma in situ, minimally invasive adenocarcinoma, and lepidic-predominant adenocarcinoma had few nodal metastases and an approximately 100% 5-year survival rate after complete resection. These findings suggested

that such patients are candidates for sublobar resection without nodal dissection, although pathologists cannot always exclude an invasion component on biopsy specimens or intraoperative frozen sections. The clinical behavior of solid, micropapillary, colloid-predominant, and invasive mucinous adenocarcinomas was worse, whereas that of acinar-predominant and papillary-predominant adenocarcinomas was intermediate. Some investigators have tentatively suggested that the prognosis for papillary-predominant adenocarcinomas is somewhat worse.[15,20] Patients in the poor prognostic group might be candidates for adjuvant therapy.

Individual lung adenocarcinomas are frequently heterogeneous, with individual tumors displaying various histologic subtypes. Several reports have shown that patient prognosis is closely associated with the dominant histologic subtype, which thus seems to represent a simple means of grading adenocarcinomas. Some issues regarding the 2011 proposed classification system remain unresolved. One such aspect is whether the classification is reproducible among pathology experts, because reaching interobserver and intraobserver agreement can be challenging even within small groups. Another is whether the classification is relevant to biopsy specimens or cytologic tissues in practice, because the assumption that tiny specimens of heterogeneous lung adenocarcinomas are representative of whole tumors is probably erroneous. Accurate classification should be prospectively tested in a small cytology/biopsy cohort. Another question is whether the quantitation of secondary histologic subtypes recommended in the new classification system at 5% intervals is in fact necessary. Furthermore,

Table 1
Summary of survival outcomes determined in 3 studies

	Yoshizawa et al,[13] 2011	Russell et al,[14] 2011	Warth et al,[15] 2012
	5-Year DFS (%)	5-Year OS (%)	OS/DFS (mo)
AD in situ	100 (n = 1)	100 (n = 1)	
Minimally invasive AD	100 (n = 8)	100 (n = 7)	
Lepidic-pred AD	90 (n = 29)	86 (n = 10)	78.5/72.6 (n = 41)
Acinor-pred AD	84 (n = 232)	68 (n = 84)	67.3/61.7 (n = 207)
Papillary-pred AD	83 (n = 143)	71 (n = 26)	48.9/37.7 (n = 23)
Micropapillary-pred AD	67 (n = 12)	38 (n = 14)	44.9/33.8 (n = 33)
Solid-pred AD	70 (n = 67)	39 (n = 49)	58.1/51.2 (n = 183)
Invasive mucinous AD	76 (n = 13)	51 (n = 10)	
Colloid AD	71 (n = 9)	51 (n = 9)	

Abbreviations: AD, adenocarcinoma; DFS, disease-free survival; OS, overall survival; -pred, -predominant.

the frequency of molecular alterations within the various histologic subtypes is not known, nor is whether these outcomes affect clinical behavior in a histology-dependent manner. The final matter to be resolved is whether the classification can predict responses to additional strategies such as adjuvant therapy. The predictive roles of histologic subtypes remain to be adequately tested.

SUMMARY AND CONCLUSIONS

The concept that only a diagnosis is vital in evaluating a difference between small-cell and non–small-cell carcinoma is quickly fading into oblivion from the viewpoint of lung cancer management. The distinction between squamous and nonsquamous carcinoma has recently become more crucial in the choice of chemotherapy for non–small-cell carcinoma. This review suggests the importance of histologic subtyping as an independent prognostic variable in lung adenocarcinoma, and that tumor responses to conventional and targeted therapies can be predicted based on a combination of histologic and molecular pathologic assessments. As with breast and prostate cancer, a histologic system based on predominant subtypes should support practical decision making for the management of lung adenocarcinomas in the near future.

REFERENCES

1. Noguchi M, Morikawa A, Kawasaki M, et al. Small adenocarcinoma of the lung. Histologic characteristics and prognosis. Cancer 1995;75:2844–52.

2. Travis WD, Colby TV, Corrin B, et al, In collaboration with Sobin LH and pathologists from 14 countries. World Health Organization international histological classification of lung tumours. Histological typing of lung and pleural tumors. 3rd edition. Berlin: Springer-Verlag; 1999.

3. Travis WD, Brambilla E, Muller-Hermelink HK, et al. Pathology and genetics: tumours of the lung, pleura, thymus and heart. World Health Organisation classification of tumours. Lyon (France): IARC Press; 2004.

4. Motoi N, Szoke J, Riely GJ, et al. Lung adenocarcinoma: modification of the 2004 WHO mixed subtype to include the major histologic subtype suggests correlations between papillary and micropapillary adenocarcinoma subtypes, EGFR mutations and gene expression analysis. Am J Surg Pathol 2008; 32:810–27.

5. Amin MB, Tamboli P, Merchant SH, et al. Micropapillary component in lung adenocarcinoma: a distinctive histologic feature with possible prognostic significance. Am J Surg Pathol 2002;26:358–64.

6. Miyoshi T, Satoh Y, Okumura S, et al. Early-stage lung adenocarcinomas with a micropapillary pattern, a distinct pathologic marker for a significantly poor prognosis. Am J Surg Pathol 2003;27:101–9.

7. Riquet M, Foucault C, Berna P, et al. Prognostic value of histology in resected lung cancer with emphasis on the relevance of the adenocarcinoma subtyping. Ann Thorac Surg 2006;81:1988–95.

8. Yim J, Zhu LC, Chiriboga L, et al. Histologic features are important prognostic indicators in early stages lung adenocarcinomas. Mod Pathol 2007; 20:233–41.

9. Borczuk AC, Qian F, Kazeros A, et al. Invasive size is an independent predictor of survival in pulmonary adenocarcinoma. Am J Surg Pathol 2009;33:462–9.

10. Barletta JA, Yeap BY, Chirieac LR. Prognostic significance of grading in lung adenocarcinoma. Cancer 2010;116:659–69.

11. Sica G, Yoshizawa A, Sima CS, et al. A grading system of lung adenocarcinomas based on histologic pattern is predictive of disease recurrence in stage I tumors. Am J Surg Pathol 2010;34:1155–62.

12. Travis WD, Brambilla E, Noguchi M, et al. IASLC/ATS/ERS international multidisciplinary classification of lung adenocarcinoma. J Thorac Oncol 2011;6: 244–85.

13. Yoshizawa A, Motoi N, Riely GJ, et al. Impact of proposed IASLC/ATS/ERS classification of lung adenocarcinoma: prognostic subgroups and implications for further revision of staging based on analysis of 514 stage I cases. Mod Pathol 2011;24:653–64.

14. Russell PA, Wainer Z, Wright GM, et al. Does lung adenocarcinoma subtype predict patient survival? A clinicopathologic study based on the new International Association for the Study of Lung Cancer/American Thoracic Society/European Respiratory Society international multidisciplinary lung adenocarcinoma classification. J Thorac Oncol 2011;6: 1496–504.

15. Warth A, Muley T, Meister M, et al. The novel histologic International Association for the Study of Lung Cancer/American Thoracic Society/European Respiratory Society classification system of lung adenocarcinoma is a stage-independent predictor of survival. J Clin Oncol 2012;30:1438–46.

16. Sakurai H, Dobashi Y, Mizutani E, et al. Bronchioloalveolar carcinoma of the lung 3 centimeters or less in diameter: a prognostic assessment. Ann Thorac Surg 2004;78:1728–33.

17. Tsutani Y, Miyata Y, Nakayama H, et al. Prognostic significance of using solid versus whole tumor size on high-resolution computed tomography for predicting pathologic malignant grade of tumors in clinical stage IA lung adenocarcinoma: a multicenter study. J Thorac Cardiovasc Surg 2012;143:607–12.

18. Okada M, Nakayama H, Okumura S, et al. Multicenter analysis of high-resolution computed

tomography and positron emission tomography/
computed tomography findings to choose therapeutic strategies for clinical stage IA lung adenocarcinoma. J Thorac Cardiovasc Surg 2011;141:
1384–91.

19. Nakayama H, Okumura S, Daisaki H, et al. Value of
integrated positron emission tomography revised

using a phantom study to evaluate malignancy
grade of lung adenocarcinoma: a multicenter study.
Cancer 2010;116:3170–7.

20. Aida S, Shimazaki H, Sato K, et al. Prognostic analysis of pulmonary adenocarcinoma subclassification
with special consideration of papillary and bronchioloalveolar types. Histopathology 2000;45:468–76.

Clinical Staging Strategies and Evaluation of Cardiopulmonary Function

Fast-tracking Investigation and Staging of Patients with Lung Cancer

Farid M. Shamji, MBBS, FRCS(C), FACS[a],*,
Jean Deslauriers, MD, FRCS(C)[b]

KEYWORDS

- Lung cancer • Fast-tracking investigation • Multidisciplinary integrated care

KEY POINTS

- Standardized clinical care pathways allow for reduction of time interval between referral and treatment.
- Multidisciplinary care teams are essential for modern management of patients with lung cancer.
- Investing in standardized clinical care pathways will ultimately reduce costs and improve quality of care.

INTRODUCTION

Lung cancer is by far the most common intrathoracic neoplasm and it continues to kill several million people every year worldwide. The most disturbing aspect of its management is that despite a better understanding of genetic susceptibility, heterogeneous histology, biologic activity, genetic mutations, and molecular markers, less than 15% of patients diagnosed with the disease will be expected to live more than 5 years. This rate is only a 2-fold improvement from what it was in the late 1950s when only 9% of patients with lung cancer could be cured.

Because clinical outcomes are better for patients diagnosed and treated at an earlier stage of disease, multidisciplinary standardized clinical care pathways have been developed at several institutions to provide a structured approach to those patients while at the same time preventing undesirable wait times for consultative, diagnostic, and cancer treatment services.[1,2] Ultimately, such measures are expected to prevent stage migration during the investigation, increase treatment options, and improve survival. In addition, it has been well shown that the introduction of clinical care pathways for major thoracic cases improves patient satisfaction[3] and reduces hospital costs.[4]

The success of standardized clinical care pathways relates to several factors, the most important being the design of the pathway itself and the use of multidisciplinary teams involving specialists in oncology (medical and radiation), pulmonary medicine, thoracic surgery, radiology, and pathology.[5] The core curriculum should also include provisions for the participation of allied health personnel specialized in preoperative teaching and support as well as in standardized postoperative care.[6,7]

LIFE HISTORY OF LUNG CANCER

To determine whether fast-tracking investigations and clinical pathways are effective in reducing delays in the diagnosis, staging, and treatment of lung cancer, one has to appreciate that there are 4 intervals in the life history of the disease (**Table 1**).

[a] Division of Thoracic Surgery, Ottawa Hospital, 501 Smyth Road, Room 6362, Box 708, Ottawa, Ontario K1H 8L6, Canada; [b] Division of Thoracic Surgery, Institut universitaire de cardiologie et de pneumologie de Québec (IUCPQ), 2725 chemin Sainte-Foy, Quebec City, Quebec G1V 4G5, Canada
* Corresponding author.
E-mail address: fshamji@ottawahospital.on.ca

Thorac Surg Clin 23 (2013) 187–191
http://dx.doi.org/10.1016/j.thorsurg.2013.01.012
1547-4127/13/$ – see front matter © 2013 Elsevier Inc. All rights reserved.

Table 1
Life history of lung cancer

Interval	Description	What Can be Done to Improve
First	Preclinical asymptomatic phase	Prevention of risks factors associated with lung cancer
Second	Symptomatic phase	• Education of general public and health providers
Third	Diagnosis and staging	• Use of standardized clinical care pathways • Multidisciplinary thoracic oncology clinics
Fourth	Treatment	• Improve supply (OR time and others) for existing demand • Creation of formal surgical oncology divisions

Abbreviation: OR, operating room.

The first interval is the preclinical asymptomatic phase, which begins with the first malignant changes in the bronchial epithelium. During that period, which can be quite long, not only does the tumor size increase but the lesion also has the potential for local invasion, lymphatic dissemination, and distant spread. During that preclinical phase, awareness of indicators of increased risk for developing lung cancer is important (**Table 2**).

The second interval is when patients recognize subtle changes in symptoms related to chronic obstructive lung disease or the onset of new symptoms, such as persistent cough or hemoptysis. The length of this interval is influenced by patients not seeking immediate medical attention or experiencing delays in getting a timely appointment with their family physician. This time is when educating the general public may have an impact by raising awareness for risk factors associated with lung cancer and symptoms that should be of concern. If health care providers, especially family physicians, are well aware of the early manifestations of lung cancer, this interval could be shortened, leading to a more rapid diagnosis and workup and increased resection rates.[8]

The third interval is between the time from suspicion of lung cancer by the family practitioner to patients being referred to a specialist for diagnosis,

staging, and treatment planning (**Fig. 1**). Ideally, all referrals should be triaged by a navigator nurse and investigations performed in an orderly fashion according to predetermined pathways, thus, avoiding delays and fragmented care.[9] During that interval, a treatment plan should be developed through a coordinated multidisciplinary approach.[5,10] Shortening this interval may also be beneficial to the promotion of patients' mental and physical wellness as well as alleviating the mental distress associated with long delays.

The fourth interval is between a confirmed diagnosis of lung cancer and treatment. Any significant delay encountered at this point is unacceptable and may have the counter effect of decreasing chances of survival for some patients who would otherwise be potentially curable. This decreased chance of survival is likely a reflection of the biology of exponential tumor growth and metastatic potential observed in the form of stage migration becoming more rapid with increasing tumor size and early nodal spread. The British Thoracic Society (see **Fig. 1**) recommends that there should be a maximum of 8 weeks between the first consultation with a specialist (respirologist or thoracic surgeon) and surgery in an uncomplicated case, and surgery should be performed within 4 weeks of surgical evaluation unless

Table 2
Indicators of increased risk for developing lung cancer

Cigarette smoking	• An active smoker of more than 20 cigarettes per day for 20 y has a 20- to 30-fold greater risk of developing lung cancer compared with a nonsmoker. • A person passively exposed to smoking has at least a 2- to 3-fold greater risk of developing lung cancer.
Occupational hazards	• Most industrial irritants act as cocarcinogens with smoking, increasing a smoker's risk rather than being the primary cause. • Exposure to ionizing radiation through the mining of iron, cobalt, arsenic ore, uranium, nickel, and chromium salts has been associated with an increased risk of developing lung cancer.
Environmental hazards	• They are probably important but need to be defined.

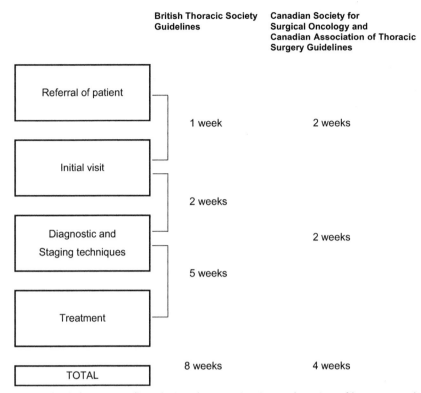

British Thoracic Society Guidelines

Canadian Society for Surgical Oncology and Canadian Association of Thoracic Surgery Guidelines

Referral of patient

1 week   2 weeks

Initial visit

2 weeks

Diagnostic and Staging techniques

2 weeks

5 weeks

Treatment

8 weeks   4 weeks

TOTAL

Fig. 1. Time-line standards for patient flow during the investigation and staging of lung cancer. (*Data from* The Lung Cancer Working Party of the British Thoracic Society Standards of Care Committee. BTS recommendations to respiratory physicians for organizing the care of patients with lung cancer. Thorax 1998;53(Suppl 1):S1–8; and Darling GE, Maziak DE, Clifton JC, et al. The practice of thoracic surgery in Canada. Can J Surg 2004;47:438–44.)

patients have to receive induction therapy.[9] Similarly, the Canadian Association of Thoracic Surgeons recommends that this delay be 4 weeks.[11] The creation of formal surgical oncology divisions with accountability for timely care may also be a good option to help decreasing waiting times during this interval.

ORGANIZATION OF STANDARDIZED CLINICAL CARE PATHWAYS FOR LUNG CANCER

Because the most effective way to improve quality is to reduce the variation in the process of providing a service, it seems that standardized clinical care pathways, formally known as physician-directed diagnostic and therapeutic plans,[12,13] are ideally suited for the investigation of patients with lung cancer. The essential components of successful standardized clinical care pathways for patients with thoracic malignancies relate to 3 important factors: (1) multidisciplinary thoracic oncology clinics, (2) streamline referral with a nurse navigator who can coordinate patient investigation through diagnostic and treatment algorithms that have been agreed on by the members of the

multidisciplinary group, and (3) adequate physical resources and funding.

Multidisciplinary Thoracic Oncology Clinics

A multidisciplinary approach to the diagnosis, staging, and treatment of patients with lung cancer is widely advocated around the globe because many patients will benefit from multimodal therapies that include medical management, surgery, chemotherapy, radiation therapy, and palliative care services.[10] Such teams should not only be multidisciplinary whereby each member provides an opinion but also interdisciplinary whereby the opinions of each member are truly integrated.

The members of that team (**Table 3**) should include thoracic oncological surgeons who are able to perform all pulmonary resectional procedures that may be required, including the resection of Pancoast tumors, tumors invading the chest wall or spine, as well as bronchoplasties and angioplasties. These surgeons should understand the role of induction and adjuvant therapies; ideally, they should probably be under one financial plan to eliminate competition for referral and operating room time. Under such an organization,

Table 3
Members of the teams involved in standardized clinical care pathways for lung cancer

Member	Expertise
Thoracic surgeons	• Able to perform all lung resectional procedures • Expertise in induction and adjuvant therapies
Medical oncologists	• Expertise with principles and indications for chemotherapy
Radiation therapists	• Expertise with latest radiation techniques and their indications
Respirologists	• Expertise in the evaluation of cardiopulmonary status and operative risk
Dedicated thoracic radiologists	• Expertise with imaging techniques used for the evaluation of patients with lung cancer
Dedicated pulmonary pathologists	• Expertise with new histologic classification of lung cancer • Ability to interpret small biopsy specimens
Allied health care personnel	• Psychologists, nutritionists, specialized thoracic nurses, physiotherapists, social workers, residents in training, and research assistants
Palliative care specialists	Expertise with palliative care for patients with advanced disease

patients are really under the care of a group rather than under the care of individual surgeons.

The team should also include medical oncologists who understand tumor biology and principles of chemotherapy as well as radiation therapists who are familiar with the latest radiation techniques, including those of stereotactic body radiation for early stage tumors. Respirologists are also important not only because they can assess cardiopulmonary function and determine operability and operative risk but also because, in most North American centers, they are the ones who carry out diagnostic bronchoscopies as well as non invasive mediastinal staging with endobronchial and endoesophageal ultrasound techniques. Dedicated thoracic radiologists are essential to the teams because they have the ability to interpret imaging studies such as computed tomography (CT) scanning, positron emission tomography (PET) scanning, and magnetic resonance imaging studies as well as being able to correlate one with the other. Most radiologists also have some degree of expertise with imaging screening programs.

The pulmonary pathologist's role is invaluable because the heterogeneity in the histology of lung cancer is now well recognized and has important implications in the management of the disease. They must understand new histologic classifications of primary lung cancer, including those of adenocarcinomas, as well as being able to interpret small biopsy specimens and be familiar with tumor banking and genetic mutations for personalized treatment.

Other people that should be part of the team include psychologists, nutritionists, specialized thoracic nurses, physiotherapists, social workers, residents in training, research assistants, and palliative care specialists. Palliative care specialists are especially important because many patients already have advanced disease at the time of presentation.

A weekly case conference should be held and attended by representatives of the previously mentioned specialties, and all cases (new and recurrent) should be presented and discussed; a tumor registry should be available and used. A standardized form should be developed for patient presentation at these weekly tumor board conferences.

Streamline Referral, Nurse Navigator, and Diagnostic Algorithms

A single-entry point of contact and a reference form should be developed similar to that of the successful Time To Treat Program implemented in Toronto in 2005 by Lo and Zeldin.[1] This program was effective in shortening the time from suspicion of lung cancer to diagnosis and it reduced time intervals at each step in the process of diagnosis, staging, and treatment. Respirologists and thoracic surgeons should agree among themselves as to which patients would be best suited to see either of them. One or 2 navigator nurses should coordinate the diagnostic workup including the facilitation of investigation bookings for CT scan, PET scan, bronchoscopy slots, and fine-needle aspiration biopsy slots. The multidisciplinary tumor boards should develop diagnostic and treatment algorithms, and these algorithms should be followed.

Physical Resources and Adequate Funding

All of these components require funding, physical resources, and committed support from hospital administrators who can provide the necessary tools for the organization and running of standardized clinical care pathways for patients with lung cancer. They must understand that ultimately, quality improvements and cost savings will result from these initiatives.

FAST-TRACKING PULMONARY RESECTIONS

Four studies[2,4,6,12] have shown that standardized clinical care pathways for postoperative management after thoracic surgical procedures have resulted in significant reductions in lengths of stay and hospital costs. In the report by Zehr and colleagues[4] from the Johns Hopkins Hospital, the greatest savings after lung resection occurred for pharmaceuticals (60%) and supplies (34%); the length of stay was significantly lower for patients in the clinical care pathway than for those who were not ($P<.002$). In the article by Wright and colleagues[2] from the Mass General Hospital, the institution of a lobectomy patient care pathway also reduced the length of stay ($P = .03$) and mean costs ($P = .47$).

SUMMARY

Lung cancer is a fatal disease with cure rates of only 15% and it remains the most common cause of cancer-related deaths in both men and women. Over the past 20 years, dramatic improvements have occurred in survival rates of patients with other solid tumors, such as breast, colorectal, prostate, and cervix, but not so in lung cancer whereby improvements have lagged behind with only a fourfold increase from the 1940s when as few as 4% of patients with lung cancer could be cured of their disease. Reducing delays for reference, investigation, and treatment through the use of standardized clinical care pathways may not improve overall long-term survival by much, but it has been well demonstrated that such a strategy is essential to improve quality of care and reduce costs through more consistent and efficient use of resources. It may also be helpful in reducing mental distress for patients and their relatives and at the end

possibly improve the cure rate beyond the current 15%. These plans are not only just a better way to practice medicine but they will also eventually be essential to the survival of health care organizations.

REFERENCES

1. Lo DS, Zeldin RA, Skrastins R, et al. Time to treat: a system re-design focusing on decreasing the time from suspicion of lung cancer to diagnosis. J Thorac Oncol 2007;2:1001–6.
2. Wright CD, Wain JC, Grillo HC, et al. Pulmonary lobectomy patient care pathway: a model to control cost and maintain quality. Ann Thorac Surg 1997;64: 299–302.
3. Shulkin DJ, Ferniany IW. The effect of developing patient compendiums for critical pathways or patient satisfaction. Am J Med Qual 1996;11:43–5.
4. Zehr KJ, Dawson PB, Yang SC, et al. Standardized clinical care pathways for major thoracic cases reduce hospital costs. Ann Thorac Surg 1998;66: 914–9.
5. Freeman RK, Van Woerkom UJ, Vyverberg A, et al. The effect of a multidisciplinary thoracic malignancy conference on the treatment of patients with lung cancer. Eur J Cardiothorac Surg 2010;38:1–5.
6. Cerfolio RJ, Pickens A, Bass C, et al. Fast-tracking pulmonary resection. J Thorac Cardiovasc Surg 2001;122:318–24.
7. Engelman RM, Rousou JA, Flack JE, et al. Fast-track recovery of the coronary bypass patient. Ann Thorac Surg 1994;58:1742–6.
8. Laroche C, Wells F, Coulden R, et al. Improving surgical resection rate in lung cancer. Thorax 1998;53:445–9.
9. The Lung Cancer Working Party of the British Thoracic Society Standards of Care Committee. BTS recommendations to respiratory physicians for organizing the care of patients with lung cancer. Thorax 1998;53(Suppl 1):S1–8.
10. Riedel RF, Wang X, McCormack M, et al. Impact of a multidisciplinary thoracic oncology clinic on the timeless of care. J Thorac Oncol 2006;1:692–6.
11. Darling GE, Maziak DE, Clifton JC, et al. The practice of thoracic surgery in Canada. Can J Surg 2004;47:438–44.
12. Tovar EA, Roethe RA, Weissig BD, et al. One-day admission for lung lobectomy: an incidental result of a clinical pathway. Ann Thorac Surg 1998;65: 803–6.
13. Musfeldt C, Hart RI. Physician-directed diagnostic and therapeutic plans: a quality care for America's health-care crisis. J Soc Health Syst 1993;4:80–7.

Performance of Integrated Positron Emission Tomography/ Computed Tomography for Mediastinal Nodal Staging in Non-Small Cell Lung Carcinoma

Stephen R. Broderick, MD*, G. Alexander Patterson, MD

KEYWORDS

- NSCLC • PET/CT • Mediastinal lymph node staging

KEY POINTS

- Positron emission tomography (PET) imaging has been shown in several trials to be superior to CT for the identification of mediastinal lymph node metastases in non-small cell lung carcinoma (NSCLC). The inclusion of PET in staging strategies reduces the number of nontherapeutic operations performed for NSCLC.
- Integrated PET/CT is superior to CT alone, PET alone, or visual correlation of PET and CT for mediastinal nodal staging.
- The clinically relevant false-positive rate of PET/CT mandates pathologic confirmation of suspected mediastinal nodal disease.

INTRODUCTION

In the last two decades positron emission tomography (PET) has become a standard component of the staging evaluation of non-small cell lung carcinoma (NSCLC). In PET, the radiolabeled glucose analog ^{18}F-flouro-2-deoxy-D-glucose (FDG) is administered to patients, undergoes cellular uptake, and is phosphorylated by hexokinase generating ^{18}F-FDG-6-phosphate. This radiolabeled metabolite accumulates in cells with relatively high rates of cellular glucose uptake and diminished dephosphorylation, such as malignant cells, and can be detected with a nuclear medicine imaging system.

The use of PET to distinguish benign and malignant pulmonary lesions or to identify sites of metastatic disease has become commonplace. Standardized quantitative criteria for abnormal PET findings are lacking. Comparison of FDG uptake to surrounding tissue or normal lung or liver provides a qualitative assessment of the metabolic activity of a given lesion. Calculation of standardized uptake values (SUV) is subject to variation across scanners, centers, and interpreting physicians. Generally, an SUV less than 2.5 is considered normal. Because PET estimates metabolic activity of tissues by assessing cellular glucose uptake, results may be falsely positive in other metabolically active lesions such as inflammatory or infectious lesions. Similarly, false-negative results may occur in slow growing or low-grade malignancies.

There is an extensive body of literature regarding the role of PET in the management of NSCLC, including its role in distinguishing benign and malignant pulmonary lesions and identification of extrathoracic metastases. This article

Division of Cardiothoracic Surgery, Department of Surgery, Washington University School of Medicine, 3108 Queeny Tower, One Barnes-Jewish Hospital Plaza, St Louis, MO 63110-1013, USA
* Corresponding author.
E-mail address: brodericks@wudosis.wustl.edu

Thorac Surg Clin 23 (2013) 193–198
http://dx.doi.org/10.1016/j.thorsurg.2013.01.014
1547-4127/13/$ – see front matter © 2013 Elsevier Inc. All rights reserved.

focuses on the use of combined PET/CT in mediastinal staging of NSCLC. **Table 1** provides evidence is to support its use and the clinical application of this modality is discussed.

PET IN MEDIASTINAL LYMPH NODE STAGING

Accurate staging of mediastinal lymph nodes is essential to appropriate management of the patient with NSCLC. The identification of metastases in mediastinal lymph nodes allows for selection of patients for stage-based treatment strategies and provides patients with the best estimate of prognosis. In the absence of extrathoracic metastases, the status of mediastinal lymph nodes is the primary determinant of resectability. Patients with mediastinal (N2) lymph node metastases are generally treated with either neoadjuvant or definitive

Table 1
Important clinical trials of PET imaging in NSCLC

Study, Year	Design	Modalities	Conclusions
Van Tinteren (PLUS trial) et al,[2] 2002	Prospective randomized multicenter	PET vs conventional staging	51% relative reduction in nontherapeutic thoracotomy Unnecessary surgery prevented in 1 of 5 subjects
Reed (ACOSOG Z0050) et al,[3] 2003	Prospective multicenter	PET vs conventional staging	Unresectable disease identified in 14% of subjects not identified by conventional staging Unnecessary surgery prevented in 1 of 5 subjects
Viney et al,[4] 2004	Prospective randomized multicenter	PET vs conventional staging	PET lead to a change in management in 13% of subjects
Lardinois et al,[6] 2003	Prospective single-center	Integrated PET/CT vs PET plus CT	PET/CT provides better diagnostic accuracy compared with visual correlation of PET and CT, PET alone, or CT alone
Cerfolio et al,[7] 2004	Prospective single-center	Integrated PET/CT vs PET alone	PET/CT provides greater sensitivity, specificity and PPV
Fischer et al,[8] 2009	Prospective randomized single-center	Integrated PET/CT vs conventional staging	PET/CT improved sensitivity of mediastinal staging 1 nontherapeutic thoracotomy avoided for every 5 PET/CT scans No difference in survival between groups
Maziak (ELPET) et al,[9] 2009	Prospective randomized multicenter	Integrated PET/CT with cranial imaging vs conventional staging with cranial imaging	PET/CT correctly upstaged a significant portion of subjects; however, 5% of subjects were incorrectly upstaged
Darling (ELPET subgroup) et al,[10] 2011	Prospective randomized multicenter	PET/CT vs mediastinoscopy or mediastinoscopy plus thoracotomy	Sensitivity, specificity, PPV and NPV of PET/CT: 70%, 94%, 64%, 95% False-positive rate is clinically relevant and confirms the need for pathologic confirmation of suspicious PET/CT findings

chemotherapy and radiotherapy, whereas those without N2 disease are candidates for primary resection.

CT provides detailed anatomic imaging of thoracic structures. The size and location of mediastinal nodes can be evaluated to identify suspicious metastatic nodal involvement. The accuracy of CT alone in identifying mediastinal lymph nodes in NSCLC is poor, with approximate sensitivity and specificity of 50% and 85%, respectively.[1] The use of PET and, subsequently, PET/CT in staging mediastinal lymph nodes has been evaluated in many studies over the last 15 years, including several randomized controlled trials.

The first randomized trial to evaluate PET in the staging of mediastinal lymph nodes was the European multicenter Pet in Lung Cancer Staging (PLUS) trial published in 2002.[2] This trial randomized 188 subjects who were scheduled for resection of suspected NSCLC to two arms: conventional staging workup or conventional staging workup with the addition of PET. The primary endpoint of the study was the number of subjects who underwent thoracotomy for benign disease, pathologic N2 disease, exploratory thoracotomy, or experienced recurrence or death within 12 months of surgery. These subjects were deemed to have had a futile thoracotomy. In the conventional staging arm, 39 of 96 (41%) subjects underwent futile thoracotomy compared with 19 of 92 (21%) with the addition of PET. The addition of PET to the conventional staging workup resulted in a 51% relative reduction in the number of futile thoracotomies and prevented unnecessary surgery in one of five subjects with suspected NSCLC.

In 2003, the American College of Surgeons Oncology Group (ACOSOG) published the results of the prospective Z0050 trial,[3] which included 303 subjects from 22 institutions with documented or suspected NSCLC deemed resectable by standard staging procedures. Radiographic staging in the Z0050 trial included CT of the chest and upper abdomen, bone scintigraphy, and CT or MRI of the head before PET. The purpose of the study was to determine whether PET identified lesions that precluded curative pulmonary resection. Despite enrolling a substantially smaller proportion of subjects with stage IIIA and IIIB disease, the results of the Z0050 trial paralleled those of the PLUS trial. Unresectable disease was identified in 43 of 303 (14.2%) subjects and potentially nontherapeutic thoracotomy was avoided in one in five subjects.

In 2004, Viney and colleagues[4] published a randomized controlled trial investigating the role of PET in early stage NSCLC. In contrast to the PLUS and Z0050 trials, this study did not demonstrate a reduction in the number of thoracotomies performed in subjects undergoing PET scan preoperatively. However, primary resection was the strategy for subjects with stage IIIA disease at the participating centers at the time of the study. Thus, identification of N2 disease on preoperative PET would not have altered the plan for thoracotomy. Had the investigators' strategy for stage IIIA disease included induction therapy or definitive chemotherapy and radiation, it is likely that PET would have prevented up to 20% of thoracotomies in the study. Regardless, PET lead to a change in stage in 18% and a change in clinical management in 13% of subjects in the study, predominantly by the identification of occult N2 disease.

INTEGRATED PET/CT

PET provides information regarding the metabolic activity of a lesion. The precise location of abnormalities identified on PET is difficult to interpret. In contrast, CT imaging provides detailed anatomic imaging without providing information on the metabolic activity of a lesion. With the presumed advantage of accurate correlation of anatomic location and metabolic activity, integrated PET/CT became available in 2000.[5]

In 2003, Lardinois and colleagues[6] compared the accuracy of integrated PET/CT with that of CT alone, PET alone, and visual correlation of CT and PET. In this prospective study of 50 subjects with known or suspected NSCLC, integrated PET/CT correctly staged the mediastinal lymph nodes in 5 of 11 subjects who were incorrectly staged by visual correlation of PET and CT. Tumor staging was more accurate than visual correlation of CT and PET, PET alone, or CT alone. Cerfolio and colleagues[7] confirmed this finding in 2004 with their prospective study demonstrating a higher sensitivity, specificity, and PPV for the identification of N2 nodal disease for PET/CT compared with PET alone. There have been two major randomized trials evaluating the utility of PET/CT in mediastinal staging of NSCLC.

Fischer and colleagues[8] randomized 189 subjects to conventional staging or conventional staging with the addition of integrated PET/CT. The primary endpoint of the study was the number of futile thoracotomies performed, defined as thoracotomy performed for stage IIIA or higher disease or a benign lesion, exploratory thoracotomy, or thoracotomy in a subject who suffered recurrence of disease or death from any cause within 12 months of surgery. Ninety four percent of subjects underwent mediastinoscopy. Twenty-one of 60 thoracotomies performed in the PET/CT group and 38 of 73 thoracotomies in the conventional staging group were considered futile. In total, 21 of 98 subjects (21%) in the PET/CT group underwent futile thoracotomy compared with 38 of 91 subjects (42%) in the conventional staging group. Just as the PLUS and ACOSOG Z0050 trials demonstrated for stand-alone PET, this study demonstrated that integrated PET/CT improved sensitivity of preoperative mediastinal staging in NSCLC. For every five PET/CT scans performed, one futile thoracotomy was avoided. The number of justified thoracotomies and survival were similar between the groups. Also, in 2009, Maziak and colleagues[9] published the results of the Early Lung PET trial (ELPET), a clinical trial comparing PET/CT with cranial imaging to conventional staging with cranial imaging. This study randomized 337 subjects and similarly found that PET/CT correctly upstaged a significant proportion of subjects by identifying N2 or extra-thoracic disease. However, in approximately 5% of subjects who underwent PET/CT, disease was incorrectly upstaged.

Although PET/CT may prevent nontherapeutic thoracotomies by identifying unrecognized N2 disease, false-positive N2 disease has the potential to deprive potentially resectable patients of curative surgery. An example of such a false-positive result is included (**Fig. 1**). A recently published subgroup analysis of the ELPET trial confirms the need for pathologic confirmation of mediastinal abnormalities identified on PET/CT.[10] In the ELPET trial, 149 subjects underwent PET/CT and subsequent mediastinoscopy or thoracotomy with lymph node sampling. The sensitivity and specificity of PET/CT for N2 disease was 70% and 94%, respectively. The positive predictive value (PPV) and negative predictive value (NPV) for PET/CT were 64% and 95%, respectively. Mediastinal N2 disease was identified by PET/CT in 22 subjects, eight of whom did not have pathologically identifiable tumor in the mediastinum. If invasive mediastinal staging had not been pursued, these eight subjects would have been deprived of potentially curative surgery, emphasizing the need for pathologic confirmation of abnormalities identified on PET/CT.

Several prospective studies have evaluated the performance of integrated PET/CT in the prediction of N2 disease in subjects with clinical T1-2 tumors. A recent meta-analysis studied the NPV of PET and CT in these subjects. The meta-analysis included 10 studies and a total of 1122 subjects. The overall NPV for PET/CT was 93%, 94% for T1 tumors, and 87% for T2 tumors. Most subjects in the included studies had T1 tumors. It should be noted that some of the included studies used visual correlation of PET and CT images, which has been shown to be inferior to integrated PET/CT. Nonetheless, the relatively high NPV across studies indicates that mediastinal metastases are unlikely with a negative PET/CT in patients with T1-2 tumors and obviates invasive preoperative mediastinal staging in these patients.[11]

RESTAGING AFTER NEOADJUVANT THERAPY

In patients with stage IIIA-N2 NSCLC, treatment with induction chemoradiotherapy followed by surgical resection has demonstrated a survival advantage compared with initial treatment with definitive chemoradiotherapy.[12] Identification of residual N2 disease following induction therapy allows for selection of patients most likely to benefit from this treatment strategy. Median survival for patients with pathologic N0 disease following induction therapy and subsequent resection for IIIA-N2 NSCLC is 28 to 30 months, whereas median survival for those patients with residual N2 disease is 9 to15 months.[13,14] Similarly, in patients with persistent N2 disease, 5-year survival ranges between 0% to 19% compared with 36% to 43% for those in whom the mediastinum were downstaged by induction therapy.[14–16]

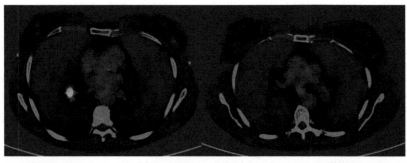

Fig. 1. Integrated PET/CT demonstrating FDG uptake in a hilar mass and false-positive uptake in subcarinal region. Suspicious FDG uptake in N2 should be confirmed by pathologic examination.

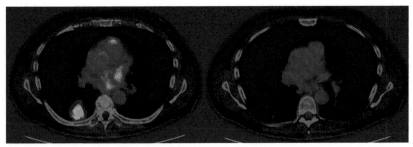

Fig. 2. Integrated PET/CT demonstrating FDG uptake in RLL mass and false-negative lack of FDG uptake in subcarinal region. This patient had level 7 lymph node metastases on pathologic examination.

Radiographic restaging of the mediastinum following induction therapy has proven to be unreliable. CT scanning alone provides scant information regarding response to treatment in lymph node metastases.[17] Likewise, PET alone has shown a high degree of variability for identification of residual N2 disease with sensitivity ranging from 20% to 67%.[18–21] Although there is some evidence that integrated PET/CT improves on the reliability of CT or PET alone, several studies have confirmed the need for pathologic confirmation of findings on PET/CT before resection after neoadjuvant therapy.[22–24] Strategies for restaging the mediastinum following induction therapy remain controversial. Initial staging with minimally invasive approaches, such as endobronchial ultrasound (EBUS) or endoscopic ultrasound (EUS), reserving mediastinoscopy to evaluate for persistent N2 disease is optimal.

SUMMARY

PET/CT is widely accepted as the standard noninvasive modality for mediastinal lymph node staging in NSCLC. In light of its ability to prevent unnecessary surgery by the identification of previously unidentified N2 disease, it is the authors' practice to obtain routine PET/CT in patients with clinical stage I-IIIA NSCLC before resection. We recommend pathologic confirmation of N2 disease identified on PET by EBUS, EUS, or mediastinoscopy when indicated. Every attempt should be made to obtain initial pathologic diagnosis of N2 disease by EBUS or EUS to reserve mediastinoscopy for the evaluation for persistent N2 disease after neoadjuvant chemoradiotherapy. We further recommend that invasive mediastinal staging be pursued in patients in whom clinical suspicion of N2 disease is high (based on presence of large, centrally located tumor or enlarged mediastinal lymph nodes), despite negative evaluation on PET/CT because false-negative results may deprive patients of an opportunity for neoadjuvant chemoradiation for stage IIIA disease (**Fig. 2**).

REFERENCES

1. Silvestri G, Gould M, Marolis M, et al. Noninvasive staging of non-small cell lung cancer: ACCP evidence-based clinical practice guidelines (2nd edition). Chest 2007;132:178S–201S.
2. van Tinteren H, Hoekstra O, Smit E, et al. Effectiveness of positron emission tomography in the preoperative assessment of patients with suspected non-small-cell lung cancer: the PLUS multicentre randomised trial. Lancet 2002;359:1388–92.
3. Reed C, Harpole D, Posther K, et al. Results of the American College of Surgeons Oncology Group Z0050 Trial: the utility of positron emission tomography in staging potentially operable non-small cell lung cancer. J Thorac Cardiovasc Surg 2003;126:1943–51.
4. Viney R, Boyer M, King M, et al. Randomized controlled trial of the role of positron emission tomography in the management of stage I and II non-small cell lung cancer. J Clin Oncol 2004;22:2357–62.
5. Beyer T, Townsend DW, Brun T, et al. A combined PET/CT scanner for clinical oncology. J Nucl Med 2000;10(Suppl 3):S377–80.
6. Lardinois D, Weder W, Hany T, et al. Staging of non-small-cell lung cancer with integrated positron-emission tomography and computed tomography. N Engl J Med 2003;348:2500–7.
7. Cerfolio RJ, Ojha B, Bryant AS, et al. The accuracy of integrated PET-CT compared with dedicated PET alone for the staging of patients with non-small cell lung cancer. Ann Thorac Surg 2004;78:1017–23.
8. Fischer B, Lassen U, Mortensen J, et al. Preoperative staging of lung cancer with combined PET-CT. N Engl J Med 2009;361:32–9.
9. Maziak D, Darling G, Inculet R, et al. Positron emission tomography in staging early lung cancer: a randomized trial. Ann Intern Med 2009;151:221–8.
10. Darling G, Maziak D, Inculet R, et al. Positron emission tomography-computed tomography compared with invasive mediastinal staging in non-small cell lung cancer: results of mediastinal staging in the early lung positron emission tomography trial. J Thorac Oncol 2011;6:1367–72.

11. Wang J, Welch K, Wang L, et al. Negative predictive value of positron emission tomography and computed tomography for stage T1-2N0 non-small cell lung cancer: a meta-analysis. Clin Lung Cancer 2012;13(2):81–9.

12. Uy KL, Darling G, Xu W, et al. Improved results of induction chemoradiation before surgical intervention for selected patients with stage IIIA-N2 non-small cell lung cancer. J Thorac Cardiovasc Surg 2007;134(1):188–93.

13. De Waele M, Serra-Mitjans M, Hendriks J, et al. Accuracy and survival of repeat mediastinoscopy after induction therapy for non-small cell lung cancer in a combined series of 104 patients. Eur J Cardiothorac Surg 2008;33(5):824–8.

14. Johnstone DW, Byhardt RW, Ettinger D, et al. Phase III study comparing chemotherapy and radiotherapy with preoperative chemotherapy and surgical resection in patients with non-small-cell lung cancer with spread to mediastinal lymph nodes (N2); final report of RTOG 89-01. Radiation Therapy Oncology Group. Int J Radiat Oncol Biol Phys 2002;54(2):365–9.

15. Bueno R, Richards WG, Swanson SJ, et al. Nodal stage after induction therapy for stage IIIA lung cancer determines survival. Ann Thorac Surg 2000; 70(6):1826–31.

16. Dooms C, Verbeken E, Stroobants S, et al. Prognostic stratification of stage IIIA-N2 non-small cell lung cancer after induction chemotherapy: a model based on the combination of morphometric-pathologic response in mediastinal nodes and primary tumor response on serial 18-fluoro-2-deoxy-glucose positron emission tomography. J Clin Oncol 2008;26(7): 1128–34.

17. De Cabanyes Candela S, Detterbeck FC. A systematic review of restaging after induction therapy for stage IIIa lung cancer: prediction of pathologic stage. J Thorac Oncol 2010;5(3):389–98.

18. Hellwig D, Graeter TP, Ukena D, et al. Value of F-18-fluorodeoxyglucose positron emission tomography after induction therapy of locally advanced bronchogenic carcinoma. J Thorac Cardiovasc Surg 2004; 128:892–9.

19. Port JL, Kent MS, Korst RJ, et al. Positron emission tomography scanning poorly predicts response to preoperative chemotherapy in non-small cell lung cancer. Ann Thorac Surg 2004;77(1):254–9.

20. Cerfolio RJ, Ojha B, Mukherjee S, et al. Positron emission tomography scanning with 2-fluoro-2-deoxy-d-glucose as a predictor of response of neoadjuvant treatment for non-small cell carcinoma. J Thorac Cardiovasc Surg 2003;125(4):938–44.

21. Ryu JS, Choi NC, Fischman AJ, et al. FDG-PET in staging and restaging non-small cell lung cancer after neoadjuvant chemoradiotherapy: correlation with histopathology. Lung Cancer 2002;35(2): 179–87.

22. De Leyn P, Stroobants S, De Wever W, et al. Prospective comparative study of integrated positron emission tomography scan compared with re-mediastinoscopy in the assessment of residual mediastinal lymph node disease after induction chemotherapy for mediastinoscopy-proven stage IIIA-N2 non-small-cell lung cancer: a Leuven Lung Cancer Group study. J Clin Oncol 2006;24: 3333–9.

23. Cerfolio RJ, Bryant AS, Ojha B. Restaging patients with N2 (stage IIIa) non-small cell lung cancer after neoadjuvant chemoradiotherapy: a prospective study. J Thorac Cardiovasc Surg 2006;132(3): 565–7.

24. Stigt JA, Oostdijk AH, Timmer PR, et al. Comparison of EUS-guided fine needle aspiration and integrated PET-CT in restaging after treatment for locally advanced non-small cell lung cancer. Lung Cancer 2009;66(2):198–204.

Relevance of Endoscopic Ultrasonography and Endobronchial Ultrasonography to Thoracic Surgeons

Kazuhiro Yasufuku, MD, PhD*

KEYWORDS

- Endobronchial ultrasonography • Endoscopic ultrasonography • Bronchoscopy • Lung cancer
- Invasive staging • Mediastinum

KEY POINTS

- Endobronchial ultrasound-guided transbronchial needle aspiration (EBUS-TBNA) has access to all of the mediastinal lymph nodes accessible by mediastinoscopy, but also extends to the N1 nodes.
- Endoscopic ultrasound fine-needle aspiration (EUS-FNA) allows access to paraesophageal and pulmonary ligament lymph nodes, which are not accessible by both mediastinoscopy and EBUS-TBNA.
- Minimally invasive endoscopic staging with EBUS-TBNA and/or EUS-FNA is the recommended choice in patients with high pretest probability of lymph node metastasis; however, all negative results should be verified by mediastinoscopy in centers with low expertise.

INTRODUCTION

Lung cancer is still the leading cause of death from malignant diseases worldwide.[1] Accurate staging of the disease is important not only to determine the prognosis but also to decide the most suitable treatment plan for non–small cell lung cancer (NSCLC). The most significant treatment decision is to distinguish those patients who can benefit from surgical resection from those who should receive chemotherapy, radiation therapy, or both. Despite advances in noninvasive radiologic staging including computed tomography (CT), positron emission tomography (PET), and PET/CT, their diagnostic accuracy is insufficient for taking clinical decisions.[2–6] Mediastinal lymph node sampling by invasive staging is recommended in the absence of distant metastases.[7–10]

Mediastinoscopy has been considered the gold standard for invasive mediastinal staging of the mediastinum. However, the emergence of new minimally invasive endoscopic techniques such as endobronchial ultrasound-guided transbronchial needle aspiration (EBUS-TBNA) and endoscopic ultrasound-guided fine-needle aspiration (EUS-FNA) has questioned the routine use of mediastinoscopy for invasive staging of NSCLC.[7–10] Both procedures are performed using a needle under real-time ultrasound guidance and can be performed under local anesthesia. EUS-FNA became an established method for examining the

Disclosure: K.Y. has received educational grants from Olympus Medical Systems Corp for CME. K.Y. has served as a consultant for Olympus America Inc and Intuitive Surgical Inc.
Division of Thoracic Surgery, Toronto General Hospital, University Health Network, University of Toronto, 200 Elizabeth Street, 9N-957, Toronto, ON M5G 2C4, Canada
* Corresponding author.
E-mail address: kazuhiro.yasufuku@uhn.ca

Thorac Surg Clin 23 (2013) 199–210
http://dx.doi.org/10.1016/j.thorsurg.2013.01.016
1547-4127/13/$ – see front matter © 2013 Elsevier Inc. All rights reserved.

mediastinum in patients with lung cancer in the early 1990s, and the role of EUS-FNA in the staging of lung cancer continues to evolve.[11–14] EUS allows ultrasonographic imaging of structures adjacent to the gastrointestinal tract, which is useful for the sampling of lymph nodes around the posterior mediastinum and upper retroperitoneum. However, the reach of EUS-FNA does not correspond completely to the reach of mediastinoscopy. On the other hand, EBUS-TBNA is a bronchoscopic modality that was initially developed in 2002 that has a reach similar to that of mediastinoscopy, but also extends to the hilar and interlobar lymph nodes (N1 nodes).[15] The combination of EBUS and EUS allows sampling of most mediastinal lymph nodes as well as N1 nodes (Fig. 1). In this article, the role of EBUS-TBNA and EUS-FNA for invasive staging of NSCLC is discussed, with emphasis on the endoscopic anatomy, procedural technique, and integration of these technologies into thoracic surgeons' practice.

BRONCHOSCOPIC ANATOMY OF THE MEDIASTINUM AND HILUM

It is extremely important to understand the anatomy of the mediastinum and the hilum before starting EBUS-TBNA or EUS-FNA. The definition of each lymph node station should be based on the newest TNM classification for lung cancer.[16] The transparent anatomy of the mediastinal structures and the lymph nodes through the different levels of the airway are illustrated in Fig. 2:

1. Lower trachea and carina (see Fig. 2A)
2. Right main bronchus (see Fig. 2B)
3. Left main bronchus (see Fig. 2C)
4. Upper trachea (see Fig. 2D)

INSTRUMENTS
EBUS-TBNA

The convex probe endobronchial ultrasound (CP-EBUS) is used for EBUS-TBNA. The CP-EBUS is an ultrasound puncture bronchoscope with a linear curved-array ultrasound transducer placed on the tip of a flexible bronchoscope (BF-UC180F-OL8; Olympus, Tokyo, Japan) (Fig. 3). Images can be obtained by directly contacting the probe or by attaching a balloon on the tip and inflating with saline. The outer diameter of the insertion tube of the CP-EBUS is 6.2 mm and that of the tip is 6.9 mm. The angle of view is 80° and the direction of view is 35° forward oblique. The inner diameter of the instrument channel is 2.2 mm. A dedicated 21-gauge or 22-gauge needle is used to perform EBUS-TBNA.

The ultrasonographic image is processed by connecting the CP-EBUS to either the dedicated ultrasound scanner (EU-C60; Olympus), the universal endoscopic ultrasound scanner with capabilities

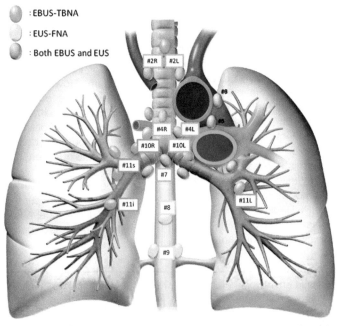

Fig. 1. Regional lymph node map for lung cancer staging. Most mediastinal lymph nodes can routinely be assessed with a combination of endobronchial ultrasound-guided transbronchial needle aspiration (EBUS-TBNA) and endoscopic ultrasound-guided fine-needle aspiration (EUS-FNA) with the exception of stations 5 and 6. EBUS-TBNA can also sample N1 nodes.

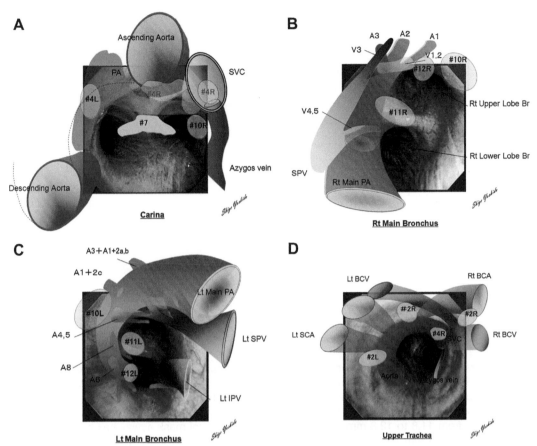

Fig. 2. Bronchoscopic anatomy of the mediastinum and hilum. (*A*) Lower trachea and carina. Anatomic landmarks of the major vessels, including the superior vena cava (SVC), azygos vein, pulmonary artery (PA), and the ascending aorta, are important for identifying lymph node stations 4R, 10R, 4L, and 7. (*B*) Right main bronchus. The interlobar pulmonary artery (PA) branching from the right main stem PA is the landmark for identifying lymph node station 11R. Lymph node station 10R is located along the lateral wall of the right main bronchus distal to the azygos vein. The lobar lymph node 12R is usually difficult to visualize with endobronchial ultrasonography. SPV, superior pulmonary vein. (*C*) Left main bronchus. Lymph node station 10L is located along the lateral wall of the left main bronchus along the left main stem pulmonary artery (PA). The interlobar lymph node station 11L lies between the bifurcation of the upper and lower lobe bronchus. IPV, inferior pulmonary vein; SPV, superior pulmonary vein. (*D*) Upper trachea. The aortic arch is the anatomic landmark for distinguishing lymph node stations 2R and 4R. BCA, brachiocephalic artery; BCV, brachiocephalic vein; SCA, subclavian artery; SVC, superior vena cava. ([*A*] *From* Yasufuku K, Nakajima T. Endobronchial Ultrasound Guided Transbronchial Needle Aspiration Manual. Tokyo: Kanehara Shuppan; 2009; with permission.)

of radial probe EBUS imaging (EU-ME1; Olympus), or the Aloka Prosound Alpha5 (Hitachi Aloka, Tokyo, Japan) for excellent image quality. The EU-ME1 is equipped with the power Doppler mode as well as the color Doppler mode. The ultrasonographic images can be captured and the size of lesions measured in 2 dimensions by the placement of cursors. The area and the circumference enclosed by caliper tracking can also be measured.

Two types of dedicated needles are available for EBUS-TBNA. The 21-gauge or the 22-gauge needle passed through the 2.2 mm instrument channel allows real-time EBUS-TBNA. This needle has various adjuster knobs, which work as a safety device to prevent damage of the channel. The maximum extruding stroke is 40 mm and to prevent excessive protrusion, a safety mechanism stops the needle at the stroke of 20 mm. The needle is also equipped with an internal sheath that is withdrawn after passing the bronchial wall, avoiding contamination during TBNA. This internal sheath is also used to clear out the tip of the needle after passing the bronchial wall.

EUS-FNA

EUS-FNA is performed by using a side-viewing dedicated videogastroscope with a dedicated

	EBUS-TBNA	EUS-FNA
Endoscope	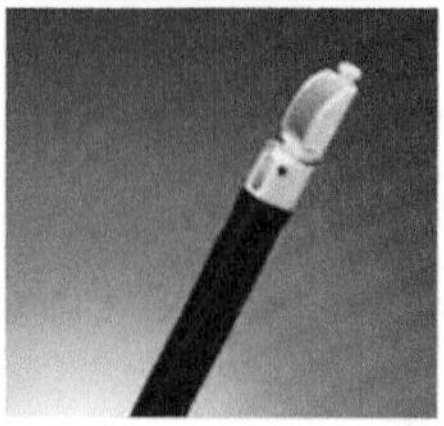	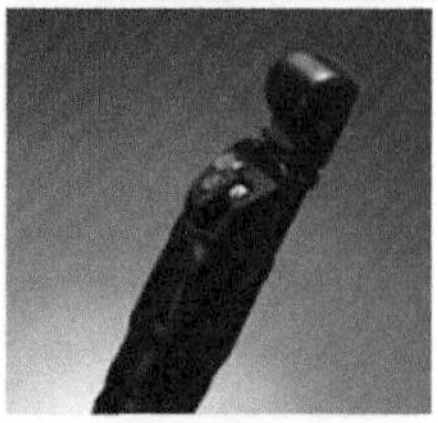
Diameter of Tip	6.9 mm	13–14.6 mm
Diameter of Endoscope	6.2 mm	11.8–12.8 mm
Scanning Range		
	50˚	120–180˚
Needle Size	21, 22G	19–25G
Channel Size	2.2 mm	2.8–3.7 mm

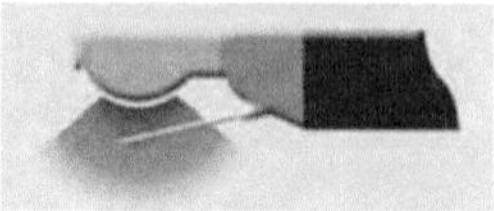

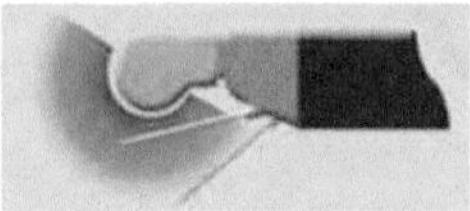

Fig. 3. Comparison of EBUS-TBNA and EUS-FNA.

curved linear-array transducer attached on the tip. Various EUS scopes from different companies are available for performing EUS-FNA (see **Fig. 3**). The outer diameter of the insertion tube of the EUS scope ranges from 11.8 to 12.8 mm, and that of the tip is 13 to 14.6 mm. The inner diameter of the instrument channel is 2.8 to 3.7 mm. The dedicated 22-gauge needles are usually used, but smaller (25-gauge) and larger (19-gauge) needles are also available.

The ultrasonographic image is processed by connecting the EUS scope to either the dedicated ultrasound scanner (EU-C60; Olympus), the universal endoscopic ultrasound scanner (EU-ME1; Olympus) or the Aloka Prosound Alpha5 (Aloka), thus enabling tissue visualization at a radius of 2 to 10 cm around the esophagus.

PROCEDURAL TECHNIQUE
Anesthesia

EBUS-TBNA and EUS-FNA can be performed on an outpatient basis under conscious sedation. For EBUS-TBNA the bronchoscope is usually inserted orally, because the ultrasound probe on the tip will limit nasal insertion. Some investigators prefer the use of the endotracheal tube or laryngeal mask airway under general anesthesia. An endotracheal tube larger than or equal to size 8 is recommended for use, relative to the size of the EBUS-TBNA scope. Cough reflex is minimal under general anesthesia, which may be an advantage during the procedure. The disadvantage of the

endotracheal tube is that is causes the bronchoscope to lie in the central position within the airway, which creates difficulty in bringing its tip in close proximity to the trachea or bronchus. The use of the laryngeal mask airway has been shown to be useful during EBUS-TBNA.[17]

EBUS-TBNA

Bronchoscopic examination of the airway should be performed with a regular flexible bronchoscope before EBUS-TBNA. After achieving local anesthesia and conscious sedation, the CP-EBUS is inserted orally and passed through the vocal cords by visualizing the anterior angle of the glottis. Once the bronchoscope is introduced into the airway until the desired lymph node station is reached (**Fig. 4**A), the balloon is inflated with normal saline to achieve a maximum contact with the tissue of interest. The tip of the CP-EBUS is flexed and gently pressed against the airway (**Fig. 4**B). Ultrasonically visible vascular landmarks are used to identify the specific lymph node stations according to the International Lymph Node Map devised by the International Association for the Study of Lung Cancer (IASLC).[16] The Doppler mode is used to confirm and identify surrounding vessels as well as the blood flow within lymph nodes. After identifying the lesion of interest, the bronchoscopic image of the airway is simultaneously visualized to localize the insertion point of the needle. Once the point of entry is decided using small landmarks on the airway,

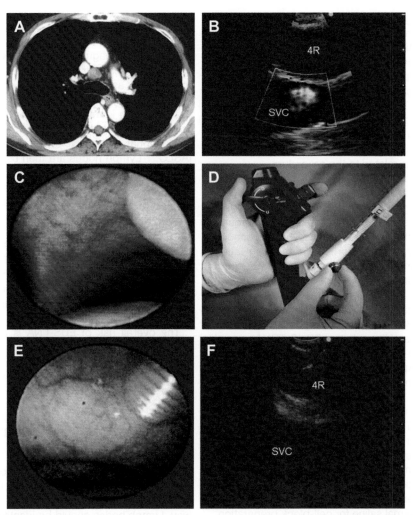

Fig. 4. EBUS-TBNA procedure. Computed tomography scan of an enlarged right lower paratracheal lymph node (*A*) and corresponding endobronchial ultrasonographic image of the right lower paratracheal lymph node (4R) and superior vena cava (SVC) confirmed by power Doppler mode (*B*). The outer sheath is adjusted and gently advanced out of the channel, which is confirmed by endoscopic image (*C, D*). The needle is passed through the intercartilage space (*E*) and into the lymph node (*F*).

the dedicated TBNA needle is fastened on to the working channel of the bronchoscope. The sheath adjuster knob is loosened and the length of the sheath is adjusted so that the sheath can be visualized on the endoscopic image (**Fig. 4**C, D). The tip of the bronchoscope is flexed up for contact and the lymph node is visualized again on the ultrasonographic image. After the needle-adjuster knob is loosened, the needle can be passed through the airway into the lymph node. The cartilaginous ring should be avoided during penetration (**Fig. 4**E). Once the needle is confirmed to be inside the lymph node (**Fig. 4**F), the internal stylet is used to clear out the internal lumen, which may become clogged with bronchial membrane. The internal stylet is then removed and negative pressure is applied with the Vaclok syringe. In the case of a hypervascular lymph node, negative pressure may cause bloody samples, therefore EBUS-TBNA can be done without suction. The needle is moved back and forth inside the lymph node to obtain samples. Finally, the needle is retrieved inside the outer sheath and the entire needle is removed from the bronchoscope.

CP-EBUS can access the upper paratracheal (stations 2R, 2L), lower paratracheal (stations 4R, 4L), subcarinal (station 7), and retrotracheal (station 3p) lymph nodes, but can also extend further to access the hilar (station 10), interlobar (station 11), and lobar (station 12) nodal stations. CP-EBUS cannot access the prevascular (station 3a), subaortic (station 5), para-aortic (station 6), paraesophageal (station 8), and pulmonary ligament (station 9) lymph nodes (see **Fig. 1**).

Complications related to EBUS-TBNA are similar to those of bronchoscopy and conventional TBNA and include pneumothorax, pneumomediastinum, hemomediastinum, mediastinitis, bacteremia, and pericarditis. To date there are no major complications reported in the literature. Although EBUS has enabled the bronchoscopist to see beyond the airway, one must be aware of the possible complications related to the procedure.

The standard EBUS classification system of sonographic features of lymph nodes is useful in predicting malignant versus benign lymph nodes. Lymph nodes larger than 1 cm in short axis, round shaped, with distinct margins, heterogeneous echogenicity, and the presence of coagulation necrosis sign and without the presence of central hilar structures, are suspicious for malignancy and need to be biopsied (**Fig. 5**).[18]

It is important to process the specimen obtained by EBUS-TBNA in a proper way to achieve maximum results. Although the EBUS-TBNA procedure can be performed successfully by following the steps explained in this article, handling of the specimen may differ between centers; as this may depend on the preference of the cytopathologist, one should follow one's own institutional standards. The internal stylet is usually used to push out samples. In the presence of a cytopathologist the first few drops are placed on the slide glass, and smears are made for rapid on-site cytologic evaluation using Diff-Quik staining. The rest of the specimen is placed in a 50-mL conical tube filled with normal saline for cell-block preparation. The remaining specimen within the needle is also washed in this conical tube.[15]

EUS-FNA

After introduction, the EUS scope is advanced into the distal esophagus and then slowly withdrawn while making circular movements. Anatomic landmarks such as the inferior vena cava, right and left atrium, azygos vein, main pulmonary artery, and aorta are identified. If present, lymph nodes are described and numbered according to the International Lymph Node Map devised by the IASLC.[16] Lymph nodes are then usually biopsied with a 22-gauge needle under real-time ultrasound guidance with monitoring of the needle during insertion and aspiration. Specimens can be judged for adequacy during the procedure, similar to EBUS-TBNA.

EUS can access the pulmonary ligament (station 9), paraesophageal (station 8), subcarinal (station 7), and paratracheal (stations 2, 4) lymph nodes. EUS usually cannot access the prevascular (station 3a), subaortic (station 5), para-aortic (station 6), and N1 lymph nodes.

The overall risk of EUS-FNA is approximately 0.5%, and may include perforation of the bowel wall or posterior pharynx, infection, hemorrhage, and cardiac or respiratory complications related to the sedation medications.

SYSTEMATIC ASSESSMENT OF MEDIASTINAL AND HILAR LYMPH NODES

During EBUS-TBNA or EUS-FNA, all of the mediastinal and hilar lymph nodes should be assessed, characterized, and documented in a systematic way. Lymph nodes should be identified according to the International Lymph Node Map devised by the IASLC.[16] The vascular anatomy is used

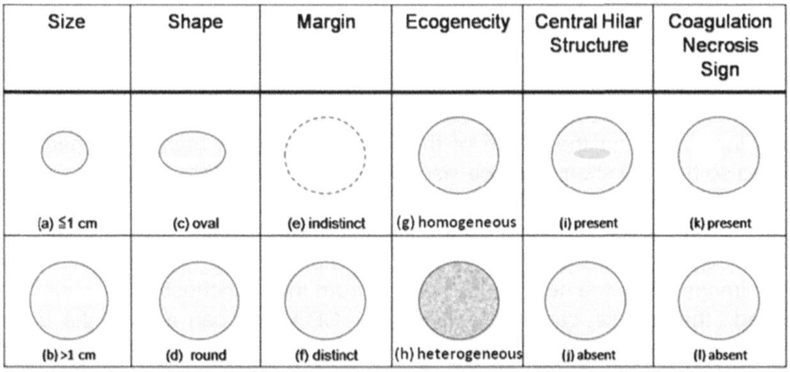

Size	Shape	Margin	Ecogenecity	Central Hilar Structure	Coagulation Necrosis Sign
(a) ≤1 cm	(c) oval	(e) indistinct	(g) homogeneous	(i) present	(k) present
(b) >1 cm	(d) round	(f) distinct	(h) heterogeneous	(j) absent	(l) absent

Fig. 5. Sonographic features of lymph nodes during endobronchial ultrasonography. Lymph nodes with the following characteristics are independent predictive factors for lymph node metastasis and should be biopsied: round shape, heterogeneous echogenicity, distinct margin, and presence of coagulation necrosis sign. (*From* Fujiwara T, Yasufuku K, Nakajima T, et al. The utility of sonographic features during endobronchial ultrasound-guided transbronchial needle aspiration for lymph node staging in patients with lung cancer: a standard endobronchial ultrasound image classification system. Chest 2010;138:641–7; with permission.)

for identification of the lymph nodes. During the initial assessment of the lymph node, the author prefers to start from the ipsilateral hilum, working up into the mediastinum, and ending in the contralateral hilum. To avoid contamination and up-staging, EBUS-TBNA and EUS-FNA should be performed from the N3 nodes, followed by N2 and N1 nodes.

Representative lymph node stations and bronchoscopic and anatomic landmarks for optimal ultrasonographic visualization are now explained in detail (**Fig. 6**).

EBUS-TBNA

Station 11R
The bronchoscope is advanced into the intermediate bronchus. Turn to the 2-o'clock position and flex the tip just distal to the bifurcation of the right upper lobe bronchus and the intermediate bronchus. Station 11R can be visualized with the interlobar pulmonary artery running distal to the lymph node.

Station 10R
Withdraw the bronchoscope to the right main bronchus. Turn the tip to the 3-o'clock position and flex the tip to visualize station 10R. Lymph nodes identified distal to the azygos vein represent station 10R.

Station 7
Station 7 can be visualized from either the right or the left main bronchus. On the right side, turn to the 12-o'clock position and flex the tip against the right main bronchus to visualize the right main pulmonary artery. After confirmation with the Doppler mode, turn the tip counterclockwise to the 9-o'clock position to visualize station 7.

Station 4R
Withdraw the bronchoscope to the trachea looking straight toward the main carina. Turn to the 2-o'clock position and flex the tip just proximal to the main carina. Visualize the superior vena cava (SVC) and the azygos vein branching from the SVC. Station 4R is located proximal to the azygos vein close to the SVC.

Station 2R
While visualizing the SVC on the ultrasonographic image, withdraw the bronchoscope maintaining contact with the trachea at the 2- to 3-o'clock position. The SVC will bifurcate to the left and right brachiocephalic veins. When the bronchoscope is further withdrawn, the innominate artery can be identified. Follow the innominate artery medially back to the aortic arch. Any lymph node proximal

to the aortic arch right side of the trachea is station 2R.

Station 2L
The aortic arch is the vascular landmark for differentiating stations 2 and 4. Lymph nodes present on the left side of the trachea above the aortic arch constitute station 2L.

Station 4L
Facing the main carina, turn the bronchoscope to the 10-o'clock position and flex the tip just proximal to the main carina, and scan the area for station 4L. The aortic arch can be followed to the aortopulmonary window.

Station 10L
Advance the bronchoscope into the left main bronchus at the 10-o'clock position by following the left pulmonary artery on the ultrasonographic image. This area is station 10L.

Station 11L
Further advancing the bronchoscope into the left lower lobe bronchus, flex the tip at the 2-o'clock position in the carina of the upper and lower lobe bronchus. Station 11L is visualized adjacent to the interlobar pulmonary artery.

EUS-FNA

Station 9
The EUS scope is advanced into the distal esophagus and then slowly withdrawn while making circular movements. The inferior vena cava can be identified. Station 9 can be visualized around the distal esophagus.

Station 8
The EUS scope is further pulled back in circular movements. The left atrium is the anatomic landmark to identify station 8.

Station 7
The right main stem pulmonary artery can be identified by further pulling back the EUS scope. High echoic bands on the right of the pulmonary artery correlate to the trachea or left main bronchus. Using slow circular movements, the EUS scope is positioned so that the high echoic band is at the further right of the monitor: this is the subcarinal space, where station 7 can be identified.

Station 4L
After visualization of the subcarinal lymph node, the EUS scope is slightly pulled back and turned counterclockwise, where station 4L can be visualized between the right main pulmonary artery and the aortic arch.

#4R (EBUS-TBNA)

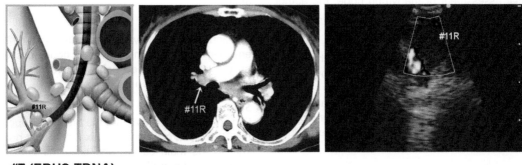

#7 (EBUS-TBNA)

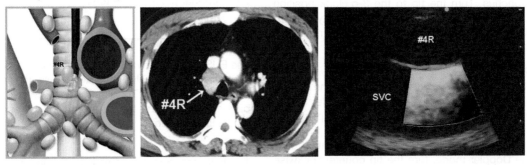

#4R (EBUS-TBNA)

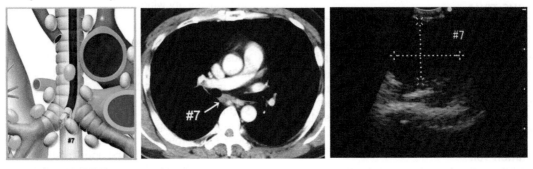

#2R (EBUS-TBNA)

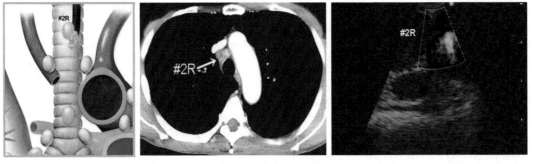

Fig. 6. Representative lymph node stations and anatomic landmarks for optimal ultrasonographic visualization.

LYMPH NODE STAGING FOR NSCLC
EBUS-TBNA

Ever since the first report of the CP-EBUS in 1994,[19] EBUS-TBNA has quickly assumed a prominent role

in lymph node staging of lung cancer.[20] Multiple studies have demonstrated high sensitivity, specificity, and diagnostic accuracy of EBUS-TBNA for mediastinal lymph node staging. One of the earlier prospective studies demonstrated sensitivity of

#4L (EBUS-TBNA)

#8 (EUS-FNA)

#7 (EUS-FNA)

#4L (EUS-FNA)

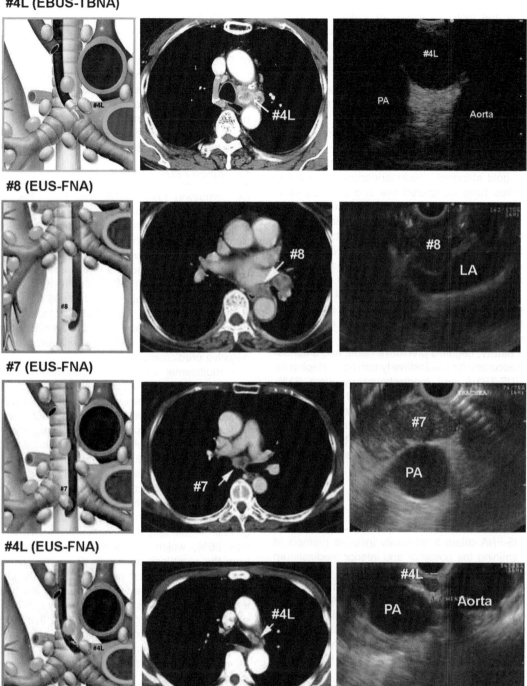

Fig. 6. *(continued)*

94.6%, specificity of 100%, positive predictive value of 100%, negative predictive value of 89.5%, and diagnostic accuracy of 96.3% for mediastinal lymph node staging. Not only did EBUS-TBNA provide reliable and pathologic staging, but it also was shown to significantly affect treatment decisions in the management of lung cancer.[21] The largest prospective study in 502 patients with lung cancer reported a sensitivity of 94%; however, given the high prevalence of malignancy in the studied population (98.2%), the negative predictive value was only 11%.[22] Furthermore, multiple prospective series and meta-analyses have demonstrated the safety, efficacy, and high diagnostic yield of EBUS-TBNA,[23–31] and it has been adopted as a modality in the American College of Chest Physicians evidence-based practice guidelines (second edition) for invasive staging of lung cancer.[9]

The ultimate question for thoracic surgeons is perhaps how EBUS-TBNA compares with the gold standard, mediastinoscopy. Only a few studies have compared the two procedures in a prospective controlled way.[32,33] A head-to-head comparison of EBUS-TBNA and mediastinoscopy in 153 potentially resectable patients with lung cancer demonstrated that EBUS-TBNA was able to sample an amount of lymph nodes equivalent to that sampled by mediastinoscopy and that in 91% of patients, there was excellent agreement between the two techniques over the stage of the mediastinum ($\kappa = 0.8$). The specificity and positive predictive value of both tests were 100%. The sensitivity, negative predictive value, and diagnostic accuracy for mediastinal lymph node staging for EBUS-TBNA and mediastinoscopy were 81%, 91%, and 93%, and 79%, 90%, and 93%, respectively, without any statistically significant differences. In a controlled setting where experienced thoracic surgeons are performing the procedure with rapid on-site cytology available, EBUS-TBNA was equivalent to mediastinoscopy for staging of the mediastinum.[33]

EUS-FNA

EUS-FNA offers a minimally invasive method of examining the posterior and inferior mediastinum in patients with lung cancer. EUS was established as a modality to evaluate the mediastinum in the early 1990s, and the role of EUS-FNA in NSCLC staging continues to evolve, with a relatively high sensitivity (74%–92%).[12,34–42] Unlike other invasive staging modalities such as EBUS-TBNA and mediastinoscopy, the sensitivity of EUS-FNA seems to be affected by variables such as size of the nodes, side of the tumor, and nodal station. EUS-FNA is reported to have a low negative predictive value of 73%, and is not a very reliable test in ruling out lymph node spread. Most investigators agree that negative results of EUS-FNA should be verified by other invasive staging modalities, especially in the presence of suggestive imaging.

EUS-FNA has also been compared with mediastinoscopy. In a prospective study of 60 patients, the sensitivity of EUS-FNA in the right paratracheal

lymph node station (station 4R) was 67%, versus 33% for mediastinoscopy. At the left paratracheal (station 4L), EUS-FNA was also more sensitive than mediastinoscopy (80% vs 33%). The sensitivity of EUS-FNA at the subcarinal station (station 7) was 100%, versus only 7% for mediastinoscopy. The results of the yield for mediastinoscopy are much lower than what has been reported in the past; however, for lymph node stations out of the reach of mediastinoscopy, EUS-FNA would seem to be the modality of choice.[39]

Combined EBUS and EUS

By combining EBUS-TBNA and EUS-FNA, the majority of the mediastinum as well as the hilar lymph nodes can be sampled. Multiple investigators have used the combined approach for invasive staging, some using a single EBUS-TBNA scope for both procedures, with excellent sensitivity ranging from 91.1% to 100% with a high negative predictive value of 91% to 95%.[43–46] To date, the combined EBUS/EUS approach has been shown to be more sensitive than EBUS or EUS independently, with a significantly better negative predictive value.

A multicenter randomized controlled trial in 241 patients with resectable NSCLC compared surgical staging alone with a combined EBUS/EUS approach followed by surgical staging if no metastases were found by endosonography.[47] Of the 123 patients who started with endosonography, 67 patients actually underwent mediastinoscopy, with nodal metastases being missed in 4 patients and a corresponding sensitivity of 94% and negative predictive value of 93%. In the mediastinoscopy-alone group, the sensitivity was 80% ($P = .04$) and the negative predictive value was 86%, which was statistically no different from the combined approach ($P = .26$). Despite the lack of difference in negative predictive value, the study demonstrated that the number of unnecessary thoracotomies was reduced by half in the combined-approach group. Based on this study, a new strategy for invasive staging was suggested, which begins with combined EBUS/EUS followed by mediastinoscopy if the lymph node metastasis is not demonstrated.

SUMMARY

EBUS-TBNA and EUS-FNA have emerged as a minimally invasive endoscopic modality for lymph node staging of NSCLC, with excellent results. There is ongoing debate about who should be performing EBUS/EUS and whether endoscopic staging should completely replace mediastinoscopy. However, the most important issue is how thoracic surgeons should incorporate the different modalities into the algorithm of mediastinal staging. Based on the current evidence, it is likely that the future of mediastinal staging lies in a combination of mediastinoscopy with EBUS and EUS. At present, not all institutions that practice thoracic surgery have the equipment, expertise, or trained personnel to safely and reliably perform endoscopic staging. Mediastinoscopy is still the gold standard for any thoracic surgeon, and should be the method of choice for invasive staging of the mediastinum in settings where endoscopic staging is not available or not optimal.

Based on the current evidence, EBUS-TBNA and EUS-FNA presents a minimally invasive procedure as an alternative to mediastinoscopy for mediastinal staging of NSCLC with discrete N2 or N3 lymph node enlargement, provided negative results are confirmed by surgical staging. If the pretest probability of lymph node metastasis is low with adequate sampling on EBUS/EUS, mediastinoscopy may not be necessary. EBUS/EUS has replaced mediastinoscopy in many patients with diffuse mediastinal adenopathy, in whom a simple tissue diagnosis is required to determine treatment. Endoscopic staging offers the advantage of obtaining a diagnosis and lymph node staging simultaneously under local anesthetic. Initial mediastinal lymph node staging by endoscopic staging will allow surgical staging to be reserved for restaging after induction treatment.

REFERENCES

1. Siegel R, Naishadham D, Jemal A. Cancer statistics, 2012. CA Cancer J Clin 2012;62:10–29.
2. Silvestri GA, Gould MK, Margolis ML, et al, American College of Chest Physicians. Non-invasive staging of non-small cell lung cancer: ACCP evidence-based clinical practice guidelines (2nd edition). Chest 2007;132:178s–201s.
3. Kramer H, Groen HJM. Current concepts in the mediastinal lymph node staging of nonsmall cell lung cancer. Ann Surg 2003;238:180–8.
4. Grondin SC, Liptay MJ. Current concepts in the staging of non-small cell lung cancer. Surg Oncol 2002;11:181–90.
5. Spiro SG, Porter JC. Lung cancer—where are we today? Current advances in staging and nonsurgical treatment. Am J Respir Crit Care Med 2002;166:1166–96.
6. Pieterman RM, van Putten JW, Meuzelaar JJ, et al. Preoperative staging of non-small cell lung cancer with positron emission tomography. N Engl J Med 2000;343:254–61.
7. Yasufuku K, Fujisawa T. Staging and diagnosis of non-small cell lung cancer: invasive modalities. Respirology 2007;12:173–83.
8. Toloza EM, Harpole L, Detterbeck F, et al. Invasive staging of Non-small cell lung cancer: a review of the current evidence. Chest 2003;123:157s–66s.
9. Detterbeck FC, Jantz MA, Wallace MB, et al. Invasive mediastinal staging of lung cancer. ACCP evidence-based clinical practice guidelines (2nd edition). Chest 2007;132:202s–20s.
10. De Leyn P, Lardinois D, Van Schil PE, et al. ESTS guidelines for preoperative lymph node staging for non-small cell lung cancer. Eur J Cardiothorac Surg 2007;32:1–8.
11. Kondo D, Imaizumi M, Abe T, et al. Endoscopic ultrasound examination for mediastinal lymph node metastases of lung cancer. Chest 1990;98:586–93.
12. Wallace MB, Silvestri GA, Sahai AV, et al. Endoscopic ultrasound-guided fine needle aspiration for staging patients with carcinoma of lung cancer. Chest 2000;117:339–45.
13. Fritscher-Ravens A, Davidson BL, Hauber HP, et al. Endoscopic ultrasound, positron emission tomography, and computerized tomography for lung cancer. Am J Respir Crit Care Med 2003;168:1293–7.
14. Eloubeidi MA, Cerfolio RJ, Chen VK, et al. Endoscopic ultrasound-guided fine needle aspiration of mediastinal lymph node in patients with suspected lung cancer after positron emission tomography and computed tomography scans. Ann Thorac Surg 2005;79:263–8.
15. Yasufuku K, Nakajima T. Endobronchial ultrasound guided transbronchial needle aspiration mannual. Tokyo: Kanehara and Co, LTD; 2009.
16. Rusch VW, Asamura H, Watanabe H, et al. The IASLC lung cancer staging project: a proposal for a new international lymph node map in the forthcoming seventh edition of the TNM classification for lung cancer. J Thorac Oncol 2009;4:568–77.
17. Sarkiss M, Kennedy M, Riedel B, et al. Anesthesia technique for endobronchial ultrasound-guided fine needle aspiration of mediastinal lymph node. J Cardiothorac Vasc Anesth 2007;21:892–6.
18. Fujiwara T, Yasufuku K, Nakajima T, et al. The utility of sonographic features during endobronchial ultrasound-guided transbronchial needle aspiration for lymph node staging in patients with lung cancer: a standard endobronchial ultrasound image classification system. Chest 2010;138:641–7.
19. Yasufuku K, Chhajed PN, Sekine Y, et al. Endobronchial ultrasound using a new convex probe—a preliminary study on surgically resected specimens. Oncol Rep 2004;11:293–6.
20. Yasufuku K, Chiyo M, Sekine Y, et al. Real-time endobronchial ultrasound-guided transbronchial needle aspiration of mediastinal and hilar lymph nodes. Chest 2004;126:122–8.
21. Yasufuku K, Chiyo M, Koh E, et al. Endobronchial ultrasound guided transbronchial needle aspiration for staging of lung cancer. Lung Cancer 2005;50:347–54.

22. Herth FJ, Eberhardt R, Vilmann P, et al. Real-time endobronchial ultrasound guided transbronchial needle aspiration for sampling mediastinal lymph nodes. Thorax 2006;61:795–8.

23. Rintoul RC, Skwarski KM, Murchison JT, et al. Endobronchial and endoscopic ultrasound-guided real-time fine-needle aspiration for mediastinal staging. Eur Respir J 2005;25:416–21.

24. Yasufuku K, Nakajima T, Motoori K, et al. Comparison of endobronchial ultrasound, positron emission tomography, and CT for lymph node staging of lung cancer. Chest 2006;130:710–8.

25. Herth FJ, Eberhardt R, Krasnik M, et al. Endobronchial ultrasound-guided transbronchial needle aspiration of lymph nodes in the radiologically and positron emission tomography-normal mediastinum in patients with lung cancer. Chest 2008;133:887–91.

26. Bauwens O, Dusart M, Pierard P, et al. Endobronchial ultrasound and value of PET for prediction of pathological results of mediastinal hot spots in lung cancer patients. Lung Cancer 2008;61:356–61.

27. Hwangbo B, Kim SK, Lee HS, et al. Application of endobronchial ultrasound-guided transbronchial needle aspiration following integrated PET/CT in mediastinal staging of potentially operable non-small cell lung cancer. Chest 2009;135:1280–7.

28. Herth FJ, Annema JT, Eberhardt R, et al. Endobronchial ultrasound with transbronchial needle aspiration for restaging the mediastinum in lung cancer. J Clin Oncol 2008;26:3346–50.

29. Gu P, Zhao YZ, Jiang LY, et al. Endobronchial ultrasound-guided transbronchial needle aspiration for staging of lung cancer: a systematic review and meta-analysis. Eur J Cancer 2009;45:1389–96.

30. Varela-Lema L, Fernandez-Villar A, Ruano-Ravina A. Effectiveness and safety of endobronchial ultrasound-transbronchial needle aspiration: a systematic review. Eur Respir J 2009;33:1156–64.

31. Adams K, Shah PL, Edmonds L, et al. Test performance of endobronchial ultrasound and transbronchial needle aspiration biopsy for mediastinal staging in patient with lung cancer: systematic review and meta-analysis. Thorax 2009;64:757–62.

32. Ernst A, Anantham D, Eberhardt R, et al. Diagnosis of mediastinal adenopathy—real-time endobronchial ultrasound guided needle aspiration versus mediastinoscopy. J Thorac Oncol 2008;3:577–82.

33. Yasufuku K, Pierre A, Darling G, et al. A prospective controlled trial of endobronchial ultrasound-guided transbronchial needle aspiration compared with mediastinoscopy for mediastinal lymph node staging of lung cancer. J Thorac Cardiovasc Surg 2011;142(6):1393–400.

34. Hawes RH, Gress F, Kesler KA, et al. Endoscopic ultrasound versus computed tomography in the evaluation of the mediastinum in patients with non-small-cell lung cancer. Endoscopy 1994;26:784–7.

35. Silvestri GA, Hoffman BJ, Bhutani MS, et al. Endoscopic ultrasound with fine-needle aspiration in the diagnosis and staging of lung cancer. Ann Thorac Surg 1996;61:1441–5.

36. Larsen SS, Krasnik M, Vilmann P, et al. Endoscopic ultrasound guided biopsy of mediastinal lesions has a major impact on patient management. Thorax 2002;57:98–103.

37. Fritscher-Ravens A. Endoscopic ultrasound evaluation in the diagnosis and staging of lung cancer. Lung Cancer 2003;41:259–67.

38. Kużdżał J, Szlubowski A. Ultrasound-guided transbronchial and transesophageal needle biopsy in the mediastinal staging of lung cancer. Thorac Surg Clin 2012;22(2):191–203.

39. Larsen SS, Vilmann P, Krasnik M, et al. Endoscopic ultrasound guided biopsy versus mediastinoscopy for analysis of paratracheal and subcarinal lymph nodes in lung cancer staging. Lung Cancer 2005;48(1):85–92.

40. Annema JT, Versteegh MI, Veselic M, et al. Endoscopic ultrasound-guided fine-needle aspiration in the diagnosis and staging of lung cancer and its impact on surgical staging. J Clin Oncol 2005;23(33):8357–61.

41. Talebian M, Bartheld von MB, Braun J, et al. EUS-FNA in the preoperative staging of non-small cell lung cancer. Lung Cancer 2010;69(1):60–5.

42. Witte B, Neumeister W, Huertgen M. Does endoesophageal ultrasound-guided fine-needle aspiration replace mediastinoscopy in mediastinal staging of thoracic malignancies? Eur J Cardiothorac Surg 2008;33(6):1124–8.

43. Vilmann P, Krasnik M, Larsen SS, et al. Transesophageal endoscopic ultrasound-guided fine-needle aspiration (EUS-FNA) and endobronchial ultrasound-guided transbronchial needle aspiration (EBUS-TBNA) biopsy: a combined approach in the evaluation of mediastinal lesions. Endoscopy 2005;37:833–9.

44. Wallace MB, Pascual JM, Raimondo M, et al. Minimally invasive endoscopic staging of suspected lung cancer. JAMA 2008;299(5):540–6.

45. Herth FJF, Krasnik M, Kahn N, et al. Combined endoscopic-endobronchial ultrasound-guided fine-needle aspiration of mediastinal lymph nodes through a single bronchoscope in 150 patients with suspected lung cancer. Chest 2010;138(4):790–4.

46. Hwangbo B, Lee GK, Lee HS, et al. Transbronchial and transesophageal fine-needle aspiration using an ultrasound bronchoscope in mediastinal staging of potentially operable lung cancer. Chest 2010;138(4):795–802.

47. Annema JT, van Meerbeeck JP, Rintoul RC, et al. Mediastinoscopy vs endosonography for mediastinal nodal staging of lung cancer: a randomized trial. JAMA 2010;304(20):2245–52.

Biomarkers and Molecular Testing for Early Detection, Diagnosis, and Therapeutic Prediction of Lung Cancer

Harvey I. Pass, MD[a],*, David G. Beer, PhD[b],
Sasha Joseph, MD[c], Pierre Massion, MD[d]

KEYWORDS

- Biomarkers • Genome sequencing • microRNA • Genomics • Proteomics • Epigenomics

KEY POINTS

- Genomic, proteomic, and epigenomic biomarkers are being investigated for the early detection, diagnosis, and prediction of therapy response in lung cancer.
- Biomarkers must be validated using one or more cohorts after discovery, ideally in blinded cohorts, and in well-controlled prospective trials.
- Although there are many studies of lung cancer biomarkers, none except for prediction of response for certain targeted therapies have been validated for clinical use.
- It is hoped that sequencing of the lung cancer genome will discover novel potential biomarkers for diagnosis, prognosis, and treatment to supplement those in clinical practice, including EGFR mutation analysis and EML4-ALK translocation fluorescence in situ hybridization.

INTRODUCTION

In the era of personalized medicine, the goal is to be able to segregate groups of patients by defining (1) a diagnosis, (2) the risk for death or recurrence of disease (prognosis), or (3) the proper therapy for the appropriate patient to maximize treatment response (prediction).[1,2] Discovery and validation of biomarkers is central to this goal. The complexity of biomarker discovery, however, is amplified by the multitude of platforms on which the biomarker will be discovered (mutational sequencing,[3-5] fluorescence in situ hybridization (FISH),[6] single-nucleotide polymorphisms (SNPs),[7] copy-number variation (CNV) of chromosomes,[8] immunohistochemistry, epigenetics including methylation studies,[9] or microRNA[10]), and by the material used (tissue, plasma, serum, urine, breath, sputum, effusion). The aim is to be able to define these biomarkers in a way whereby their use is contingent on maximal accuracy, which depends on the ability of biomarker researchers to not only put forth markers with the greatest sensitivity and specificity, but also to be able to validate these biomarkers in a methodologic algorithm that will satisfy regulatory bodies including the Food and Drug Administration (FDA) in the United States as well as other agencies abroad.

Where do thoracic surgeons fit in this complicated scheme and what are the basic principles to comprehend in this continuously changing fund of knowledge? For patients with early disease

[a] Department of Cardiothoracic Surgery, NYU Langone Medical Center, 530 First Avenue, 9V, New York, NY 10016, USA; [b] Section of Thoracic Surgery, Department of Surgery, University of Michigan Health System, 2120 Taubman Center, Ann Arbor, MI 48109-5344, USA; [c] Division of Medical Oncology, Department of Medicine, 550 First Avenue, NYU Langone Clinical Cancer Center, New York, NY 10016, USA; [d] Vanderbilt-Ingram Cancer Center, 640 PRB, 2220 Pierce Avenue, Nashville, TN 37232, USA
* Corresponding author.
E-mail address: Harvey.Pass@nyumc.org

Thorac Surg Clin 23 (2013) 211–224
http://dx.doi.org/10.1016/j.thorsurg.2013.01.002
1547-4127/13/$ – see front matter © 2013 Elsevier Inc. All rights reserved.

amenable to surgery, the bare essentials for thoracic surgeons include the realization that they are on the front line in (1) procuring the necessary materials for potentially determining whether a patient is a candidate for novel targeted therapies, and (2) biomarker discovery along with molecular pathologists and other investigators. In addition, thoracic surgeons must be prepared to provide the necessary demographic data to aid in the documentation of the fidelity of a marker for defining, for example, time to progression or death. These correlative data, and the compulsion with which they are recorded, are only partially answered by large databases such as the Society of Thoracic Surgery Database, because recurrence and survival data for the treatment of lung cancer are not part of its fields. Robust discovery and validation can only be accomplished with databases that are prospectively maintained, updated, and constantly queried for errors. Finally, in some geographic regions, surgeons are charged with the treatment of patients who qualify for adjuvant therapy without the involvement of medical oncologists, and thus must be familiar with the biomarkers already validated for use in this setting, the tissue requirements for their investigation, and the limitations of the presently available molecular tests. Independent of whether they will be charged with the final decision regarding which drug to use based on which biomarker, thoracic surgeons in 2013 are a key element of multidisciplinary lung cancer tumor boards, and should be well versed with common molecular tests.

This field is changing so rapidly, is so complex, and can be so deeply confusing that any manuscript on the subject is outdated before it is published. Hence, in the spirit of Bob Ginsberg who, despite an astounding familiarity with many subjects, insisted on focusing on the big picture instead of extraneous nonsense, this contribution is designed as a basic primer of molecular testing and biomarkers for the busy (but interested!) thoracic surgeon so that he or she will be well armed with the basic details necessary to speak up (or at least ask reasonable questions) about the subject at any tumor board. To do this a "grocery list" of all the markers or platforms that have ever been investigated, as appears in many reviews, is not provided. Only the relevant ones are discussed in a systematic way. Three large classes of biomarkers are discussed: (1) early detection/diagnosis, (2) prognostic, and (3) predictive. It is important, however, to have a basic knowledge of the technologic platforms that have been used either to discover these markers or are used in specialized, government-approved laboratories (clinical laboratory improvement amendments [CLIA]) to generate reports back to physicians regarding these markers. For the discussion of the particular biomarkers or molecular tests, this article briefly concentrates on the role they play in the carcinogenesis of lung cancer and how they are measured, followed by a review of only the seminal publications that affirm the present or future utility of the biomarker in the management of patients.

PLATFORMS USED TO MEASURE BIOMARKERS

Biomarkers can be measured from many sources including tissue, blood elements (plasma, serum, and mononuclear cells), effusions, urine, and even breath.[11,12] Ideally the biomarkers in tissue are measured in formalin-fixed paraffin-embedded tissue to avoid the use of "snap-frozen" or "fresh" specimens. The platforms that are used for these measurements are generally categorized as genomic, epigenomic, and proteomic.

Genomics

Genomics represents the analyses of genetic material (ie, DNA and RNA) in a multiplexed method, enabling the testing of multiple "genes" at the same time.

The most common method used for the discovery of biomarkers involves the use of gene-expression microarrays as a laboratory on a glass or silicon chip.[13] Each DNA spot (probe) represents a specific DNA sequence that could be a short section of a gene or other portion of DNA. The probes are joined to complementary pieces of nucleic acid material (derived from the specimen being investigated, called the target) that has been labeled so that the number of probe-target interactions can be quantitated. Individual genes can be quantitated by using specific probes for that gene instead of using the whole microarray through the process of quantitative polymerase chain reaction (qPCR).[13] qPCR is used to simultaneously amplify and quantify a DNA molecule as an absolute number of copies of that DNA or as a ratio normalized to other genes. Cutoff levels based roughly on the number of amplifications of the DNA allows for classification of genes as high expression or low expression. Using a process called real-time PCR, multiple sequences can be quantitated simultaneously.

Individual chromosomal quantitation of gains and deletions of portions of chromosomes can be performed using the technique of CNV,[14] and these techniques have been applied to microarray technologies. For an even more specific method of looking at specific gene amplifications, deletions, translocations, or fusions, FISH is performed.[6] By using probes that bind with the specific region of the chromosome where the gene is located, as well as using probes to mark specific regions of a specific chromosome, the number of copies of a specific gene can be quantitated.

In addition to knowing that the expression of a gene is abnormally increased or decreased, it is important to understand whether the reason for aberrant expression is based on a specific mutation or mutations of that gene.[5] It is not difficult to conceptualize that a mutation in one or both alleles of a gene would downregulate the expression of that particular gene; however, a new concept that must be understood is that of mutations causing oncogene addiction. This concept was introduced to emphasize the apparent dependency of some cancers on one or a few genes or proteins for the maintenance of the malignant phenotype. The reasons for this phenomenon are multifaceted, but the theory is that this important gene is a master controller of one or more crucial pathways for the cell to avoid self-destruction by apoptosis, and the mutation alters the balance of control of these pathways. Hence, the search for any and all mutations in lung cancer, searching for crucial genes that may be targeted for therapeutic intervention by small molecules or other means, has led to mutation testing.[15] To interpret mutations in the genome one must first have the normal sequence of the human genome, and the magnitude of this effort is evident when one considers that this involved 3.2 billion base pairs and 25,000 expressed genes (which in reality represents only 2% of the genome).[16] The original cost of the project was US$70 million; the genome can now be commercially sequenced using next-generation techniques (NGS) for approximately $4,000. NGS and "massive-parallel" DNA sequencing are high-throughput DNA sequencing technologies that sequence large numbers of different DNA sequences in a single reaction (ie, in parallel). All NGS technologies monitor the sequential addition of nucleotides to immobilized and spatially arrayed DNA templates, but differ substantially in how these templates are generated and how they are interrogated to reveal their sequences.

Another rapidly accelerating aspect of genomics is the measurement of microRNAs. MicroRNAs, or mirs, are a species of small (19–22 nucleotides) noncoding single-stranded RNA molecules that can interact with target mRNA molecules. Different microRNAs may function as tumor suppressors or oncogenes, and the deregulation of their expression is associated with the initiation and progression of cancers through activation and/or repression of controlling pathways.[17]

Epigenomics

Epigenomics refers to changes in the expression of genes caused by mechanisms other than changes in the underlying DNA sequence that will result in functionally relevant genomic modifications without changing the nucleotide sequence. These changes are generally classified as promoter methylation or histone modification.[18] DNA methylation involves promoter regions that are the sites of transcription initiation, and causes a repression of gene expression. Unmethylated promoter regions are associated with actively expressed genes. Histones, the most prevalent protein in protein-DNA complexes (chromatin), are responsible for condensing and packaging DNA. By remodeling chromatin structure through histone modification and changing the density of DNA packaging, gene expression can thus be modulated. A variety of posttranslational mechanisms can alter histones, leading to altered gene activation.[18]

Proteomics

Proteomics is the study of the proteome (the entire complement of proteins) including the modifications made to a particular set of proteins, and the goal of proteomic technologies is to find those very low-abundance proteins or their modifications that are specifically associated with malignancy.[19] The study of proteins may have advantages over genomic or epigenomic techniques, because (1) many proteins are modified, such as by phosphorylation that alters their activity; (2) different splice variants exist for proteins, which may have alternative activities in different states of disease; and (3) many proteins can only function when they form complexes with other proteins or nucleic acids. The binding of specific nucleic acid moieties to proteins has been exploited as a novel proteomic technique known as Aptamer or SomaMer (Slow Off Rate Modified Aptamers) technology.[20] Most techniques for biomarker discovery in proteomics, however, involve the use of mass spectroscopy with sequencing of peptide fragments to detect low-abundance proteins. Proteomics also involves the use of antibodies for the identification of novel biomarkers. These antibodies can be used in tissue using specific and sensitive immunohistochemical techniques. For serum of plasma measurements of a particular protein, the use of 2 or more antibodies to a particular protein, known as an enzyme-linked immunosorbent assay (ELISA), is one of the most common first-order methods for discovery and validation of potential protein. Another aspect of proteomics involves the measurement of autoantibodies generated as a response in the serum to a cancer as foreign (antigenic) phenomenon, and autoantibody arrays are presently being evaluated for this purpose.[21–24]

SPECIFIC BIOMARKERS OR PROFILES IN LUNG CANCER

For the busy thoracic surgeon, it is important to limit the discussion to those biomarkers that are most recent and have been at least partially validated by using a training and test set. This first step is the easiest by which to evaluate the robustness of a biomarker profile, and simply involves dividing from the outset all specimens in the experiment (ie, cases and controls) into a discovery set (training) and a test set (validation). The test set is put aside and is not evaluated until the biomarker panel is "locked in" from statistical and bioinformatics analyses of the discovery set. These markers are then ready to move on to a blinded validation using the identical types of materials harvested at another institution or institutions (which may have been archived or obtained in the context of a previously completed prospective trial). This section discusses the biomarkers that satisfy these requirements, according to the type of biomarker (early detection/diagnosis; prognostic; predictive of tumor response) and the type of material for biomarker exploration (tissue or blood elements).

Biomarkers for Early Detection and Diagnosis

Two broad categories of clinical relevance, early detection and diagnosis, can be addressed by biomarkers, and these categories may indeed be investigated as single markers or combinations of markers. The markers of early diagnosis may not necessarily be the same as those for diagnosis. Early-detection biomarkers address the risk of developing lung cancer or to have an early stage lung cancer and should be able to complement other methods for the early detection of lung cancer, specifically low-dose helical computed tomography (CT) scanning.[1] The ultimate goal is to decrease the number of unnecessary radiologic tests that must be performed and to present an enriched population of at-risk individuals for CT evaluation who have been found to have a biomarker profile which, with high sensitivity and specificity, either places them at risk for the development of lung cancer or signals the presence of an existing lung cancer. Diagnostic biomarkers would, it is hoped, reduce the number of abortive thoracotomies/thoracoscopies/needle or core biopsies by having high specificity for distinguishing a malignant nodule from a benign nodule. In this context the individual presents to the physician with an undiagnosed indeterminate

nodule seen on radiographic imaging that ideally is between 0.8 and 2 cm, and the biomarker would aid the physician in suggesting the next part of a diagnostic or therapeutic algorithm to follow.[25] Most studies in the literature have analyzed biomarkers from cohorts of patients with proven lung cancer with nodules of a given size range, compared with individuals who are age-matched and sex-matched smokers from the same institution, or with individuals having abortive thoracotomies (obviously a more difficult cohort to have suitable archived reagents). There are studies, however, which have taken advantage of patients in protocol-based screening studies of lung cancer to query the existence of early detection and diagnostic biomarkers (as well as prognostic biomarkers; see later discussion).[26]

As seen in **Table 1**, a variety of studies have been published that use different platforms in search of single or multiplexed markers of early disease or nodule differential diagnosis, and at present it is impossible to predict which ones will be successful in prospective validations.[19,20,22–36] Some of the more novel approaches include Spira's attempts to define a risk profile by using surrogate airway tissue gene expression (proximal airway biopsies) to see if they reflect the presence of a lung cancer, and his work is now being extended to studies of the more proximal respiratory tree, including nasal swab profiling.[29] Using proteomic techniques, Rahman and colleagues[30] were able successfully validate a prediction model that was diagnostic of lung cancer from bronchial biopsies by using a signature consisting of 9 matrix-assisted laser desorption/ionization mass spectrometry (MALDI-MS) mass-to-charge ratio features. Despite having some similarity in the pathways identified in these 2 studies, there is no overlap between the proteomic signature genes and the mRNA identified in the study by Spira and colleagues.[29] A less invasive approach for early detection would involve biomarker discovery using blood elements, specifically serum and plasma, and a variety of proteomic techniques (autoantibody, MALDI, Luminex, Aptamer) have defined various profiles with first-order validation (see **Table 1**). Despite excellent accuracy of the autoantibody platforms, only Annexin 1 has been found to be commonly expressed in 2 of the 4 methods.[22,24] The MALDI-MS platform originally described by Yildiz and colleagues[35] has now been refined to examine the proteome in a much deeper fashion, and future studies will describe newer, less abundant, but possibly more specific peptides for subsequent validation. The Aptamer/SomaMer platform, which apparently has a wider range and lower coefficient of variation for

Table 1
Early detection and diagnostic biomarkers for lung cancer

Authors,Ref. Year	Specimen	Type of Marker	Marker(s)	No. of Markers	Platform	Train (n)	Test (n)	Sensitivity (%)	Specificity (%)	AUC
Schmidt et al,[27] 2010	Bronchial aspirates	DNA methylation	SHOX2	1	PCR	n/a	523	68	95	86
Richards et al,[28] 2011	Tumors, normal tissues	DNA methylation	TCF21	1	PCR	42	63	76	98	n/a
Spira et al,[29] 2007	Airway epithelium	mRNA	Gene expression signature	80	Affy array	77	52	80	84	n/a
Rahman et al,[30] 2005	Bronchial biopsies	MALDI signature	TMLS4, ACBP, CSTA, cytoC, MIF, ubiquitin, ACBP, Des-ubiquitin	9	MALDI-MS	51	60	66	88	77
Zhong et al,[21] 2006	Serum	AutoAB	Phage peptides	5	ELISA	46	56	91	91	99
Qiu et al,[22] 2008	Serum	AutoAB	Annexin I, 14-3-3 theta, LAMR1	3	Protein array		170	51	82	73
Wu et al,[31] 2012	Serum	AutoAB	Phage peptide clones	6	ELISA	20	180	92	92	96
Boyle et al,[24] 2011	Serum	AutoAB	p53, NY-ESO-1, CAGE, GBU4-5, Annexin-1 and SOX2	6	ELISA	241	255	32	91	64
Begum et al,[32] 2011	Serum	DNA Methylation	APC, CDH1, MGMT, DCC, RASSF1A, AIM	6	qPCR	32–369	106	84	57	n/a
Chen et al,[33] 2012	Serum	MicroRNA	miRNA signature	10	qRT-PCR	310	310	93	90	97
Bianchi et al,[34] 2011	Serum	MicroRNA	miRNA signature	34	qRT-PCR	64	64	71	90	89
Yildiz et al,[35] 2007	Serum	Protein	MALDI-MS signature	7	MALDI-MS	185	106	58	86	82
Ostroff et al,[20] 2010	Serum	Aptamers	Aptamer Signature	12	Aptamers	985	341	89	83	90
Lee et al,[36] 2012	Serum	Luminex proteomics	AIAT, CYFRA 21-1, IGF-1, RANTES, AFP	5	Luminex	347	49	80.3	99.3	99.1
Shen et al,[37] 2011	Plasma	MicroRNA	miRNA-21, -126, -210, -486-5p	4	qRT-PCR	28	87	86	97	93
Kneip et al,[38] 2011	Plasma	DNA methylation	SHOX2	1	qPCR	40	371	60	90	78
Boeri et al,[26] 2011	Plasma	MicroRNA array and qRT-PCR	15 miRNA signature	15	miRNA array and qRT-PCR	20	15	80	90	85
Boeri et al,[26] 2011	Plasma	MicroRNA array and qRT-PCR	13 miRNA signature	13	miRNA array and qRT-PCR	19	16	75	100	88

Abbreviations: Affy, Affymetrix; AUC, area under the receiver-operating curve; ELISA, enzyme-linked immunosorbent assay; MALDI-MS, matrix-assisted laser desorption/ionization mass spectrometry; n/a, no data available; (q)PCR, Real Time PCR; (q)RT (quantitative) reverse transcription; Test, test or validation set; Train, training set.

discovery than other proteomic techniques, is limited by the number of nucleic acid aptamers synthesized to bind selectively to proteins in serum. Nevertheless, in a large multicenter study, excellent specificity and sensitivity distinguished lung cancer nodules for patients without nodules or with benign nodules.[20] The Luminex technique, essentially multiplexing multiple antibodies with serum or plasma using a beading technology, also has had promising validation of a 5-protein and 10-protein profile in two separate studies with one common marker, CYFRA 21.1.[36]

Probably the most rapidly advancing discipline for early diagnosis and detection has been the study of microRNAs in serum and plasma, aided by commercially available microarrays that can quantify the expression of the mature species. Although there are presently more than 1800 mature human microRNAs, most of the data have been generated from microarrays capable of detecting 400 to 800 microRNAs, and the number of mature human microRNAs is increasing with novel methods of discovery, including RNAseq.[39] The 5 studies in **Table 1** all have striking sensitivities and specificities for validation sets using signatures that range from 4 to 34 microRNAs; however, it is disappointing that only 2 studies[26,37] share 1 species (mir-21), which is commonly upregulated in malignancy. The study by Boeri and colleagues[26] is notable because of its use of two Italian screening protocols, one for discovery and the other for validation, and the investigators were able to describe reproducible signatures for high risk of lung cancer, diagnosis, and prognosis (see below).

Prognostication of Lung Cancer

Molecular prognostication of lung cancer could potentially predict those patients who, independent of stage, would be at higher risk for either recurrence or death following therapy. Possibly its greatest use would be in the delineation of patients with completely resected Stage I lung cancer who may need adjuvant therapy despite the small size of their malignancy. The studies to date have used single or multiple immunohistochemical markers, "best-guess" genes or combination of genes measured in tissue of blood, or expression microarray data using standard or custom oligochips to delineate individuals with short time to recurrence/death from those with long time to recurrence/death who are of the same pathologic stage (**Table 2**).

Lung tumors have significant morphologic and molecular heterogeneity[58] and, because of the large number of genetic alterations, development of lung carcinoma likely requires alterations of multiple pathways and genes. Individual markers are unlikely to be present in all tumors. There have been many articles documenting univariate and multivariate analyses for possible single markers, the majority of which have been assayed using immunohistochemical techniques. Immunohistochemistry results can be inconsistent or contradictory depending on the specificity of the antibodies, and immunohistochemical scoring is semiquantitative and subjective in determining the intensity of staining, the percentage of tumor cells stained, and cellular localization. Unfortunately, very few of these have gone on to independent validation, and some have been found to be part of multiplexed profiles.

Gene signatures are limited by inconsistent reproducibility in independent validation sets, and have been investigated using reverse transcription–polymerase chain reaction (RT-PCR) or expression arrays. Aside from the molecular heterogeneity of non–small cell lung cancer (NSCLC), the pathways involved may be more important than the specific genes because overexpression of different genes in the same pathway may have similar effects. Gene-expression profiling using microarrays allows the analysis of thousands of genes simultaneously to identify potential gene signatures for classifying patients with different clinical outcomes. Probably the most representative study involving a multi-institutional effort evaluated 442 lung adenocarcinomas through a consortium including the University of Michigan, Moffitt Cancer Center, Memorial Sloan-Kettering, the University of Toronto, and the Dana-Farber Cancer Institute, using common protocols, reagents, and a microarray platform. The complexity of this study is illustrated by that fact that there were 8 classifiers developed using various methods including gene clustering and univariate testing on a training set composed of samples from 2 of the institutions. It is both interesting and sobering that most of the models performed better when combined with clinical covariates, as previously described in prostate and breast cancers.[48] Other genomic profiles that have had impressive validation and are moving to prospective validation include those by Zhu and colleagues[51] and Kratz and colleagues.[53] Both studies were able to stratify adenocarcinoma patients into good or poor risk for survival cohorts. The study by Kratz and colleagues is remarkable for its series of large validation studies in formalin-fixed paraffin tissue as well as the international nature of the datasets.

Proteomic approaches have also involved the use of MALDI-MS technology in both tissue and blood. Yanagisawa and colleagues[59] described a proteomic classifier comprising 15 MALDI-MS signals that was able to classify American patients into good-prognosis and poor-prognosis groups, which included thymosin B10, thymosin B4, and calmodulin. Following up on this study, the same group used MALDI-MS to derive a prognosis-associated proteomic signature from 174 specimens from Japanese NSCLC tumors and 27 specimens from normal lung tissue, which were randomly divided into a training set (116 NSCLC and 20 normal lung specimens) and an independent, blinded validation set (58 NSCLC and 7 normal lung specimens).[60] Signals from the training set that were associated with specimens from relapsed patients who died within 5 years of surgical treatment were compared with those individuals who were alive with no symptoms of relapse after a median follow-up of 89 months. A signature of 25 signals was associated with both relapse-free survival and overall survival, also including thymosin B10 and thymosin B4. Xu and colleagues[61] expanded on these observations and further evaluated calmodulin, thymosin B4, and thymosin B10 for their prognostic values using immunohistochemistry (IHC). The combined IHC scores of the proteins were found to be correlated with NSCLC patient survival ($P = .004$). These data are encouraging for the initiation of future validation studies.

MicroRNA expression profiles have also been explored for prognostication of NSCLC, and a few of the studies have had validation with separate cohorts. Yanaihara and colleagues[54] used a microRNA microarray to determine profiles that correlated with survival in a cohort including Stage I lung adenocarcinomas. High levels of hsa-mir-155 and low hsa-let-7a-2 were correlated with poor survival, and these results were validated in an independent data set. Yu and colleagues[55] used RT-PCR to determine microRNA expression in 112 NSCLCs divided into training and test sets of 56 tumors each. A 5-microRNA signature was found to be an independent predictor of cancer recurrence and survival, and was validated in an independent set of 62 tumors. Two microRNAs, hsa-mir-221 and hsa-let-7a, were protective, whereas hsa-mir-137, hsa-mir-372, and hsa-mir-182 were associated with decreased overall and disease-free survival. The study by Saito and colleagues[57] was novel in that 3 separate geographically distinct cohorts were used to validate a predetermined 3-microRNA signature, and only mir-21 successfully predicted survival in all 3 cohorts. Finally, one of the more influential studies in the field has been the examination of prognostic microRNA profiles in the plasma from 2 Italian screening studies.[39] Using a microRNA microarray

in tissue and plasma from one cohort, the signature was validated for successful prognostication in the other. With all of the validated microRNA studies, a variety of microRNAs have been found to be associated with the signatures; however, the most common associating microRNAs have been the let-7 family, mir-221, and mir-21. Let-7 has been linked to ras,[62] and mir-21 acts as an anti-apoptotic factor and promotes cell proliferation.[63]

BIOMARKERS, MUTATIONS, AND PREDICTION OF TREATMENT RESPONSE

Mutational analysis of NSLCs has become increasingly important; not only for the treatment of disease but also for its prognostic and predictive value. In less than a decade, molecular profiling of NSCLC has become the standard of care. This section briefly discusses notable mutations in NSCLC, commenting on their significance for treatment (predictive value) and the prognostic value they provide the patient.

EGFR

Epidermal growth factor receptor (EGFR) is a receptor tyrosine kinase that is part of the same family of tyrosine kinase signaling receptors that include Her2 (a known target in breast cancer). Once activated, these tyrosine kinases drive both the RAS and the PI3 kinase pathways, allowing for cell proliferation and suppression of apoptosis.[64] Both overexpression of EGFR and activating mutations in the kinase domain of the intracellular portion of the receptor kinase have been demonstrated in lung malignancies. EGFR mutations in NSCLC most often occur in young, female nonsmokers of Asian ancestry. In Caucasian populations, EGFR mutations occur in 10% to 15% of NSCLC. EGFR-mutated NSCLC tend to have a better prognosis than other NSCLC, especially KRAS-mutated NSCLC.[65] PCR mutational analysis of EGFR focuses primarily on 2 mutations. The first, and more common, is in exon 19 and the second is in exon 21. It is important to remember that in metastatic NSCLC, the exon-19 mutation carries a more favorable prognosis than exon 21, as exon-21 mutations have a shorter duration of response to EGFR tyrosine kinase inhibitors.[66,67]

Over the last decade the main focus of targeted therapy in lung cancer has been this EGFR pathway, and mutational analysis of EGFR has become the biomarker standard for lung cancer therapy. With treatment options targeting the receptor on both sides of the cell membrane, there are effective ways to blockade EGFR. Erlotinib and gefitinib are small-molecule tyrosine kinase

Table 2
Prognostic biomarkers for lung cancer

Authors,[Ref.] Year	Platform	Histology/Stage	Train (n)	Test (n)	Findings
Skrzypski et al,[40] 2008	RT-PCR	SCC Stages I–IIIA	66	26	3-gene prognosis in SCC
Chen et al,[41] 2007	Customized array, RT-PCR	ADC, SCC, Stages I–III	125	New 65, in silico 86 (Beer[42])	5-gene independent predictor of TTP and OS
Beer et al,[42] 2002	Oligochip	ADC Stages I/II	43	43, in silico 84	50-gene prognostic signature for ADC
Raponi et al,[43] 2006	Oligochip	ADC	43 + 83 in silico	In silico 72	50-gene prognostic signature for ADC
Lu et al,[44] 2006	Oligochip	NSCLC Stage I	197 in silico	In silico 64	64-gene signature for OS. Nine genes part of previous databases
Larsen et al,[45] 2007	Oligochip	ADC Stages I/IIA	48	In silico 95	54-gene signature for TTP
Bianchi et al,[46] 2007	In silico discovery	NSCLC Stage I	101 in silico	70 new, 45 in silico	10-gene signature stratified patients by OS
Guo et al,[47] 2008	In silico discovery	ADC, SCC Stages I–III	170	Three in silico validation: 111, 24, 129	Independent 35-gene signature stratified patients by OS, including Stage I
Shedden et al,[48] 2008	Multi-institutional Oligochip	ADC	442	Separate discovery and validation sets	8 different classifiers
Sun et al,[49] 2008	In silico discovery, Oligochip validation	ADC, SCC Stages I–IV	In silico: 86 ADC, 129 SCC	Two sets: 84 ADC, 45 ADC and 45 SCC	Two 50-gene signatures separated OS for ADC and SCC despite few overlapping genes
Boutros et al,[50] 2009	qRT-PCR	ADC, SCC Stages I/II	147	11 public databases	6-gene signature stratifies by risk of death

Study	Method	Type/Stage			Result
Zhu et al,[51] 2010	Oligochip	ADC Stages IB/II	133	In silico: 356 Stage IB/II patients	15-gene signature stratified OS and OS after ACT in high-risk patients
Chen et al,[52] 2011	Oligochip	NSCLC	In silico 442	In silico × 2; 117, 133	Breast cancer gene signature stratified OS of early-stage NSCLC and OS after ACT in high-risk patients
Kratz et al,[53] 2012	RT-PCR	ADC Stages I–III	361	Two validation sets: 433, 1006	14-gene expression stratifies for OS for stage I. FFPE specimens uniquely used
Yanaihara et al,[54] 2006	mir array	ADC Stages I–IV	32 ADC	32 ADC	hsa-mir-155, ahsa-let-7a-2 stratify OS
Yu et al,[55] 2008	mir array, RT-PCR	NSCLC Stages I–III	112 NSCLC	62 NSCLC	miRNA signature for TTP and OS (hsa-let-7a, hsa-mir-221, hsa-miR-137, hsa-mir-372, hsa-mir-182)
Landi et al,[56] 2010	mir array	SCC Stages I–IIIA	125	Two SCC validation cohorts: 49, 76	miR-638 and miR-107 prognostic in SCC
Saito et al,[57] 2011	mir-17, mir-21, mir-155, PCR	ADC Stages I–II	USA (89), Norway (37), Japan (191)		miR-21 stratifies OS
Boeri et al,[26] 2011	mir array, qRT-PCR	ADC, SCC Stages I–IV	40	34	mir-221, mir-660, mir-486-5p, mir-28-3p, mir-197, mir-106a, mir-451, mir-140-5p, and mir-16 stratify for OS

Abbreviations: ACT, adjuvant chemotherapy; ADC, adenocarcinoma; FFPE, formalin-fixed paraffin embedded; In silico, performed on computer or via computer simulation; mir, microRNA; NSCLC, non–small cell lung cancer; OS, overall survival; SCC, squamous cell carcinoma; TTP, time to progression.

inhibitors that selectively block EGFR signaling. The Iressa Pan Asia Study (IPASS), which compared the efficacy of gefitinib with carboplatin/paclitaxel cytotoxic chemotherapy in pulmonary adenocarcinomas, demonstrated gefitinib's superiority over first-line chemotherapy in the subset of patients with EGFR mutations.[68] It is interesting that in patients without EGFR mutations, chemotherapy was of greater benefit than gefitinib. The OPTIMAL study, comparing erlotinib with gemcitabine/carboplatin in Chinese patients with untreated EGFR-mutated NSCLC, found a considerable time-to-progression advantage for the erlotinib arm compared with chemotherapy.[69] EGFR targeting with immunotherapy has been achieved with cetuximab, and has been shown to be of benefit in tumors that overexpress EGFR on the cell surface.[70] Although these studies have shown the potential of EGFR targeted therapy in the metastatic setting, targeted therapy against EGFR has not been proved effective in the adjuvant setting for early-stage NSCLC. However, between 30% and 35% of patients with resected early-stage lung cancers will have either local or distant relapse of disease within 5 years of surgery; therefore, reflex mutational testing of all resected tumors may allow for prompt initiation of therapy for patients with early-stage NSCLC on relapse.

KRAS

KRAS (V-Ki-ras2 Kirsten rat sarcoma viral oncogene homologue) mutations occur in 20% to 30% of patients with adenocarcinomas, and are thought to impart a worse prognosis than those with wild-type (nonmutated) KRAS.[65,71] Unlike EGFR mutations, KRAS mutations tend to occur in patients with a prior smoking history.[65] Although targeted therapy has become increasingly important over the last decade, treatment for KRAS-mutated NSCLC remains limited to standard platinum doublet chemotherapy. Unfortunately, efforts to target KRAS directly have not been successful. The future of treatment for KRAS mutations most likely will not target KRAS itself, but rather target the signaling pathway downstream of KRAS.

EML4-ALK and ROS1 Fusion Proteins

EML4-ALK is a fusion protein created by an inversion in chromosome 2p, leading to the fusion of the echinoderm microtubule-associated protein-like 4 (EML4) gene and the anaplastic lymphoma kinase (ALK) gene. Using FISH, this fusion can be recognized in lung cancer cells. This fusion protein accounts for 2% to 7% of all NSCLC and has been successfully targeted with a small-molecule inhibitor.[72] The actual function of the fusion protein is still under investigation; however, ALK itself is a target of interest in numerous malignancies and has been shown to partner with other genes to create novel proteins that are implicated in tumorigenesis.[73]

ROS1 fusion proteins involve the rearrangement of the v-ros gene, a receptor tyrosine kinase of the insulin receptor family, and numerous partners.[74] As with ALK fusion proteins, ROS1 fusion proteins are associated with other malignancies and are most notably found in glioblastoma. Similar to EGFR mutations, ROS1 rearrangements occur in NSCLC adenocarcinomas, and patients are more likely to be young and never smokers. Thus far it appears that ROS1 rearrangements occur in 1% to 2% of NSCLC.[73]

Crizotinib, a small-molecule tyrosine kinase inhibitor targeting ALK and c-MET, binds the adenosine triphosphate (ATP) binding site of the ALK enzyme, preventing ATP from binding and autophosphorylating the fusion protein. It is highly selective for these tyrosine kinases, and in phase II trials it has been shown to be effective in the treatment of NSCLC patients with EML4-ALK as well as ROS1 fusion proteins.[72,74,75]

ERCC1

Excision repair cross-complementation group 1 (ERCC1) is involved in nucleotide base excision repair. Specifically, it recognizes and repairs DNA damage similar to the damage created by platinum chemotherapy.[64] As such, ERCC1 has been investigated as a predictive biomarker for platinum sensitivity; however, its importance is a matter of debate. Most studies exploring the link between ERCC1 and platinum sensitivity have been small, with fewer than 100 patients enrolled. The largest study, a landmark article by Olaussen and colleagues,[76] is a retrospective analysis of the International Adjuvant Lung Cancer Trial (IALT). This study has provided the most convincing evidence that patients with high ERCC1 expression tend to have a worse overall survival when treated with platinum chemotherapy than those with low ERCC1 expression. Several meta-analyses of studies addressing this question have also concluded that there is evidence to support the claim that high ERCC1 expression predicts a poor response to platinum chemotherapy.[77–80]

In early-stage or chemotherapy-naïve patients, ERCC1 expression was thought to have prognostic value on overall survival. In 2005, Simon and colleagues[81] provided evidence suggesting chemotherapy-naïve patients with high ERCC1 expression have a longer overall survival than those with low ERCC1 expression. This finding

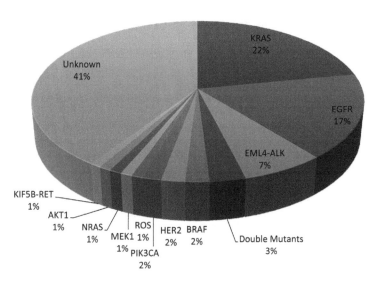

Fig. 1. Approximate frequency of major driving mutations in non–small cell lung cancer (NSCLC). Pie chart shows the approximate percentage distribution of clinically relevant driver mutations identified to date in individuals with NSCLC adenocarcinomas. The chart was generated using data presented by The Lung Cancer Mutation Consortium from 2011, augmented by published data on novel driving mutations.

was confirmed by Olaussen's retrospective analysis of the IALT trial.[64,76] Surprisingly, meta-analyses of studies exploring the prognostic value of ERCC1 have resulted in starkly differing conclusions.[79,80] These meta-analyses noted the major obstacles in making their assessment as a lack of uniformity in defining high ERCC1 expression and the methodology used to assess ERCC1 expression. Therefore larger, prospective trials specifically addressing the prognostic value of ERCC1 in early-stage NSCLC are required.

RRM1

Ribonucleotide reductase messenger 1 (RRM1) is the regulatory component of a multifunctional enzyme ribonucleotide reductase. This enzyme suppresses cell migration by inducing the PTEN (phosphatase and tensin homologue) pathway while also aiding in DNA synthesis and repair.[64] In early-stage lung cancers, high RRM1 expression may be prognostic of improved survival. Zheng and colleagues[82] reported that overall survival was longer than 120 months in patients with high RRM1 expression, compared with 60 months for those with low RRM1 expression. Conversely, several studies suggest that low RRM1 levels are predictive of longer survival with chemotherapy when compared with high RRM1 in advanced lung cancer.[83–85] Of note, RRM1 is a known target of gemcitabine chemotherapy. A meta-analysis of NSCLC patients treated with gemcitabine confirmed that those with low RRM1 expression had increased time to progression, higher response rates, and improved overall survival compared with those with high RRM1.[86] Small investigations suggest that using RRM1 expression to determine choice of chemotherapy may

be of value, with low-RRM1–expressing NSCLC deriving greater benefit with gemcitabine chemotherapy. However, it is important to recognize that these findings need to be validated in larger, prospective studies.

FUTURE DIRECTIONS

The Lung Cancer Mutation Consortium, made up of 14 cancer centers around the United States, was set up specifically to "identify prognostic markers, define predictive markers of response/resistance to new therapies, and identify new targets." Through their efforts and others, treatment of NSCLC is transitioning from a "one size fits all" model, using the same type of treatment plan for all NSCLC, to a more thoughtful, personalized model that seeks to provide refined prognostic information to patients and use targeted agents to treat NSCLC. As the cost of high-throughput whole-genome sequencing becomes more affordable, it may become the ideal modality with which to screen mutational differences and identify rare genetic variants in malignancies to further individualize the management of these patients. At present, around 40% of lung adenocarcinomas do not have identified driving mutations (**Fig. 1**).[87] The promise of whole-genome sequencing lies in the identification of novel driving mutations. As these novel mutations are discovered and subsequently targeted for treatment, a growth in the understanding of NSCLC and the armamentarium with which to fight the disease will transpire.

REFERENCES

1. Hassanein M, Callison JC, Callaway-Lane C, et al. The state of molecular biomarkers for the early

detection of lung cancer. Cancer Prev Res (Phila) 2012;5(8):992–1006.

2. Lin J, Beer DG. Molecular predictors of prognosis in lung cancer. Ann Surg Oncol 2012;19(2):669–76.

3. Hammerman PS, Hayes DN, Wilkerson MD, et al. Comprehensive genomic characterization of squamous cell lung cancers. Nature 2012;489(7417):519–25.

4. Peifer M, Fernandez-Cuesta L, Sos ML, et al. Integrative genome analyses identify key somatic driver mutations of small-cell lung cancer. Nat Genet 2012;44(10):1104–10.

5. Imielinski M, Berger AH, Hammerman PS, et al. Mapping the hallmarks of lung adenocarcinoma with massively parallel sequencing. Cell 2012;150(6):1107–20.

6. Halling KC, Kipp BR. Fluorescence in situ hybridization in diagnostic cytology. Hum Pathol 2007;38(8):1137–44.

7. LaFramboise T, Weir BA, Zhao X, et al. Allele-specific amplification in cancer revealed by SNP array analysis. PLoS Comput Biol 2005;1(6):e65.

8. John T, Liu G, Tsao MS. Overview of molecular testing in non-small-cell lung cancer: mutational analysis, gene copy number, protein expression and other biomarkers of EGFR for the prediction of response to tyrosine kinase inhibitors. Oncogene 2009;28(Suppl 1):S14–23.

9. Tessema M, Belinsky SA. Mining the epigenome for methylated genes in lung cancer. Proc Am Thorac Soc 2008;5(8):806–10.

10. Jiang YW, Chen LA. microRNAs as tumor inhibitors, oncogenes, biomarkers for drug efficacy and outcome predictors in lung cancer [review]. Mol Med Report 2012;5(4):890–4.

11. Mazzone PJ, Wang XF, Xu Y, et al. Exhaled breath analysis with a colorimetric sensor array for the identification and characterization of lung cancer. J Thorac Oncol 2012;7(1):137–42.

12. Phillips M, Altorki N, Austin JH, et al. Detection of lung cancer using weighted digital analysis of breath biomarkers. Clin Chim Acta 2008;393(2):76–84.

13. Zhu CQ, Pintilie M, John T, et al. Understanding prognostic gene expression signatures in lung cancer. Clin Lung Cancer 2009;10(5):331–40.

14. Zhao X, Li C, Paez JG, et al. An integrated view of copy number and allelic alterations in the cancer genome using single nucleotide polymorphism arrays. Cancer Res 2004;64(9):3060–71.

15. Bunn PA Jr, Doebele RC. Genetic testing for lung cancer: reflex versus clinical selection. J Clin Oncol 2011;29(15):1943–5.

16. Collins FS, Morgan M, Patrinos A. The human genome project: lessons from large-scale biology. Science 2003;300(5617):286–90.

17. Mallick R, Patnaik SK, Yendamuri S. MicroRNAs and lung cancer: biology and applications in diagnosis and prognosis. J Carcinog 2010;9:1–10.

18. Wen J, Fu J, Zhang W, et al. Genetic and epigenetic changes in lung carcinoma and their clinical implications. Mod Pathol 2011;24(7):932–43.

19. Meyerson M, Carbone D. Genomic and proteomic profiling of lung cancers: lung cancer classification in the age of targeted therapy. J Clin Oncol 2005;23(14):3219–26.

20. Ostroff RM, Bigbee WL, Franklin W, et al. Unlocking biomarker discovery: large scale application of aptamer proteomic technology for early detection of lung cancer. PLoS One 2010;5(12):e15003.

21. Zhong L, Coe SP, Stromberg AJ, et al. Profiling tumor-associated antibodies for early detection of non-small cell lung cancer. J Thorac Oncol 2006;1(6):513–9.

22. Qiu J, Choi G, Li L, et al. Occurrence of autoantibodies to annexin I, 14–3–3 theta and LAMR1 in prediagnostic lung cancer sera. J Clin Oncol 2008;26(31):5060–6.

23. Wu L, Chang W, Zhao J, et al. Development of autoantibody signatures as novel diagnostic biomarkers of non-small cell lung cancer. Clin Cancer Res 2010;16(14):3760–8.

24. Boyle P, Chapman CJ, Holdenrieder S, et al. Clinical validation of an autoantibody test for lung cancer. Ann Oncol 2011;22(2):383–9.

25. Pecot CV, Li M, Zhang XJ, et al. Added value of a serum proteomic signature in the diagnostic evaluation of lung nodules. Cancer Epidemiol Biomarkers Prev 2012;21(5):786–92.

26. Boeri M, Verri C, Conte D, et al. MicroRNA signatures in tissues and plasma predict development and prognosis of computed tomography detected lung cancer. Proc Natl Acad Sci U S A 2011;108(9):3713–8.

27. Schmidt B, Liebenberg V, Dietrich D, et al. SHOX2 DNA methylation is a biomarker for the diagnosis of lung cancer based on bronchial aspirates. BMC Cancer 2010;10:600.

28. Richards KL, Zhang B, Sun M, et al. Methylation of the candidate biomarker TCF21 is very frequent across a spectrum of early-stage nonsmall cell lung cancers. Cancer 2011;117(3):606–17.

29. Spira A, Beane JE, Shah V, et al. Airway epithelial gene expression in the diagnostic evaluation of smokers with suspect lung cancer. Nat Med 2007;13(3):361–6.

30. Rahman SM, Shyr Y, Yildiz PB, et al. Proteomic patterns of preinvasive bronchial lesions. Am J Respir Crit Care Med 2005;172(12):1556–62.

31. Wu X, Chen H, Wang X. Can lung cancer stem cells be targeted for therapies? Cancer Treat Rev 2012;38(6):580–8.

32. Begum S, Brait M, Dasgupta S, et al. An epigenetic marker panel for detection of lung cancer using cell-free serum DNA. Clin Cancer Res 2011;17(13):4494–503.

33. Chen X, Hu Z, Wang W, et al. Identification of ten serum microRNAs from a genome-wide serum micro-RNA expression profile as novel noninvasive bio-markers for nonsmall cell lung cancer diagnosis. Int J Cancer 2012;130(7):1620–8.

34. Bianchi F, Nicassio F, Marzi M, et al. A serum circulating miRNA diagnostic test to identify asymptomatic high-risk individuals with early stage lung cancer. EMBO Mol Med 2011;3(8):495–503.

35. Yildiz PB, Shyr Y, Rahman JS, et al. Diagnostic accuracy of MALDI mass spectrometric analysis of un-fractionated serum in lung cancer. J Thorac Oncol 2007;2(10):893–901.

36. Lee HJ, Kim YT, Park PJ, et al. A novel detection method of non-small cell lung cancer using multi-plexed bead-based serum biomarker profiling. J Thorac Cardiovasc Surg 2012;143(2):421–7.

37. Shen J, Todd NW, Zhang H, et al. Plasma micro-RNAs as potential biomarkers for non-small-cell lung cancer. Lab Invest 2011;91(4):579–87.

38. Kneip C, Schmidt B, Seegebarth A, et al. SHOX2 DNA methylation is a biomarker for the diagnosis of lung cancer in plasma. J Thorac Oncol 2011; 6(10):1632–8.

39. Boeri M, Pastorino U, Sozzi G. Role of microRNAs in lung cancer: microRNA signatures in cancer prognosis. Cancer J 2012;18(3):268–74.

40. Skrzypski M, Jassem E, Taron M, et al. Three-gene expression signature predicts survival in early-stage squamous cell carcinoma of the lung. Clin Cancer Res 2008;14(15):4794–9.

41. Chen HY, Yu SL, Chen CH, et al. A five-gene signature and clinical outcome in non-small-cell lung cancer. N Engl J Med 2007;356(1):11–20.

42. Beer DG, Kardia SL, Huang CC, et al. Gene-expression profiles predict survival of patients with lung adenocarcinoma. Nat Med 2002;8(8):816–24.

43. Raponi M, Zhang Y, Yu J, et al. Gene expression signatures for predicting prognosis of squamous cell and adenocarcinomas of the lung. Cancer Res 2006;66(15):7466–72.

44. Lu Y, Lemon W, Liu PY, et al. A gene expression signature predicts survival of patients with stage I non-small cell lung cancer. PLoS Med 2006;3(12):e467.

45. Larsen JE, Pavey SJ, Passmore LH, et al. Gene expression signature predicts recurrence in lung adenocarcinoma. Clin Cancer Res 2007;13(10): 2946–54.

46. Bianchi F, Nuciforo P, Vecchi M, et al. Survival prediction of stage I lung adenocarcinomas by expression of 10 genes. J Clin Invest 2007;117(11):3436–44.

47. Guo NL, Wan YW, Tosun K, et al. Confirmation of gene expression-based prediction of survival in non-small cell lung cancer. Clin Cancer Res 2008; 14(24):8213–20.

48. Shedden K, Taylor JM, Enkemann SA, et al. Gene expression-based survival prediction in lung adenocarcinoma: a multi-site, blinded validation study. Nat Med 2008;14(8):822–7.

49. Sun Z, Wigle DA, Yang P. Non-overlapping and non-cell-type-specific gene expression signatures predict lung cancer survival. J Clin Oncol 2008; 26(6):877–83.

50. Boutros PC, Lau SK, Pintilie M, et al. Prognostic gene signatures for non-small-cell lung cancer. Proc Natl Acad Sci U S A 2009;106(8):2824–8.

51. Zhu CQ, Ding K, Strumpf D, et al. Prognostic and predictive gene signature for adjuvant chemotherapy in resected non-small-cell lung cancer. J Clin Oncol 2010;28(29):4417–24.

52. Chen DT, Hsu YL, Fulp WJ, et al. Prognostic and predictive value of a malignancy-risk gene signature in early-stage non-small cell lung cancer. J Natl Cancer Inst 2011;103(24):1859–70.

53. Kratz JR, He J, Van Den Eeden SK, et al. A practical molecular assay to predict survival in resected non-squamous, non-small-cell lung cancer: development and international validation studies. Lancet 2012;379(9818):823–32.

54. Yanaihara N, Caplen N, Bowman E, et al. Unique microRNA molecular profiles in lung cancer diagnosis and prognosis. Cancer Cell 2006;9(3):189–98.

55. Yu SL, Chen HY, Chang GC, et al. MicroRNA signature predicts survival and relapse in lung cancer. Cancer Cell 2008;13(1):48–57.

56. Landi MT, Zhao Y, Rotunno M, et al. MicroRNA expression differentiates histology and predicts survival of lung cancer. Clin Cancer Res 2010;16(2):430–41.

57. Saito M, Schetter AJ, Mollerup S, et al. The association of microRNA expression with prognosis and progression in early-stage, non-small cell lung adenocarcinoma: a retrospective analysis of three cohorts. Clin Cancer Res 2011;17(7):1875–82.

58. Kadota K, Suzuki K, Kachala SS, et al. A grading system combining architectural features and mitotic count predicts recurrence in stage I lung adenocarcinoma. Mod Pathol 2012;25(8):1117–27.

59. Yanagisawa K, Shyr Y, Xu BJ, et al. Proteomic patterns of tumour subsets in non-small-cell lung cancer. Lancet 2003;362(9382):433–9.

60. Yanagisawa K, Tomida S, Shimada Y, et al. A 25-signal proteomic signature and outcome for patients with resected non-small-cell lung cancer. J Natl Cancer Inst 2007;99(11):858–67.

61. Xu BJ, Gonzalez AL, Kikuchi T, et al. MALDI-MS derived prognostic protein markers for resected non-small cell lung cancer. Proteomics Clin Appl 2008;2(10–11):1508–17.

62. Johnson SM, Grosshans H, Shingara J, et al. RAS is regulated by the let-7 microRNA family. Cell 2005; 120(5):635–47.

63. Hatley ME, Patrick DM, Garcia MR, et al. Modulation of K-Ras-dependent lung tumorigenesis by Micro-RNA-21. Cancer Cell 2010;18(3):282–93.

64. Coate LE, John T, Tsao MS, et al. Molecular predictive and prognostic markers in non-small-cell lung cancer. Lancet Oncol 2009;10(10):1001–10.

65. Johnson ML, Sima CS, Chaft J, et al. Association of KRAS and EGFR mutations with survival in patients with advanced lung adenocarcinomas. Cancer 2013;119(2):356–62.

66. Li M, Zhang Q, Liu L, et al. The different clinical significance of EGFR mutations in exon 19 and 21 in non-small cell lung cancer patients of China. Neoplasma 2011;58(1):74–81.

67. Sun JM, Won YW, Kim ST, et al. The different efficacy of gefitinib or erlotinib according to epidermal growth factor receptor exon 19 and exon 21 mutations in Korean non-small cell lung cancer patients. J Cancer Res Clin Oncol 2011;137(4): 687–94.

68. Mok TS, Wu YL, Thongprasert S, et al. Gefitinib or carboplatin-paclitaxel in pulmonary adenocarcinoma. N Engl J Med 2009;361(10):947–57.

69. Zhou C, Wu YL, Chen G, et al. Erlotinib versus chemotherapy as first-line treatment for patients with advanced EGFR mutation-positive non-small-cell lung cancer (OPTIMAL, CTONG-0802): a multi-centre, open-label, randomised, phase 3 study. Lancet Oncol 2011;12(8):735–42.

70. Pirker R, Pereira JR, Szczesna A, et al. Cetuximab plus chemotherapy in patients with advanced non-small-cell lung cancer (FLEX): an open-label randomised phase III trial. Lancet 2009;373(9674): 1525–31.

71. Janne PA, Engelman JA, Johnson BE. Epidermal growth factor receptor mutations in non-small-cell lung cancer: implications for treatment and tumor biology. J Clin Oncol 2005;23(14):3227–34.

72. Kwak EL, Bang YJ, Camidge DR, et al. Anaplastic lymphoma kinase inhibition in non-small-cell lung cancer. N Engl J Med 2010;363(18): 1693–703.

73. Johnson JL, Pillai S, Chellappan SP. Genetic and biochemical alterations in non-small cell lung cancer. Biochem Res Int 2012;2012:940405.

74. Bergethon K, Shaw AT, Ou SH, et al. ROS1 rearrangements define a unique molecular class of lung cancers. J Clin Oncol 2012;30(8):863–70.

75. Shaw AT, Yeap BY, Solomon BJ, et al. Effect of crizotinib on overall survival in patients with advanced non-small-cell lung cancer harbouring ALK gene rearrangement: a retrospective analysis. Lancet Oncol 2011;12(11):1004–12.

76. Olaussen KA, Dunant A, Fouret P, et al. DNA repair by ERCC1 in non-small-cell lung cancer and cisplatin-based adjuvant chemotherapy. N Engl J Med 2006;355(10):983–91.

77. Chen S, Zhang J, Wang R, et al. The platinum-based treatments for advanced non-small cell lung cancer, is low/negative ERCC1 expression better than high/positive ERCC1 expression? A meta-analysis. Lung Cancer 2010;70(1):63–70.

78. Roth JA, Carlson JJ. Prognostic role of ERCC1 in advanced non-small-cell lung cancer: a systematic review and meta-analysis. Clin Lung Cancer 2011; 12(6):393–401.

79. Jiang J, Liang X, Zhou X, et al. ERCC1 expression as a prognostic and predictive factor in patients with non-small cell lung cancer: a meta-analysis. Mol Biol Rep 2012;39(6):6933–42.

80. Hubner RA, Riley RD, Billingham LJ, et al. Excision repair cross-complementation group 1 (ERCC1) status and lung cancer outcomes: a meta-analysis of published studies and recommendations. PLoS One 2011;6(10):e25164.

81. Simon GR, Sharma S, Cantor A, et al. ERCC1 expression is a predictor of survival in resected patients with non-small cell lung cancer. Chest 2005;127(3):978–83.

82. Zheng Z, Chen T, Li X, et al. DNA synthesis and repair genes RRM1 and ERCC1 in lung cancer. N Engl J Med 2007;356(8):800–8.

83. Rosell R, Danenberg KD, Alberola V, et al. Ribonucleotide reductase messenger RNA expression and survival in gemcitabine/cisplatin-treated advanced non-small cell lung cancer patients. Clin Cancer Res 2004;10(4):1318–25.

84. Ceppi P, Volante M, Novello S, et al. ERCC1 and RRM1 gene expressions but not EGFR are predictive of shorter survival in advanced non-small-cell lung cancer treated with cisplatin and gemcitabine. Ann Oncol 2006;17(12):1818–25.

85. Boukovinas I, Papadaki C, Mendez P, et al. Tumor BRCA1, RRM1 and RRM2 mRNA expression levels and clinical response to first-line gemcitabine plus docetaxel in non-small-cell lung cancer patients. PLoS One 2008;3(11):e3695.

86. Gong W, Zhang X, Wu J, et al. RRM1 expression and clinical outcome of gemcitabine-containing chemotherapy for advanced non-small-cell lung cancer: a meta-analysis. Lung Cancer 2012;75(3):374–80.

87. Pao W, Hutchinson KE. Chipping away at the lung cancer genome. Nat Med 2012;18(3):349–51.

Prognostic Implications of Treatment Delays in the Surgical Resection of Lung Cancer

William K. Evans, MD, FRCPC

KEYWORDS

- Lung cancer • Prognosis • Diagnosis • Wait times

KEY POINTS

- The early diagnosis of lung cancer is infrequent because of tumor biology (long natural history and high metastatic potential), few early symptoms, and patient delay in seeking medical attention.
- Lack of an organized system to diagnose and stage lung cancer contributes to delays in treatment.
- Strategies to reduce delays in diagnosis lead to higher surgical resection rates.
- The literature is not convincing that reducing diagnostic and treatment delays improves survival in symptomatic lung cancer probably because the usual delay represents only a very small component of the natural history of the typical lung cancer.

INTRODUCTION

Every publication on lung cancer (LC) begins with a recitation of the terrible toll that lung cancer takes in the author's jurisdiction. This article is no different; the author sadly acknowledges that despite the fact that Canada has led the world in smoking cessation initiatives, there will still be an estimated 25 600 new cases of diagnosed LCs and 20 100 deaths in 2012.[1] In both Canadian men and women, LC is the second-most common cancer after prostate and breast, respectively. In total, the number of LC cases exceeds the combined number of breast, colon, and prostate cancer cases. Importantly, the 5-year survival of patients diagnosed with LC remains poor. Despite recent improvements in the therapy for surgically resected, locally advanced, and metastatic disease, the overall 5-year survival for LC in Canada remains abysmally poor at 16%.[1] The survival of patients with non–small cell lung carcinoma (NSCLC) by stage according to the seventh edition TNM classification is shown in **Table 1**.[2]

This poor 5-year survival rate is largely attributable to the fact that LC typically presents in an advanced stage, with 60% of NSCLC and 84% of small-cell LCs diagnosed as either stage III or IV in the province of Ontario, Canada's largest province (Cancer Care Ontario Informatics 2010, personal communication). Other factors, such as age, sex, performance status, and comorbidities, play a role in prognosis but are not amenable to any clinical intervention. Many tumor factors have been shown in at least one study to have independent prognostic significance. These factors include histologic features; clinical chemistry and serum tumor markers; markers of tumor proliferation; markers of cellular adhesion; molecular regulators of cellular growth (eg, ras oncogene or protein, epidermal growth factor receptor, Erb-b2, motility-related protein-1, and hepatocyte growth factor); regulators of the metastatic cascade (eg, tissue polypeptide antigen, cyclin D-1 and cathepsin); and regulators of apoptosis (p53 and bcl-2), among others.[3]

THE CHALLENGE OF DIAGNOSING LC EARLY

It is well recognized that the only real opportunity to cure LC occurs with surgical resection, but

Juravinski Cancer Centre, 699 Concession Street, Hamilton, Ontario L8V 5C2, Canada
E-mail address: Bill.Evans@jcc.hhsc.ca

Thorac Surg Clin 23 (2013) 225–232
http://dx.doi.org/10.1016/j.thorsurg.2013.01.006
1547-4127/13/$ – see front matter © 2013 Elsevier Inc. All rights reserved.

Table 1
Median survival of NSCLC by TNM stage (seventh edition)

Stage	Median Survival (mo)
IA	59
IB	48
IIA	30
IIB	24
IIIA	14
IIIB	9
IV	4

Data From Groome PA, Bolejack V, Crowley JJ, et al. The IASLC Lung Cancer Staging Project: validation of the proposals for the revision of the T, N, and M descriptors and consequent stage groupings in the forthcoming (seventh) edition of the TNM classification of malignant tumors. J Thorac Oncol 2007;2(8):694–705.

relatively few patients present with disease that is amenable to surgery. The reasons for this are multiple. In the first instance, it is generally thought that tumors grow exponentially and that from the time of the first malignant cell until the tumor mass reaches 1 cm, it has passed through more than 30 doublings. Based on a mean LC tumor cell doubling time of between 160 and 400 days depending on cell type, approximately 8 to 10 years have passed before a LC is clinically detectable.[4,5] This time is ample for malignant cells with metastatic potential to disseminate via the bloodstream or lymphatics to distant sites. So, even if the primary tumor is relatively small (1–2 cm) and resected, there may already be micrometastatic spread. Typically, this metastatic disease becomes apparent within 2 to 3 years, explaining why even the 5-year survival of surgically resected LC is generally less than 50%. The exponential nature of tumor growth also means that toward the end of a tumor's natural life cycle, it will typically seem to increase in size dramatically and may move a patient's stage of disease from one that was potentially resectable to one that is not.[6]

Secondly, the pulmonary symptoms from the LC are often difficult to differentiate from other respiratory symptoms in a current or former smoker and can easily be mistaken for an acute exacerbation of bronchitis or confused with pneumonia. Symptoms resulting from metastatic disease are also often confused with other common illnesses if the primary tumor is asymptomatic. Headaches, vague symptoms of indigestion, fatigue, and bone pain can all be the first signs of metastatic cancer.

Patients can delay seeking medical attention for a variety of reasons, including difficulty accessing a family physician, fear of receiving a diagnosis with a poor prognosis, or other factors. The stigma that is now associated with being a cigarette smoker may also be a factor in the delay to seek medical attention. The mean delay from initial symptoms to a first visit to a general practitioner (GP) is in the range of 60 days.[7–15] Once patients present to their family physician, the median time to referral to a specialist can vary from 14 to 33 days[16]; the total interval from first symptoms to treatment can range from 3 to 7 months.[7,9,17]

BARRIERS TO PROMPT DIAGNOSIS AND TREATMENT

Although there is little that can be done to overcome patient delays and nothing to do to change the biology of LC and its often silent and sinister presentation, once there is suspicion of LC, numerous reports document the fact that there is often a significant delay to definitive treatment. That is something that can be addressed by improvements in the organization of the health care system. Shortening the time to treatment and increasing the proportion of patients who are candidates for surgical resection could conceivably improve survival. Some, if not most, of the delay in getting to a diagnosis can be attributed to the complexity of the health care system itself and the lack of an organized system to get the multiplicity of tests needed to establish a diagnosis and stage LC done. Every experienced oncologist has witnessed patients whose diagnosis has been delayed through inappropriate courses of antibiotics or diagnostic testing. In some of these cases, there can be little doubt that poor clinical management has led to a treatment delay that has prevented a potentially curative treatment approach. An efficient system to diagnose LC might increase the probability of a potentially curative intervention.

Certainly there is ample evidence of treatment delays for elective surgery, including surgery for LC, in many different countries and health systems.[18] As it relates specifically to LC, Billing and Wells[19] studied delays in diagnosis in patients with LC who underwent surgical treatment in Cambridge, United Kingdom in 1996. The mean time from presentation to surgery was 109 days among 39 patients undergoing surgical resection.

In 2005, Salomaa and colleagues[16] described results from a retrospective review of 132 patients seen in several Finnish hospitals. The median delay from patient reported symptoms to assessment by a GP was 14 days and the referral from the GP to a specialist took a further 24 days. It then took a median of 15 days for the specialist to establish the diagnosis and a further 15 days to begin treatment. Overall, the median delay from symptoms to treatment was almost 4 months. Thirty percent of patients received treatment within 1 month from the first visit to the consultant and 61% received treatment within 2 months. Treatment delays were actually shorter in patients with advanced disease, perhaps because the extent of disease was more evident and fewer tests were required to establish the diagnosis and stage. The investigators attributed some of the diagnostic delay to the large number of consecutive diagnostic procedures commonly used in the diagnosis and staging of LC. Longer specialist delay correlated with better survival in patients with advanced disease in this relatively small study. Diagnostic delay did not seem to lead to a worse prognosis, although the investigators speculated that this may not be true in patients with early stage disease.

In a study of 256 patients seen in hospitals in Montreal, Canada between 1993 and 2002, Liberman and colleagues[20] noted significant delays at multiple steps in the journey of patients with LC. Overall, the mean and median times from symptoms or initial contact to surgery were 208 and 109 days, respectively. There was a surprisingly long interval between radiological diagnosis and surgery (mean 135 days, median 80 days). The time from contact with a thoracic surgeon and surgery was also long at 104 days (mean) and 82 days (median). The investigators attribute much of the delay to lack of resources, including access to computed tomography (CT) scans and positron emission tomography for diagnosis and to operating room blocks for definitive surgery.

So, access to the diagnostic and staging tests, to health care professionals, and to surgical resources can all contribute to delays in getting to definitive treatment.

WAIT-TIME DELAYS AND SURGICAL RESECTION RATES

It is intuitive to think that a shorter time to diagnosis would translate to a greater proportion of early stage disease being amenable to surgical resection. From the work of Naruke and colleagues[21] from Japan and others, it is clear that patients with stage I NSCLC have significantly better survival than those with higher-stage tumors. It follows that efforts to identify LC at an earlier stage should allow higher resection rates and achieve better outcomes.

Murray and colleagues[22] from the United Kingdom recognized that the surgical resection rates for NSCLC were low in the United Kingdom,

with rates ranging between 5% and 10%[23–25] compared with approximately 25% in the United States and Europe. To see if the resection rate could be improved by overcoming access barriers, they evaluated a rapid 2-stop diagnostic system in a pilot study compared with the conventional method of undertaking diagnostic investigations in 3 district general hospitals. Eighty-eight patients were enrolled prospectively and randomized to the conventional approach or to a centralized rapid diagnostic system at the Royal Marsden Hospital. They noted a 4-week improvement in the time to first treatment in the rapid diagnostic assessment arm of the pilot, with 13 out of 30 patients (43%) proceeding to radical treatment compared with 9 out of 27 patients (33%) in the conventional arm. Not surprisingly, patients were more satisfied with their care experience in the rapid assessment arm of the study ($P = .01$).

The elements of the central assessment approach were rapid access to CT scans and a same-day decision on the most appropriate route to obtain a tissue diagnosis. The recommended procedure was undertaken that same day. Patients were reviewed after 3 working days at a multidisciplinary meeting, which included thoracic surgeons, clinical oncologists, a radiologist, a palliative care team representative, and the study coordinator. At this meeting, a management plan with a decision on the treatment intent was made for each patient. Overall, the pilot study showed a 10% higher radical treatment rate (not statistically significant) and there was higher patient satisfaction. Patients discussed at the multidisciplinary meeting were also more likely to receive chemotherapy and to use less primary care resources. However, these investigators recognized that to demonstrate whether a higher radical treatment rate can result in a 5% to 10% improvement in survival rate would require a study of about 600 patients; to date, such a study has not been undertaken.

In 1995, Laroche and colleagues[26] also implemented a quick-access 2-stop investigation service at Papworth, United Kingdom to investigate all patients presenting to any one of 3 surrounding health districts with suspected LC. Once staging was complete, the patients were reviewed by a multidisciplinary team, which included a thoracic surgeon and an oncologist. Of 181 patients with NSCLC, 47 (25%) underwent successful surgical resection: 59% had stage I and 21% had stage II disease. The median time from presentation to the peripheral clinic to surgical resection was 5 weeks (range 1–13 weeks). The investigators concluded that the quick-access investigation, routine CT scanning, and the review of every patient with a confirmed diagnosis of LC by a thoracic surgeon led to a substantial increase in the surgical resection rate compared with the experience before the introduction of the quick-access clinic. The investigators expressed concern that many potentially operable patients were being denied the chance of curative surgery in the absence of expedited access to diagnosis and surgical consultation but could not prove that survival was actually increased by surgery at an earlier stage.

Dransfield and colleagues[27] reported that resection rates in the Birmingham Veterans Affairs Medical Center (BVAMC), part of the Veterans Affairs health care system in the United States, had typically been low. Based on registry data from their institution in 1993, the surgical resection rate was only 12.6%.[27] This finding was consistent with data from the larger regional Veterans Integrated Service Network, which resected only 15.3% of patients diagnosed with NSCLC[28] but lower than the US resection rates at that time (25%–28%).[29,30] Following the implementation of a specialized Lung Mass Clinic, the resection rate for 156 patients with NSCLC at the BVAMC increased to 20%. The investigators noted that the overall survival of these patients was comparable with other reports at 65% at 3 years; but again, as in other studies, they could not prove that the higher resection rate resulted in improved survival.

BUT DOES REDUCING DELAYS YIELD A BETTER PROGNOSIS?

The results described earlier suggest that strategies to facilitate prompt access to diagnostic and staging investigations can increase resection rates, particularly if the rates have been low in a particular institution or jurisdiction. However, because of their design, none of these studies have been able to definitively demonstrate a beneficial impact of earlier diagnosis on survival.

In a 2008 systematic review, Olsson and colleagues[10] identified 15 studies that looked at the effect of timeliness of treatment and outcome. The review gave mixed results, with 8 studies showing no association.[16,31–37] Only 3 studies demonstrated a worse survival in patients who had delays in diagnosis and treatment.[38–40] Two of these studies included patients who were identified through mass-screening studies.[39,40] An interesting observation made in the study of Kashiwabara and colleagues[40] was that tumors that were initially missed on screening but identified a year later at the time of repeat screening had a worse median survival than those that were followed up promptly, and survival correlated

with increases in tumor size. The hazard of death increased by 5.5% for each additional 1 mm in tumor size at the time of diagnosis.[40] Kanashiki and colleagues[39] found that survival was worse in patients whose diagnosis was made more than 4 months after an initial abnormal chest radiograph.

Four studies included in the systematic review actually showed that patients who had less timely access to care actually had a better survival.[11–13,41] Comber and colleagues[11] noted better LC-specific survival in patients with longer time intervals to treatment compared with those who waited less than 1 month. Myrdal and colleagues[13] noted that patients with more advanced disease had shorter times to diagnosis and treatment. Neal and colleagues[12] reported that survival was worse in patients who were urgently referred and that patients with urgent referrals had more advanced disease at diagnosis. Although these observations may seem counterintuitive, it may simply reflect the urgency commonly given to patients who present with more advanced, nonsurgical disease and the sense that they must be given priority access to diagnostic tests to expedite treatment.

Since the Olsson systematic review, 2 further retrospective studies of all LC cases presenting to a defined health area have been published. A Spanish study of 415 patients with LC concluded that an overall delay was associated with longer survival, probably reflecting the fact that patients with more advanced and symptomatic disease are treated more rapidly.[14] A retrospective study of 271 patients from the Norwegian Cancer Registry concluded that survival time was not influenced by diagnostic delay.[15]

The reality probably is that for many, if not most patients, the magnitude of the delay in the usual diagnostic workup of symptomatic patients for treatment does not constitute a major amount of the total lifespan of a LC and, therefore, has little impact on prognosis. However, the observations from the Kashiwabara study indicate that when the delay is substantial, as in a missed small lesion in a screening study, the impact on survival can be significant.

The fact that screen-detected clinical stage I LC has an extremely good prospect of 10-year survival supports the view that interventions early in the natural history of the disease can lead to better outcomes. The large collaborative trial led by Henschke[42] screened 31 567 asymptomatic patients at risk for LC using low-dose CT performed at intervals of 7 to 18 months. A total of 484 LCs were detected, 412 (80%) of which were clinical stage I. This group had an estimated

10-year survival rate of 88% (95% confidence interval [CI], 84%–91%). Of those who underwent resection within 1 month of the diagnosis, the survival rate was reported to be 92% (95% CI, 88%–95%). Although this study elicited controversy when published because of its design and other factors, these investigators' observations have now been confirmed by the large randomized trial conducted by the large National Lung Screening Trial (NLST), which observed a significant stage shift (**Table 2**) that resulted in an impressive 20% reduction in LC mortality at 6 years.[43] Clearly, the potential exists to improve the prognosis of LC, if only it can be identified early enough.

WAIT-TIME REDUCTION WOULD STILL BE IMPORTANT EVEN IF IT DID NOT AFFECT PROGNOSIS

The psychological impact of a presumptive diagnosis of cancer cannot be underestimated. Although it is recognized that there are sociodemographic and clinical variables that may contribute to patients delaying to seek medical attention for symptoms, fear seems to be an important psychological factor that can lead either to help-seeking behavior or to delay.[44] Prompt determination of the correct diagnosis with relief of anxiety for those who do not have a malignant diagnosis and supportive communication about the disease and the consequences of the diagnosis for those that do would seem to be the best strategy. Evidence supports the approach of providing patients with information that will prepare them for an aversive situation because it generally enables them to cope more effectively.[45]

Waiting for care has also become a highly political issue in many countries, particularly those with publically funded health care systems. A wide variety of policies have been implemented to reduce wait times to diagnosis and treatment in the Organization for Economic Cooperation and Development countries and are well described in a 2005 article by Siciliani and Hurst.[18] Increasingly, the public reporting of wait times and the linkage of funding to good performance are additional reasons to have systems in place that shorten the time from symptoms to diagnosis and treatment.

IMPROVING ACCESS TO DIAGNOSIS AND CARE

The recognition of the system bottlenecks causing patient delays has incented numerous innovative approaches and a growing movement toward creating diagnostic assessment clinics or programs. One example of an innovation recently described by Lo and colleagues[46] is a Time to Treat Program at the Toronto East General Hospital, Toronto, Ontario. Key elements of their approach to rapid diagnosis were the establishment of a single point of contact for LC referrals and a referral form specially designed to define the urgency of the referral and the most appropriate specialist for patients to see. Referral forms are faxed to a central booking clerk who acts as the navigator to coordinate the care of the patients during their diagnostic workup. Other features of the Time to Treat Program are a standardized workup according to a defined lung cancer pathway and dedicated CT scan and bronchoscopy slots. Following the implementation of these measures, the median time from suspicion of LC to referral to a specialist consultation decreased from 20 days to 6 days and the median time from referral to actual consultation decreased from 17 days to 4 days. The median time from specialist consultation to CT scan decreased from 52 days to 3 days and the median time from CT scan to diagnosis decreased from 128 days to 20 days. The investigators comment that the earlier diagnosis of LC may allow increased

Table 2
Stage distribution in the NLST in comparison with usual stage distribution in Canada

Stage	NLST T_0 (%)	NLST T_1 (%)	NLST T_2 (%)	NLST Overall (%)	NSCLC Usual Canadian Stage Distribution (%) All Ages	55–74 y
I	60	64	70	64	17	20
II	8	10	6	8	4	6
III	20	16	13	17	26	25
IV	12	10	11	11	53	49

Data from The National Lung Screening Trial Research Team. Reduced lung-cancer mortality with low-dose computed tomographic screening. N Engl J Med 2011;365:395–409; and Canadian Cancer Registry and the Canadian Partnership Against Cancer's Cancer Risk Management Model, unpublished data.

treatment options for patients and may improve outcomes, although they were not able to offer definitive proof.

DIAGNOSTIC ASSESSMENT UNITS/ PROGRAMS

The idea of consolidating the diagnostic assessment activities for LC in a 1- or 2-stop ambulatory clinic is gaining momentum. Assessment clinics were initially introduced for breast cancer where there is good evidence that they reduce wait times and patient anxiety while increasing patient satisfaction. However, in 2004, when Gagliardi and colleagues[47] undertook a systematic review of diagnostic assessment units, they found that more than half of the 20 reports described experience with breast assessment centers and there were no reports of lung diagnostic assessment units (DAUs) at that time. The reports in the review also failed to evaluate the utility of these units apart from identifying a generally high level of patient satisfaction with the efficiency of the diagnostic workup.

Despite the lack of formal evaluation, including whether DAUs improve the prognosis for patients with LC, the value of these units is supported by the medical literature that demonstrates the value of concentrating clinical expertise within multi-disciplinary teams[48,49] for appropriate decision making and by the volume-outcome literature.[50,51]

Organizational standards for diagnostic assessment programs (DAP) have recently been recommended by Cancer Care Ontario.[52] The key purpose of a DAP is to provide timely and equitable access to high-quality diagnostic care. The diagnostic workup needs to include coordinated referral and follow-up, and the workup should be conducted according to disease-specific protocols with wait-time benchmarks. Through a recent Lung Cancer Disease Pathway Initiative, standard diagnostic pathways for small-cell LC and NSCLS have been developed and are available on the Cancer Care Ontario Web site.[53]

Targets for the wait times for diagnosis and treatment of LC should be embedded within these DAPs, but what these targets should be is a matter of opinion but not grounded in science. Several bodies have made recommendations for these targets. In the United Kingdom, where patients with cancer have been more commonly diagnosed in an advanced stage, referral guidelines have been introduced to reduce diagnostic delays and increase the proportion of early stage cancer. These UK government policies guarantee that everyone suspected of cancer should be able to see a hospital doctor within 2 weeks of their primary care provider deciding that they need to be seen urgently.[54,55] The National Health Service - National Cancer Plan targets a maximum interval of 1 month from diagnosis to treatment. The British Thoracic Society and the Joint Collegiate Council for Oncology recommend a maximum time from referral to first respiratory specialist visit of 7 days and a maximum of 56 days from specialist consultation to surgery.[56] The recommendations of the Swedish Lung Cancer Study Group are that 80% of patients should have their diagnostic tests completed within 4 weeks of the initial consultation with a specialist and that treatment should start within 2 weeks of test completion.[13] The RAND Corporation recommends a maximum of 6 weeks from diagnosis to treatment.[57] Canadian recommendations are a maximum of 4 weeks between the first visit to a family physician and diagnosis and the waiting time for surgery should not exceed 2 weeks.[58]

SUMMARY

The prognosis of LC is poor because most cases present in an advanced stage. Few things can be done to alter this reality. Screening holds the greatest promise, and it is evident that small tumors found through screening have an excellent prognosis. For the typical patient with symptomatic LC, delays in the diagnostic workup of a few weeks are very unlikely to have much impact on prognosis; but more substantial delays may result in the disease progressing from a potentially resectable stage to one that is not. Resectability does not necessarily lead to long-term survival because that will be determined by the underlying biology of the cancer and its propensity to metastasize. However, only surgery with or without adjuvant chemotherapy can offer a real chance of long-term survival, so it is important to maximize the potential for surgical resection by organizing the health care system in such a way that the diagnostic workup can be completed promptly. At the very least, a rapid diagnostic workup will help patients and their family members cope with the understandable anxiety of not knowing whether they have cancer and if they have cancer, what treatment will be offered. Lung DAUs or virtual programs with patient navigation will maximize the potential for early diagnosis and the best currently possible outcomes.

REFERENCES

1. Canadian Cancer Society's Steering Committee on Cancer Statistics. Canadian cancer statistics 2012. Toronto: Canadian Cancer Society; 2012. ISSN 0835–2976.

2. Groome PA, Bolejack V, Crowley JJ, et al, on behalf of the International Staging Committee, Cancer Research and Biostatistics, Observers to the Committee and Participating Institutions. The IASLC lung cancer staging project: validation of the proposals for revision of the T, N, and M descriptors and consequent stage groupings in the forthcoming (seventh) edition of the TNM classification of malignant tumors. J Thorac Oncol 2007;2(8): 694–705.

3. Brundage M, Davies D, Mackillop WJ. Prognostic factors in non-small cell lung cancer. A decade of progress. Chest 2002;122:1037–57.

4. Arai T, Kuroishi T, Saito Y, et al. Tumour doubling time and prognosis in lung cancer. Jpn J Clin Oncol 1994;24(4):199–204.

5. Honda O, Johkoh T, Sekiguchi J, et al. Doubling time of lung cancer determined using three-dimensional volumetric software: comparison of squamous cell carcinoma and adenocarcinoma. Lung Cancer 2009;66(2):211–7.

6. Radzikowska E, Roszkowowski-Sliz K, Glaz P. The impact of timeliness of care on survival in non-small cell lung cancer. Pneumonol Alergol Pol 2012;80(5): 422–9.

7. Radzikowska E, Glaz P, Roszkowski K. Lung cancer management and prognosis. Pneumonol Alergol Pol 2001;69:600–10.

8. Fergusson RJ, Gregor A, Dodds R, et al. Management of lung cancer in South East Scotland. Thorax 1996;51:569–74.

9. Koyi H, Hillerdal G, Branden E. Patient's and doctor's delays in the diagnosis of chest tumours. Lung Cancer 2002;35:53–7.

10. Olsson JK, Schultz EM, Gould MK. Timeliness of care in patients with lung cancer: a systematic review. Thorax 2009;64:749–56.

11. Comber H, Korin DP, Deady S, et al. Delays in treatment in the cancer services: impact on cancer stage and survival. Ir Med J 2005;98:238–9.

12. Neal RD, Allgar VL, Ali N. Stage, survival and delays in lung cancer, colorectal, prostate and ovarian cancer: comparison between diagnostic routes. Br J Gen Pract 2007;57:212–9.

13. Myrdal G, Lambe M, Hillerdal G, et al. Effect of delays on prognosis in patients with non-small cell lung cancer. Thorax 2004;59:45–9.

14. Gonzalez-Barcala FJ, Garcia-Prim JM, Alvarez-Dobano JM, et al. Effects of delays on survival in patients with lung cancer. Clin Transl Oncol 2011; 12:836–42.

15. Skaug K, Eide GE, Gulsvik A. Predictors of long term survival of lung cancer patients in Norwegian community. Clin Respir J 2011;5:50–8.

16. Salomaa ER, Sallinen S, Hiekkanen H, et al. Delays in the diagnosis and treatment of lung cancer. Chest 2005;128:2282–8.

17. Porta M, Gallen M, Malats N, et al. Influence of "diagnostic delay" upon cancer survival: an analysis of five tumour sites. J Epidemiol Community Health 1991;45:225–30.

18. Siciliani L, Hurst J. Tackling excessive waiting times for elective surgery: a comparative analysis of policies in 12 OECD countries. Health Policy 2005;72:201–15.

19. Billing JS, Wells FC. Delays in the diagnosis and surgical treatment of lung cancer. Thorax 1996;51: 903–6.

20. Liberman M, Liberman D, Sampalis JS, et al. Delays to surgery in non-small-cell lung cancer. Can J Surg 2006;49:31–6.

21. Naruke T, Tsuchiya R, Kondo H, et al. Prognosis and survival after resection for bronchogenic carcinoma based on the 1997 TNM staging classification: the Japanese experience. Ann Thorac Surg 2001;71: 1759–64.

22. Murray PV, O'Brien ME, Sayer R, et al. The pathway study: results of a pilot feasibility study in patients suspected of having lung carcinoma investigated in a conventional chest clinic setting compared to a centralized two-stop pathway. Lung Cancer 2003;42:283–90.

23. Kesson E, Bucknall CE, McAlpine LG, et al. Lung cancer – management and outcome in Glasgow, 1991-92. Br J Cancer 1998;78(10):1391–5.

24. Watkin SW, Hayhurst GK, Green JA. Time trends in the outcome of lung cancer management: a study of 9,090 cases diagnosed in the Mersey Region 1974-86. Br J Cancer 1990;61:590–6.

25. Gregor A, Thomson CS, Brewster DH, et al. Management and survival of patients with lung cancer in Scotland diagnosed in 1995: results of a national population based study. Thorax 2001;56:212–7.

26. Laroche C, Wells F, Coulden R, et al. Improving surgical resection rate in lung cancer. Thorax 1998;53:445–9.

27. Dransfeld MT, Lock BJ, Garver RI. Improving the lung cancer resection rate in the US Department of Veterans Affairs health system. Clin Lung Cancer 2006;7(4):268–72.

28. United States Department of Veterans Affairs. Available at: http://www.va.gov. Accessed November 4, 2005.

29. Humphrey E, Smart C, Winchester D, et al. National survey of the pattern of care for carcinoma of the lung. J Thorac Cardiovasc Surg 1990;100:837–43.

30. Fry W, Menck H, Winchester D. The national cancer database report in lung cancer. Lung Cancer 1996; 77:1947–55.

31. Ringbaek T, Borgeskov S, Lange P, et al. Diagnostic and therapeutic process and prognosis in suspected lung cancer. Scand Cardiovasc J 1999; 33:337–43.

32. Pita-Fernandez S, Montero-Martinez C, Pertega-Diaz S, et al. Relationship between delayed

diagnosis and the degree of invasion and survival in lung cancer. J Clin Epidemiol 2003;56: 820–5.

33. Loh LC, Chan LY, Tan RY, et al. Effect of time delay on survival in patients with non small cell lung cancer – a Malaysian study. Asia Pac J Public health 2006;18:69–71.

34. Bozcuk H, Martin C. Does treatment delay affect survival in non-small cell lung cancer? A retrospective analysis from a single UK centre. Lung Cancer 2001;34:243–52.

35. Aragoneses FG, Moreno N, Leon P, et al. Influence of delays on survival in the surgical treatment of bronchogenic carcinoma. Lung Cancer 2002;36: 59–63.

36. Kashiwabara K, Koshi S, Ota K, et al. Outcome in patients with lung cancer found retrospectively to have had evidence of disease on past lung cancer mass screening roentgenograms. Lung Cancer 2002;35:237–41.

37. Quarterman RL, McMillan A, Ratcliffe MB, et al. Effect of preoperative delay on prognosis for patients with early stage non-small cell lung cancer. J Thorac Cardiovasc Surg 2003;125:108–13.

38. Buccheri G, Ferrigno D. Lung cancer: clinical presentation and specialist referral time. Eur Respir J 2004;24:898–904.

39. Kanashiki M, Satoh H, Ischikawa H, et al. Time from finding abnormality on mass-screening to final diagnosis for lung cancer. Oncol Rep 2003;10: 649–52.

40. Kashiwabara K, Koshi S, Itonaga K, et al. Outcome in patients with lung cancer found on lung cancer mass screening roentgenograms, but who did not subsequently consult a doctor. Lung Cancer 2003; 40:67–72.

41. Annakkaya AN, Arbal P, Balbay O, et al. Effect of symptom-to-treatment interval on prognosis in lung cancer. Tumori 2007;93:61–7.

42. International Early Lung Cancer Action Program Investigators, Henschke CI, Yankelevitz DF, Libby DM, et al. Survival of patients with stage I lung cancer detected on CT screening. N Engl J Med 2006;355(17):1763–71.

43. The National Lung Screening Trial Research Team. Reduced lung-cancer mortality with low-dose computed tomographic screening. N Engl J Med 2011; 365:395–409.

44. Dubayova T, van Dijk JP, Nagyova I, et al. The impact of the intensity of fear on patient's delay regarding health care seeking behaviour: a systematic review. Int J Public Health 2010;55:459–68.

45. Dracup K, Moser D. Beyond socio-demographic: factors influencing to seek treatment for symptoms of acute myocardial infarction. Heart Lung 1997; 26:253–62.

46. Lo DS, Zeldin RA, Skrastins R, et al. Time to treat: a system redesign focusing on decreasing the time from suspicion of lung cancer to diagnosis. J Thorac Oncol 2007;2:1001–6.

47. Gagliardi A, Grunfeld E, Evans WK. Evaluation of diagnostic assessment units in oncology: a systematic review. J Clin Oncol 2004;22:1126–35.

48. Clausen J, Hsieh YC, Acharaya S, et al. Results of the Lynn Sage Second-Opinion Program for local therapy in patients with breast carcinoma: changes in management and determinants of where care is delivered. Cancer 2002;94:889–94.

49. Staradub VL, Messenger KA, Hao N, et al. Changes in breast cancer therapy because of pathology second opinions. Ann Surg Oncol 2002;9:982–7.

50. Birkmeyer JD, Siewers A, Finlayson EV, et al. Hospital volume and surgical mortality in the United States. N Engl J Med 2002;346:1128–37.

51. Birkmeyer JD, Stukel TA, Siewers AE, et al. Surgeon volume and operative mortality in the United States. N Engl J Med 2003;349:2117–27.

52. Brouwers M, Crawford J, Elison P, et al. Organizational standards for diagnostic assessment programs. Available at: http://www.cancercare.on.ca/ toolbox/qualityguidelines/other-reports/collaborative-pr-ebs/. Accessed October 10, 2012.

53. Available at: https://www.cancercare.on.ca/ocs/qpi/ dispathmgmt/disease_pathway_maps/. Accessed October 15, 2012.

54. Department of Health. Referral guidelines for suspected cancer. London: Department of Health; 2000.

55. Department of Health. The NHS cancer plan. London: Department of Health; 2000.

56. British Thoracic Society. BTS recommendations to respiratory physicians for organizing the care of patients with lung cancer: the Lung Cancer Working Party of the British Thoracic Society Standards of Care Committee. Thorax 1998;53(Suppl 1):S1–8.

57. Reifel J. Lung cancer. In: AQsch S, Kerr E, Hamilton E, et al, editors. Quality of care for oncologic conditions and HIV: a review of the literature and quality indicators. RAND Corporation; 2000. Available at: http://www.rand.org/pubs/monograph_reports/MR1281. Accessed October 10, 2012.

58. Simunovic M, Gagliardi A, McCready D, et al. A snapshot of waiting times for cancer surgery provided by surgeons affiliated with regional cancer centres in Ontario. CMAJ 2001;165:421–5.

Physiology and Clinical Applications of Cardiopulmonary Exercise Testing in Lung Cancer Surgery

Nha Voduc, MD, FRCPC

KEYWORDS

- Preoperative assessment • Exercise physiology • Cardiopulmonary exercise testing
- Vo_2 (oxygen uptake)

KEY POINTS

- Cardiopulmonary exercise testing (CPET) permits measurement of oxygen uptake (Vo_2), an indicator of overall cardiopulmonary fitness and a useful measurement in the assessment of operative risk for lung resection patients.
- CPET should be considered for the risk stratification of potential lung resection patients with FEV_1 (forced expiratory volume in first second of expiration) or diffusion capacity of carbon monoxide of less than 80% predicted.
- Predicted postoperative peak Vo_2 measurements of less than 10 mL/kg/min are associated with significantly increased risk of mortality and morbidity after lung resection.
- CPET is not indicated or appropriate for all patients; clinicians ordering CPET should be aware of the contraindications and limitations of this test.

INTRODUCTION

Pulmonary resection is the cornerstone of management for patients with localized primary lung cancer. However, given that tobacco smoking is a common risk factor for lung cancer, chronic obstructive pulmonary disease, and cardiovascular disease, many patients who have lung cancer have preexisting cardiorespiratory disease. Consequently, many patients with surgically resectable lung cancer disease may not be operable. The surgeon must weigh the potential benefits of surgery with the risk of postoperative complications.

Cardiopulmonary exercise testing (CPET) has been shown to be an invaluable diagnostic tool in the preoperative assessment of the patient who has lung cancer. It can be used to measure disability, distinguish between cardiovascular and respiratory causes of exercise limitation, and aid in the risk stratification of potential candidates for pulmonary resection. Exercise is unique in that it simultaneously places demands on both the cardiovascular and respiratory systems. This characteristic makes exercise testing an ideal tool for evaluating cardiovascular and respiratory function. However, CPET is neither required by nor applicable to all patients who have lung cancer. This article provides an overview of cardiopulmonary exercise physiology, describes the nature of CPET, and discusses the evidence supporting its role in the preoperative assessment of the patient who has lung cancer. It also discusses the contraindications and limitations to CPET, the effects of surgical resection on exercise physiology, and potential alternatives to formal CPET.

Division of Respirology, University of Ottawa, Ottawa Hospital, General campus, 501 Smyth Road, Mailbox 211, Ottawa, Ontario K1H 8L6, Canada
E-mail address: nvoduc@Ottawahospital.on.ca

Thorac Surg Clin 23 (2013) 233–245
http://dx.doi.org/10.1016/j.thorsurg.2013.01.005
1547-4127/13/$ – see front matter © 2013 Elsevier Inc. All rights reserved.

thoracic.theclinics.com

BASICS OF EXERCISE PHYSIOLOGY

Under normal circumstances, our cardiovascular and respiratory systems have tremendous capacity to respond to the increased metabolic demands associated with physical activity. At rest, an individual uses only a small fraction of their potential cardiovascular and respiratory output. Therefore, it is not surprising that many patients with clinically significant respiratory or cardiac disease may not have clinically obvious findings at rest. By increasing demands on both the cardiovascular and respiratory systems, exercise testing represents a useful modality for uncovering the presence of disease and assessing disability.

Arguably, the single best measurement of overall cardiopulmonary fitness is the maximum oxygen uptake (Vo_2 max). This measurement is often expressed as milliliters of oxygen (uptake) per minute. Oxygen is required to meet the increased energy requirements of exercise, and consequently the body must increase its oxygen uptake. The process requires the coordinated function of multiple systems. Oxygen uptake is determined by multiple factors: respiratory function, cardiac function, oxygen-carrying capacity in the blood, distribution of blood, and extraction and use of oxygen in the peripheral tissues.

Theoretically, impairment of any of these systems can impair the uptake and use of oxygen. However, in health, the relative capacity or reserve of the respiratory system is greater than the cardiovascular reserve. At the maximum exercise, the average healthy individual is limited by their cardiovascular system (oxygen transport and use) and uses only 60% to 70% of their maximum ventilatory capacity. Ventilatory limitation to exercise occurs only in patients with respiratory disease or in elite athletes. Elite athletes' cardiovascular systems may have greater than normal capacity, resulting in use of their entire respiratory capacity at peak exercise.

The fact that only a portion of the respiratory capacity is used at peak exercise for most healthy individuals has major clinical implications. First, this situation means that mild respiratory disease is not associated with a reduction in exercise capacity. It also means that interventions that reduce lung function, such as pulmonary resection, do not necessary have a proportional impact on overall functional capacity.

PRINCIPLES OF CPET

CPET differs from conventional cardiac stress testing in that it uses a pneumotachograph and gas analyzers, which enable the measurement of key metabolic variables: ventilation, oxygen production, and carbon dioxide. These variables, in addition to heart rate, provide the cornerstones for CPET. They allow CPET to simultaneously assess cardiovascular and respiratory responses during exercise. This section reviews selected cardiopulmonary exercise measurements and principles that are essential for the preoperative assessment of the patient undergoing thoracic surgery. Those readers interested in other applications of CPET or more details on the methodology and interpretation of CPET are referred to the American Thoracic Society (ATS)/American College of Chest Physicians (ACCP) guidelines for CPET and as well as an excellent textbook edited by Weisman and Zeballos.[1]

Key Exercise Measurements

Vo_2

Possibly the most important and unique feature of CPET is that it permits direct measurement of Vo_2. Vo_2 max refers to the highest Vo_2 attainable by the patient. Provided that exercise testing is conducted under consistent conditions, Vo_2 max is a highly reproducible measurement.[2] During exercise, Vo_2 increases with work load. Vo_2 max is attained when further increases in work load are no longer associated with any further increases in work load (a plateau is seen on the Vo_2 vs work graph). Consequently, determination of the Vo_2 max requires significant effort on behalf of the patient: the patient has to continue exercising at their maximum capacity for long enough to visualize this plateau. Although this goal can be accomplished by highly motivated patients (particularly those who exercise regularly and who are accustomed to experiencing significant levels of dyspnea and fatigue), many patients are not able to sustain exercise long enough to discern a clear Vo_2 max. For these patients, the term peak Vo_2 is conventionally used. Peak Vo_2 is the highest Vo_2 measured during the exercise test. If a patient shows evidence of approaching cardiovascular or respiratory limitation, the peak Vo_2 obtained is likely close to the patient's maximum Vo_2.

Maximum Vo_2 is influenced by patient size and muscle mass used during exercise, as well as fitness; larger individuals have a higher Vo_2 than smaller individuals. To help standardize Vo_2 for individuals of different sizes and make it a better reflection of relative fitness, Vo_2 is often reported as Vo_2 per kilogram. This strategy has obvious limitations: the Vo_2/kg is disproportionally low in obese individuals and disproportionally high in patients who are underweight. Alternative estimates of fitness have been suggested, such as

V_{O_2}/height, V_{O_2}/body mass index, or even V_{O_2}/lean body weight. None of these alternatives have been formally evaluated in the preoperative literature.

Heart rate and cardiovascular limitation

As work load demands increase during exercise, cardiovascular output must increase. During early exercise, this goal is accomplished by increases in both heart rate and stroke volume. Stroke volume reaches a plateau early, and subsequent increases in cardiac output are reflected by linear increases in heart rate. For most individuals, the cardiac output is limited by heart rate. The maximum attainable heart rate can be predicted using the equation: $210 - (0.65 \times age)$, although there is some degree of variation between individuals. At the end of exercise, if a patient's heart rate is at least 90% of their predicted maximum heart rate, it is reasonable to conclude that their exercise capacity is limited by cardiovascular factors.

Other signs of cardiovascular limitation include arrhythmias or decreases in systolic blood pressure. During exercise, systolic blood pressure increases, reflecting increases in stroke volume. A drop in systolic blood pressure is an ominous sign and may reflect failure of the cardiac pump or severe pulmonary vascular disease.

Patients with heart disease or conditions that reduce oxygen transport or use (such as anemia or deconditioning), typically show proportionally greater heart rate increases for a given V_{O_2} (increased HR/V_{O_2} slope).

Ventilation and ventilatory limitation

Another of the unique measurements obtained during CPET is minute ventilation. Ventilation must increase during exercise, to meet the increased metabolic need for oxygen and to eliminate carbon dioxide. In health, the main stimulus for ventilation is carbon dioxide production. Increases in ventilation are accomplished by increases in both tidal volume and respiratory rate. Similar to stroke volume, the increase in tidal volume reaches a plateau early during exercise, after which further increases in ventilation are reflected by increases in respiratory rate. The peak tidal volume attained during exercise is influenced by lung mechanics and respiratory muscle strength. It is approximately 60% of the resting vital capacity.

Maximum ventilatory capacity during exercise can be estimated using a variety of predictive equations. Exercise is limited by ventilatory factors if peak ventilation attained during exercise is at least 85% of the predicted maximum ventilation. The reliability of predictive equations for maximum ventilation is variable, depending on the equation

used and patient population. Flow volume loop assessments can also be obtained during exercise testing and may potentially offer a more reliable method of identifying ventilatory limitation. The interested reader is referred to the ATS/ACCP guidelines for CPET[2] for an overview of alternative methods of assessing ventilatory limitation.

Lung disease may have 2 potential effects on ventilatory responses during exercise. Alterations in lung mechanics seen in either obstructive or restrictive lung diseases lead to reductions in the maximum ventilatory capacity. If severe enough, these reductions result in early exercise limitation. Furthermore, lung disease may also be associated with increased physiologic dead space, which must be compensated for by increases in ventilation. This situation is reflected by an increased ventilation/V_{O_2} slope during exercise.

Anaerobic threshold

As exercise intensity increases, aerobic mechanisms for energy production are not adequate and anaerobic mechanisms must be recruited to meet metabolic energy demands. The disadvantage to anaerobic energy pathways is the production of lactic acid, which is metabolized to CO_2 and water. The CO_2 produced by anaerobic mechanisms stimulates increased ventilation. The term anaerobic threshold (AT) refers to the point at which there is a rapid increase in arterial lactate levels. Although it is possible to directly measure lactate levels by blood tests performed during exercise, this is not typically measured in clinical settings. The AT is most often estimated to occur when there is a change in the V_{O_2}/VCO_2 slope during exercise (V-slope method).

The AT is expressed as a percentage of the predicted maximum V_{O_2}, and typically occurs at 40% to 70% of the predicted maximum V_{O_2}. Work loads lower than the AT can be sustained indefinitely (provided there are adequate energy stores), whereas work loads greater than AT cannot be sustained.

Any condition that could impair oxygen transport or use could potentially affect the AT. Common causes of a reduced AT include deconditioning and cardiovascular disease. Anemia or, rarely, mitochrondial myopathies may also be associated with reductions in AT. AT is an appealing measurement because it reflects overall cardiovascular fitness and its determination does not require a maximal effort from the patient. However, it does have limitations: a clear AT may not be discernable from the exercise data for all patients. Furthermore, patients with severe respiratory disease may be limited by respiratory factors before attaining an AT.

Exercise Methodology

To conduct CPET, an exercise machine is used to provide a standardized resistance. The 2 most widely used exercise devices for this purpose are a treadmill and cycle ergometer. Although both modalities have their proponents, one is not necessary superior to the other for all patients, and it is important to be aware of their relative strengths and weaknesses.

Treadmill testing is advantageous because it uses motions that are familiar to almost all patients: walking/running. Because the work load on treadmill exercise is shared among more muscle groups than cycling, patients are able to achieve a 10% higher Vo_2 and are less likely to terminate treadmill exercise because of quadriceps fatigue.[3,4] On occasion, it may be advantageous for the patient to achieve a higher Vo_2 to detect certain physiologic abnormalities (eg, ischemic heart disease). Given the ubiquitous nature of cardiac stress testing, which primarily uses treadmill exercise, most hospitals already have a treadmill available. The disadvantages to treadmills include no direct measurement of work load, increased motion artifact, and (theoretically) reduced safety. For treadmill testing, a work load is established by adjusting the treadmill speed and incline. However, for a given speed, there can be significant variations in the work load placed on the patient, depending on gait and length of stride. When patients are running on a treadmill, there is greater body motion, which can potentially affect the quality of electrocardiographic (EKG) tracings and make the measurement of blood pressure more challenging (this can be offset by the use of automated blood pressure cuffs). Treadmill exercise does place greater demands on patients' coordination and balance than a stationary cycle ergometer. This situation may be problematic for more elderly and frail patients.

Cycle ergometry is advantageous because it provides a more stable platform for exercise than treadmill testing. Because patients exercise in a seated position on a stationary cycle, there is generally less motion artifact and fewer demands on the coordination of the patient. Furthermore, because the patient's weight is supported, cycle ergometry can be used to measure exercise performance in patients whose exercise capacity is too low to permit ambulation. Cycle exercise for CPET is typically performed on an electronically braked cycle ergometer, which allows the work load to be directly set by the laboratory personnel. The software in the cycle ergometer varies the resistance based on the cycling speed, to maintain a specified work load. The disadvantage to cycle ergometry is that the motion may not be as familiar as walking for some patients.

Regardless of which exercise modality is used, it is important for the clinician to be aware that peak Vo_2 measured on cycle ergometry is typically lower than the peak Vo_2 measured during treadmill testing. Although normal ranges for exercise parameters such as Vo_2 and V_E have been established specifically for cycle ergometry, this discrepancy makes it difficult to compare results for cycle ergometry with treadmill testing for a given patient. Most studies evaluating CPET in preoperative risk assessment used cycle ergometry.

Most clinical CPETs should be symptom limited to record the highest attainable results for metabolic measurements. This criterion means that during the test, the patient is given standardized verbal encouragement to exercise as long as possible. The test is usually terminated only when the patient cannot exercise further because of intolerable symptoms (usually leg fatigue or dyspnea). On occasion, CPET may be stopped by the laboratory personnel before the development of symptom limitation because of safety concerns. Indications to stop CPET include significant ventricular arrhythmias, severe hypertension, hypotension, reduced consciousness, inability to follow commands, and profound oxygen desaturation (**Box 1**). This situation emphasizes the need for clinical CPET to be conducted by

---

Box 1
Indications for exercise termination

Chest pain suggestive of ischemia

Ischemic EKG changes

Complex ectopy

Second-degree or third-degree heart block

Decrease in systolic pressure by more than 20 mm Hg from highest value during test

Hypertension (>250 mm Hg systolic and >120 mm Hg diastolic)

Severe desaturation (<80%)

Sudden pallor

Loss of coordination

Mental confusion

Dizziness or presyncope

Signs of respiratory failure

Data from American Thoracic Society, American College of Chest Physicians. ATS/ACCP Statement on cardiopulmonary exercise testing. Am J Respir Crit Care Med 2003;167:211–77.

appropriately trained medical personnel who are capable of recognizing the need for early termination of the test.

A variety of exercise protocols have been established for CPET. These protocols vary in rate of increase in work load (or increase in speed and incline in treadmill protocols) and how much time is spent at a given work load (duration of each stage). The choice of protocol should be dictated by the patient population and clinical circumstances. For most clinical CPETs, there is no need to compare CPET results between different patients, and consequently a protocol is chosen by the laboratory personnel before the exercise test, based on estimations of the patient's exercise capacity. Ideally, the duration of exercise should be 8 to 12 minutes.[2,5] Tests that are shorter than 8 minutes may not provide enough exercise data (although this might be unavoidable in patients with severe cardiac or respiratory disease). In contrast, tests that are too long may result in patients terminating exercise because of muscle fatigue, before cardiovascular or pulmonary limits can be reached.

In cycle ergometry, most clinical CPETs are conducted using a simple incremental program: the work load is increased by 5 to 20 W, every 1 or 2 minutes. Given that most patients with lung resection undergoing exercise testing have comorbidities, a work load increase of 10 W/min (or 20 W increases at 2-minute intervals) has been typically used in the preoperative literature. A 2-minute warm-up period with pedaling at a low resistance (20 W) may be used.

CPET IN PREOPERATIVE ASSESSMENT
Relationship Between Exercise Parameters and Operative Risk

Numerous studies have established a link between cardiopulmonary fitness, as measured by peak Vo_2 and poor surgical outcomes. The first study to show this relationship for patients with pulmonary resection was published by Eugene in *Surgery Forum* in 1982.[6] This study reported that a low peak Vo_2 was associated with increased postoperative mortality in patients with pulmonary resection. The investigators retrospectively reviewed preoperative peak Vo_2 measurements in 19 patients who went on to undergo pneumonectomy. These investigators found that that a peak Vo_2 of less than 1 L/min was associated with 100% mortality, whereas no mortality was identified in patients who achieved a peak Vo_2 of more than 1 L/min. Furthermore, the investigators also did not identify a relationship between preoperative FEV_1 (forced expiratory volume [FEV] in first

second of expiration) and surgical outcome. Despite the small sample size and retrospective nature of this study, its results did provoke significant interest in the role of CPET for the evaluation of patients undergoing thoracic surgery.

In 1984, Smith and colleagues[7] reported that Vo_2 was also able to predict the likelihood of postoperative complications. These investigators evaluated 22 patients undergoing lung resection surgery. In contrast to the Eugene study, Smith and colleagues did standardize Vo_2 for patient size. They found that a Vo_2/kg of less than 15 mL/kg/min was associated with a 100% complication rate whereas a Vo_2/kg of more than 20 was associated with only a 10% complication rate. Bechard and Wetstein[8] reported similar results when they compared pulmonary function and exercise parameters in 50 patients undergoing lung surgery who did and did not experience postoperative complications. These investigators found no difference in mean FEV_1 between the 2 groups but significant differences in exercise performance. The group who developed complications had a significantly lower peak Vo_2 than the group who did not. There were no complications in patients with a peak Vo_2/kg greater than 20 mL/kg/min, whereas patients with a peak Vo_2/kg of less than 10 had a 71% complication rate. In addition, the only deaths in their study occurred in patients with a peak Vo_2 of less than 10 (mortality was 29% for patients with a peak Vo_2/kg <10).

Not all studies have reported an association between exercise performance and risk of operative complications. However, a meta-analysis of 14 studies performed by Benzo and colleagues[9] reported differences in peak Vo_2 (as well as peak Vo_2/kg) in patients with lung resection who did and did not develop postoperative complications.

Although peak Vo_2/kg is a good reflection of exercise capacity, it is also dependent on age and is affected by obesity. It is possible that using peak Vo_2/kg as the only measure of operability may unfairly bias the assessment against older or obese individuals. Bolliger and colleagues[10] evaluated the % predicted peak Vo_2 as an alternative measure. They compared the receiver-operator curves for Vo_2/kg and percent predicted Vo_2 against complication rates. Because the patient's results are compared against a predicted reference based on their age, age was excluded as a factor. Similarly, the results are not directly affected by the patient's weight. Bolliger and colleagues found that the area under the curve (AUC) for % predicted Vo_2 was slightly greater than the AUC for Vo_2/kg. A peak Vo_2 greater than 75% predicted was associated with only a 10% complication rate. One limitation to this approach is that most patients for whom exercise testing is conducted have a peak V_{O_2} that is less than 75% of predicted. Despite evaluating a relatively healthy patient population (mean FEV_1 and diffusion capacity of carbon monoxide [DLCO] were >80% for the study group), only 49% of their patients attained a peak V_{O_2} of more than 75% of predicted.

One of the key studies to establish the role of CPET in the preoperative evaluation of the high-risk patient undergoing thoracic surgery was published by Morice and colleagues.[11] These investigators prospectively performed CPET in 37 high-risk patients. These patients were all deemed high-risk because of preexisting respiratory impairment, at least by traditional standards. To be included in the study, all patients had to have either: FEV_1 less than 40%, a predicted postoperative FEV_1 of less than 33% or a respiratory acidosis (P_{CO_2} [partial pressure of carbon dioxide] >43). Eight of 37 patients showed a peak V_{O_2} of greater than 15 mL/kg/min, despite their baseline respiratory impairment. Those patients were offered surgery (lobectomy or segmentectomy) and had a 0% postoperative mortality. This study showed that CPET was able to identify a subset of high-risk patients who could still undergo surgical resection safely.

AT has also been evaluated as a predictor of postoperative complications, and may further refine the predictive results obtained by peak V_{O_2}/kg measurements. Torchio and colleagues[12] found that among patients with a peak V_{O_2}/kg of less than 20 mL/kg/min, no patients with an AT of more than 14.5 mL/kg/min experienced severe complications, whereas 92% of patients with an AT less than 14.5 mL/kg/min experienced severe complications. The main limitation of using AT is that it may not be identifiable in all patients. Bechard and Wetstein[8] previously recognized an association between AT and postoperative complications but did not focus on AT, because they found that it could be identified in only 58% of their patients.

There has been little study on the association between ventilatory limitation during exercise testing and risk of operative complications. Dales and colleagues[13] in a retrospective analysis found that a ventilatory reserve of less than 25 L at peak exercise was associated with an increased risk of respiratory complications, but this has not been validated in a prospective study.

Preoperative Assessment Algorithms

Traditionally, CPET was used a last resort test in the preoperative evaluation of the patient with lung resection. CPET was performed only on high-risk patients, with the goal of identifying the subset of patients who could still undergo surgery with a low risk of complications. CPET was not used unless patients had already undergone pulmonary function testing (PFT) and quantitative perfusion scanning and if their postoperative predicted (ppo) FEV_1 or DLCO was less than 40%.[14,15]

Over the last decade, this approach has been challenged. Wyser and Bolliger[16] evaluated the usefulness of an algorithm that used CPET before nuclear perfusion scanning. When they compared their algorithm with the traditional approach, they found that both approaches excluded a comparable number of patients, but the algorithm using CPET immediately after PFTs and before nuclear scanning was associated with a lower complication rate. Because of these results, recent guidelines have adopted this algorithm.[17] The 2009 European Respiratory Society (ERS)/European Society of Thoracic Surgeons guidelines for radical therapy in lung cancer, suggested the following approach for the respiratory evaluation of potential patients for lung resection (**Fig. 1**):

1. Measurement of FEV_1 and DLCO. If both are greater than 80%, may proceed to surgery.
2. If either FEV_1 or DLCO is less than 80%, CPET should be performed. If the peak V_{O_2} is greater than 75% of predicted or V_{O_2}/kg is greater than 20 mL/kg/min, then may proceed to surgery.
3. If peak V_{O_2} less than 35% of predicted or V_{O_2}/kg is less than 10, surgical resection is not recommended.
4. If the V_{O_2} or V_{O_2}/kg are between theses ranges, then ppo values for FEV_1, DLCO, and peak V_{O_2} should be calculated. Surgical resection that leaves a ppo FEV_1 and ppo DLCO both greater than 30% and a ppo V_{O_2} greater than 10 mL/kg/min may proceed.

Safety and Clinical Limitations of CPET

Clinicians ordering CPET must be familiar with the potential complications and contraindications to CPET. Exercise testing is generally safe, with severe complication rates of less than 1:10 000[10]. Absolute contraindications to CPET include severe or uncontrolled cardiac disease (cardiomyopathy, unstable angina, and arrhythmias), uncontrolled asthma, significant infection or metabolic derangement, or an uncooperative patient (**Box 2**). Consequently, CPET should not be ordered before a clinical assessment.

CPET can diagnose cardiac disease, but CPET may be less sensitive and specific than other forms of cardiac stress testing. The diagnosis of ischemic heart disease with CPET (as with conventional

ERS/ESTS TASK FORCE

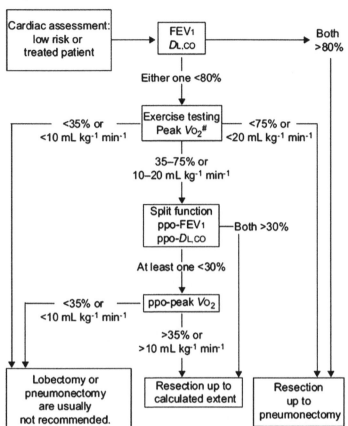

Fig. 1. ERS/ESTS preoperative assessment algorithm. (*From* Bolliger CT, Perruchoud AP. Functional evaluation of the lung resection candidate. Eur Respir J 1998;11:206; with permission from the European Respiratory Society.)

cardiac stress testing) is based on the presence of ST depressions on EKG tracings. Gianrossi and colleagues[18] published a meta-analysis of 147 studies comparing exercise-induced ST abnormalities with coronary angiography. They found a substantial variation in the published literature, but the overall sensitivity and specificity of ST changes for significant coronary artery disease was 68% and 77%, respectively. CPET can detect other abnormalities associated with cardiac disease, such as an increased heart rate to Vo_2 slope and a reduced AT. However, these CPET measurements are not specific to cardiac disease: they can be affected by other conditions that reduce oxygen delivery or use, such as deconditioning or anemia. Consequently, if the clinical preoperative evaluation suggests a high likelihood of cardiac disease, the patient should be sent for more specific testing, such as a dobutamine echocardiogram, in addition to PFT and CPET.

Not all patients undergoing thoracotomy are capable or willing to perform preoperative exercise testing, but this factor itself may be a harbinger of increased risk. Epstein and colleagues[19] prospectively evaluated 74 thoracotomy cases at their center. Nineteen percent were unable to undergo CPET. These patients had similar resting pulmonary function compared with most who underwent CPET, but scored higher on the cardiac risk index (described later). They had significantly more complications and significantly higher mortality.

ALTERNATIVES TO CPET FOR PREOPERATIVE EVALUATION

Compared with other forms of exercise testing, CPET is the most resource intensive, and consequently, CPET is not available in all centers performing lung resection. Other forms of exercise testing have been used for preoperative evaluation.

Stair Climbing

Stair climbing has been used for preoperative assessment for decades. For this test, the patient is asked to climb as many flights of stairs as possible. The test is self-paced: there is no

---

Box 2
Absolute and relative contraindications for CPET

Absolute:

Myocardial infarction within previous 3 to 5 days

Unstable angina

Uncontrolled arrhythmias, causing symptoms or hemodynamic instability

Syncope

Active endocarditis, myocarditis, or pericarditis

Symptomatic aortic stenosis

Uncontrolled heart failure or pulmonary edema

Acute pulmonary embolus or pulmonary infarction

Thrombosis of lower extremities

Suspected dissecting aneurysm

Uncontrolled asthma

Respiratory failure

Acute noncardiopulmonary disorder, which may affect exercise performance or be aggravated by exercise

Room air oxygen saturation less than 85% at rest

    NB: although CPET can be performed with supplemental oxygen in these cases, reliable measurement of Vo_2 is not possible with supplemental oxygen use

Relative:

Left main coronary stenosis or equivalent

Moderate stenotic valvular disease

Severe untreated systemic hypertension (>200 mm Hg systolic, >120 mm Hg diastolic)

Tachyarrhythmias or bradyarrhythmias

High-degree atrioventricular block

Hypertrophic cardiomyopathy

Significant pulmonary hypertension

Advanced or complicated pregnancy

Electrolyte abnormalities

Orthopedic impairment that compromises exercise performance

Data from American Thoracic Society, American College of Chest Physicians. ATS/ACCP Statement on cardiopulmonary exercise testing. Am J Respir Crit Care Med 2003;167:211–77.

---

required speed or time limitation. The primary measurement is number of flights of stairs climbed. In 1968, Van Nostrand and colleagues[20] published a chart review of patients undergoing pneumonectomy and found that inability to climb 2 flights of stairs without severe dyspnea was associated with a 50% mortality after pneumonectomy. Although this study is widely cited, among the 91 patients with stair climbing data, only 4 were unable to climb 2 or less flights of stairs with severe dyspnea.

Stair climbing is appealing because of its simplicity, but it is difficult to standardize, for both the patient and the health facility conducting the test. There are no well-accepted standards for details such as climbing pace, use of railing for support, height of each step, or numbers of stairs in each flight. There are no established normal ranges for stair-climbing distance. Furthermore, stair climbing provides no direct physiologic information. Pollock and colleagues[21] did report an approximate correlation between number of stairs climbed and peak V_{O_2} measured via cycle ergometer but did not specifically assess for a relationship between stair-climb results and operative outcomes. Brunelli and colleagues[22] have published several studies on stair climbing in patients undergoing thoracic surgery. Brunelli and Salati[23] evaluated prospectively 160 patients and found that altitude attained on stair climbing was a superior predictor of postoperative complications than either resting FEV_1 or predicted postoperative FEV_1. Only 6.5% of patients able to climb 14 m of stairs developed postoperative complications, whereas 50% of patients who climbed 12 m or less developed complications. This study did not directly compare stair climbing with formal CPET. Because of the low cost and simplicity of stair climbing, Brunelli and Salati have suggested stair climbing be used before CPET during preoperative evaluation. In their algorithm, patients who were able to climb 22 m (or climb at least 12 m and had ppo FEV_1 and ppo DLCO >40%) could proceed to operation without need for CPET. CPET would be used only for patients who were unable to climb 22 m and had a ppo FEV_1 or ppo DLCO of less than 40%. Although this approach is appealing, its usefulness requires validation.

Six-Minute Walk Test

The conduct of the 6-minute walk test (6MWT) is reflected in its name: the patient is asked to walk as far as possible over a period of 6 minutes. The primary outcome of interest is distance walked. The concept and usefulness of a timed walking test were originally validated by Cooper[24] with the 12-minute walk test; however, Butland and colleagues[25] subsequently reported close correlation between results from a 6MWT and a 12-minute walk test. They also reported slightly less variance in the results of the 6MWT on repeated testing. Consequently, the 6MWT has largely replaced its longer counterpart. Similar to stair climbing, the 6MWT does not provide direct physiologic information, although the distance walked during a 6MWT has been shown to correlate with quality of life measures as well as aerobic capacity (V_{O_2}) in patients with lung disease.[26,27] Furthermore, standardized protocols have been published to improve the reproducibility of 6MWT.[28]

The 6MWT can be used to assess responses to therapy (particularly pulmonary rehabilitation) and is validated as a prognostic indicator for chronic lung disease. Holden and colleagues[29] found a significant difference in preoperative 6MWT distance between patients who died within 90 days of surgery compared with those who survived. However, data for 6MWT in preoperative patients are limited and inconsistent. Consequently, it is not recommended for preoperative assessment.[17,30]

Risk Indices

Some investigators have suggested the use of scoring systems for assessing the risk of postoperative complications. One of the first to be specifically developed for patients with lung resection and possibly the most widely cited was published by Epstein and colleagues.[31] They combined the cardiac risk index developed by Goldman with additional respiratory factors to create the cardiopulmonary risk index (CPRI). Patients received a CPRI score of 1 to 10, based on the sum of their cardiac risk index score (1–4; 1 for a Goldman score of 0–5, 2 for 6–12, 3 for 12–25, and 4 for >25) and pulmonary risk index score (1 point each for the presence of obesity, smoking within 8 weeks of surgery, productive cough within 5 days of surgery, diffuse wheezing within 5 days of surgery, FEV_1/FVC (forced vital capacity) <0.7, and $Paco_2$ [partial pressure of carbon dioxide, arterial] >45 mm Hg). These investigators found that patients with a CPRI of 4 or greater were more likely to experience postoperative complications (positive predictive value of 79% and negative predictive value of 86%). In addition, when CPRI score and peak V_{O_2} were evaluated in a multiple regression model, peak V_{O_2} did not add any additional predictive value for postoperative complications. The limitations to using the CPRI are its relative complexity as well as reliance on some subjective factors. A subsequent study by Ferguson confirmed a difference in mean CPRI scores for patients who did and did not experience postoperative complications but found that the difference was small (less than half a point on the 10-point CPRI scale).[32]

More recently, Falcoz and colleagues[33] derived a scoring system designed to predict in-hospital mortality for thoracic surgery. Their system (Thoracoscore) was based on the outcomes of 15,183 patients from 59 French hospitals between 2002 and 2005. These investigators found that the following factors were associated with an increased risk of mortality: age, sex, American Society of Anesthesiologists score, performance status, dyspnea score, priority of surgery (urgent or not), procedure (pneumonectomy or other), diagnosis (benign or malignant), and number of comorbidities score (0, 1–2, or 3+). The Thoracoscore has been validated in other hospital settings.[34] As with Epstein's CPRI, the limitations of the Thoracoscore are its complexity and use of potentially subjective factors (eg, priority of surgery, number of comorbidities). However, it is appealing, because it can provide an estimation of mortality risk.

POSTOPERATIVE OUTCOMES

Although CPET is not routinely used after lung resection surgery, a few studies have used CPET in the postoperative period to assess the effect of surgery on exercise capacity. Brunelli and colleagues[35] performed CPETs on patients undergoing lobectomy and pneumonectomy at discharge and 1 month and 3 months after resection. Lobectomy was associated with a 12% reduction in peak Vo_2 at discharge, but this improved to 3% at 3 months (not statistically different from preoperative exercise capacity). Pneumonectomy was associated with an 18% reduction in peak Vo_2 at time of discharge. Three months later, patients who underwent a pneumonectomy still had a peak Vo_2 that was 11% lower than their preoperative measurements. Although statistically significant, the reduction in peak Vo_2 is smaller than reductions in lung function after pneumonectomy (at 3 months after pneumonectomy, FEV_1 and DLCO was still 34% and 20% lower than preoperative values).

Bolliger and colleagues[36] compared postoperative Vo_2/kg with predictions of postoperative Vo_2/kg calculated using the same methodology as ppo FEV_1: ppo Vo_2/kg = preoperative Vo_2 × (1 − number of segments to be resected/19). These investigators found that calculations of ppo Vo_2/kg significantly overestimated the degree of exercise capacity loss after an operation. At 6 months after surgery, the loss in exercise capacity was only about half the loss predicted by equation. This finding is not surprising, because the relationship between Vo_2 loss and lung function loss is not linear. Although Bolliger and colleagues did not find that ppo Vo_2/kg accurately predicted postoperative exercise capacity, they did find that it was the best predictor for both postoperative morbidity and mortality. Mortality in patients with a ppo Vo_2 of less than 10 mL/kg/min (3 of 25 patients studied) was 100%.

Although preoperative peak Vo_2/kg measurements can help predict likelihood of complications in the postoperative period, its value in the prediction of long-term outcomes or postoperative disability has not been well established. Beccaria and colleagues[37] reviewed the outcomes of 62 patients with lung cancer resection. Seven patients had a ppo FEV_1 of less than 40% but underwent surgical resection because their peak Vo_2/kg was greater than 10 mL/kg/min. Of these 7 patients, 2 became oxygen-dependent and experienced marked limitation of daily living.

CONTROVERSIES AND LIMITATIONS OF THE EXISTING RESEARCH

Although a preponderance of data and expert opinion support a role for CPET in the evaluation of the preoperative patient, there are limitations to the existing literature and controversies with this approach.

Lack of Focus on High-Risk Patients

Most of the exercise literature does not focus specifically on the higher-risk patient. Current practice recommendations suggest CPET be used only on higher-risk patients (who are believed to be at increased risk for poor outcomes because of low ppo lung function). Most studies performed CPET on all patients undergoing resection, regardless of their preoperative risk. Only a few studies focused exclusively on high-risk patients.[11,16] Although this oversight is understandable for studies published before the role of CPET in preoperative evaluation became well established, more modern studies still remain too inclusive in their study population.

Extent of Surgical Resection

Much of the existing literature does not take into account the extent of surgical resection. For example, the original article by Eugene[6] as well as the more recent study by Wyser[16] included patients undergoing segmentectomy, single lobectomy, bilobectomy, and pneumonectomy. The physiologic impact and risk from a segmentectomy would be expected to be less than a pneumonectomy, and so it would intuitively be expected to use different peak Vo_2/kg thresholds, depending on the extent of surgery. These thresholds remain to be established. The use of a ppo Vo_2/kg greater than 10, as suggested by Bolliger and colleagues,[10] may represent the best method of taking into account the extent of surgical resection, but this requires confirmation.

Long-Term Outcomes

It remains to be proved whether preoperative exercise performance has any influence on long-term clinical outcomes. Most of the literature has focused on clinical outcomes within 30 days of surgery. Long-term outcomes are more likely to be dependent on factors other than cardiopulmonary physiology. Therefore, it may be unrealistic to expect pre-Vo_2 (or any other exercise finding) to have any major predictive value in long-term outcomes.

Clinical Relevance of Postoperative Complications

There has been an attempt by many investigators to use a consistent definition for postoperative complications. The original study establishing a link between peak Vo_2/kg and complications by Smith[7] focused on cardiopulmonary complications: $Paco_2$ greater than 45 mm Hg, greater than 48 hours' mechanical ventilation, myocardial infarction, arrhythmias, pneumonia, lobar atelectasis, pulmonary embolus, and death. Many subsequent investigators have used similar definitions for postoperative complications in their studies.[10–12] Studies that have included a broader range of complications such as excessive blood loss or wound infection have not identified a relationship between complications and exercise performance.[38]

The clinical significance of these cardiopulmonary complications is highly variable. For example, postoperative atelectasis may have no adverse long-term sequelae, even if bronchoscopy is required in the postoperative period. Most of the complications are likely preferable to unresected lung cancer, provided that the patient is not left with major permanent disability. Consequently, some investigators have argued that it would be incorrect to exclude patients solely because of an increased risk of complications.[39]

Consequences of Not Operating

Much of the existing literature focuses on the outcomes of patients who undergo surgery, without the context of clinical outcomes for early-stage cancer that is left unresected. Consequently, it is difficult to establish what mortality or complication rate should be prohibitive for surgery. Although a patient with moderate chronic obstructive pulmonary disease may be at increased risk for postoperative complications and even mortality, it is difficult to know at what point these risks outweigh the potential benefits of cancer resection. A recent study by Loewen and colleagues[40] showed the value and limitations of CPET in patients undergoing surgery for lung cancer. They used an algorithm similar to that suggested by Wyser and colleagues. Patients with a ppo FEV_1 less than 33% or greater than 900 mL underwent CPET. If their peak Vo_2/kg was at least 15, the patient was offered surgery. If the peak Vo_2/kg was less than 15, patients were categorized as very high risk. These patients could still undergo surgery depending on the discretion of the thoracic surgeon (the use of additional testing such as DLCO or perfusion scanning was not described). Of the 403 patients with adequate data, 86 were categorized as very high risk (ppo FEV_1 <33% or <900 mL and peak Vo_2 <15). Of these patients, 68 underwent some form of thoracotomy. Although the study did confirm that peak Vo_2 was a predictor of both postoperative complications and poor outcome (death or respiratory failure), the mortality in the subset of the very-high-risk patient group was only 4% (3 of 68). Although the selection of patients for surgery was not randomized (thus leaving the outcomes vulnerable to confounding by other patient factors), the investigators did note that the 5-year survival of the 68 high-risk patients who underwent surgery was superior to that of patients who did not undergo resection. This study shows the importance of not basing operative decisions solely on a fixed threshold value for peak Vo_2. The threshold for operating is a moving target; it is influenced by improvements in surgical technique and postoperative care as well as the development and refinement of effective nonsurgical treatment of early-stage lung cancer (eg, radical radiotherapy).

SUMMARY

CPET is a valuable tool in the preoperative assessment of the patient who has lung cancer. It can identify patients at increased risk for mortality as well as postoperative complications. However, it is neither required nor appropriate for all patients. It should not be a substitute for a careful clinical assessment. The results obtained from cardiopulmonary exercise should be used to aid, not replace, clinical judgment. As with any other diagnostic test in medicine, its value is dependent on the ability of the clinician to use it judiciously.

REFERENCES

1. Weisman IM, Zeballos RJ. Clinical exercise testing. Progress in Respiratory Research, vol. 32. Basel (Switzerland): Karger; 2002.
2. American Thoracic Society, American College of Chest Physicians. ATS/ACCP statement on cardiopulmonary exercise testing. Am J Respir Crit Care Med 2003;167:211–77.
3. Miyamura M, Honda Y. Oxygen intake and cardiac output during maximal treadmill and bicycle exercise. J Appl Physiol 1972;32(2):185–8.
4. Hermansen L, Saltin B. Oxygen uptake during maximal treadmill and bicycle exercise. J Appl Physiol 1969;26(1):31–7.
5. Balady GJ, Arena R, Sietsema K, et al. Clinician's guide to cardiopulmonary exercise testing in adults: a scientific statement from the American Heart Association. Circulation 2010;122(2):191–225.

6. Eugene J, Brown SE, Light RW, et al. Maximum oxygen consumption: a physiologic guide to pulmonary resection. Surg Forum 1982;33:260–2.

7. Smith TP, Kinasewitz GT, Tucker WY, et al. Exercise capacity as a predictor of post-thoracotomy morbidity. Am Rev Respir Dis 1984;129(5):730–4.

8. Bechard D, Wetstein L. Assessment of exercise oxygen consumption as preoperative criterion for lung resection. Ann Thorac Surg 1987;44(4):344–9.

9. Benzo R, Kelley GA, Recchi L, et al. Complications of lung resection and exercise capacity: a meta-analysis. Respir Med 2007;101(8):1790–7.

10. Bolliger CT, Jordan P, Solèr M, et al. Exercise capacity as a predictor of postoperative complications in lung resection candidates. Am J Respir Crit Care Med 1995;151(5):1472–80.

11. Morice RC, Peters EJ, Ryan MB, et al. Exercise testing in the evaluation of patients at high risk for complications from lung resection. Chest 1992; 101(2):356–61.

12. Torchio R, Gulotta C, Parvis M, et al. Gas exchange threshold as a predictor of severe postoperative complications after lung resection in mild-to-moderate chronic obstructive pulmonary disease. Monaldi Arch Chest Dis 1998;53(2):127–33.

13. Dales RE, Dionne G, Leech JA, et al. Preoperative prediction of pulmonary complications following thoracic surgery. Chest 1993;104(1):155–9.

14. Gilbreth EM, Weisman IM. Role of exercise stress testing in preoperative evaluation of patients for lung resection. Clin Chest Med 1994;15(2): 389–403.

15. Datta D, Lahiri B. Preoperative evaluation of patients undergoing lung resection surgery. Chest 2003; 123(6):2096–103.

16. Wyser C, Stulz P, Solèr M, et al. Prospective evaluation of an algorithm for the functional assessment of lung resection candidates. Am J Respir Crit Care Med 1999;159(5 Pt 1):1450–6.

17. Brunelli A, Charloux A, Bolliger CT, et al. ERS/ESTS clinical guidelines on fitness for radical therapy in lung cancer patients (surgery and chemo-radiotherapy). Eur Respir J 2009;34(1):17–41.

18. Gianrossi R, Detrano R, Mulvihill D, et al. Exercise-induced ST depression in the diagnosis of coronary artery disease. A meta-analysis. Circulation 1989; 80(1):87–98.

19. Epstein SK, Faling LJ, Daly BD, et al. Inability to perform bicycle ergometry predicts increased morbidity and mortality after lung resection. Chest 1995;107(2):311–6.

20. Van Nostrand D, Kjelsberg MO, Humphrey EW. Pre-resectional evaluation of risk from pneumonectomy. Surg Gynecol Obstet 1968;127(2):306–12.

21. Pollock M, Roa J, Benditt J, et al. Estimation of ventilator reserve by stair climbing. Chest 1993;104: 1378–83.

22. Brunelli A, Al Refai M, Monteverde M, et al. Stair climbing test predicts cardiopulmonary complications after lung resection. Chest 2002;121(4): 1106–10.

23. Brunelli A, Salati M. Preoperative evaluation of lung cancer: predicting the impact of surgery on physiology and quality of life. Curr Opin Pulm Med 2008;14(4):275–81.

24. Cooper KH. A means of assessing maximal oxygen intake. Correlation between field and treadmill testing. JAMA 1968;203(3):201–4.

25. Butland RJ, Pang J, Gross ER, et al. Two-, six-, and 12-minute walking tests in respiratory disease. Br Med J (Clin Res Ed) 1982;284(6329):1607–8.

26. Guyatt GH, Townsend M, Keller J, et al. Measuring functional status in chronic lung disease: conclusions from a randomized control trial. Respir Med 1991;85(Suppl B):17–21 [discussion: 33–7].

27. Cahalin L, Pappagianopoulos P, Prevost S, et al. The relationship of the 6-min walk test to maximal oxygen consumption in transplant candidates with end-stage lung disease. Chest 1995;108(2):452–9.

28. ATS Committee on Proficiency Standards for Clinical Pulmonary Function Laboratories. ATS statement: guidelines for the six-minute walk test. Am J Respir Crit Care Med 2002;166(1):111–7.

29. Holden DA, Rice TW, Stelmach K, et al. Exercise testing, 6-min walk, and stair climb in the evaluation of patients at high risk for pulmonary resection. Chest 1992;102(6):1774–9.

30. Brunelli A, Pompili C, Salati M. Low-technology exercise test in the preoperative evaluation of lung resection candidates. Monaldi Arch Chest Dis 2010;73(2):72–8.

31. Epstein SK, Faling LJ, Daly BD, et al. Predicting complications after pulmonary resection. Preoperative exercise testing vs a multifactorial cardiopulmonary risk index. Chest 1993;104(3):694–700.

32. Ferguson MK, Durkin AE. A comparison of three scoring systems for predicting complications after major lung resection. Eur J Cardiothorac Surg 2003;23(1):35–42.

33. Falcoz PE, Conti M, Brouchet L, et al. The Thoracic Surgery Scoring System (Thoracoscore): risk model for in-hospital death in 15,183 patients requiring thoracic surgery. J Thorac Cardiovasc Surg 2007; 133(2):325–32.

34. Chamogeorgakis T, Toumpoulis I, Tomos P, et al. External validation of the modified Thoracoscore in a new thoracic surgery program: prediction of in-hospital mortality. Interact Cardiovasc Thorac Surg 2009;9(3):463–6.

35. Brunelli A, Xiumé F, Refai M, et al. Evaluation of expiratory volume, diffusion capacity, and exercise tolerance following major lung resection: a prospective follow-up analysis. Chest 2007; 131(1):141–7.

36. Bolliger CT, Wyser C, Roser H, et al. Lung scanning and exercise testing for the prediction of postoperative performance in lung resection candidates at increased risk for complications. Chest 1995;108(2): 341–8.

37. Beccaria M, Corsico A, Fulgoni P, et al. Lung cancer resection: the prediction of postsurgical outcomes should include long-term functional results. Chest 2001;120(1):37–42.

38. Colman NC, Schraufnagel DE, Rivington RN, et al. Exercise testing in evaluation of patients for lung resection. Am Rev Respir Dis 1982; 125(5):604–6.

39. Lim E, Beckles M, Warburton C, et al. Cardiopulmonary exercise testing for the selection of patients undergoing surgery for lung cancer: friend or foe? Thorax 2010;65(10):847–9.

40. Loewen GM, Watson D, Kohman L, et al. Preoperative exercise Vo2 measurement for lung resection candidates: results of Cancer and Leukemia Group B Protocol 9238. J Thorac Oncol 2007; 2(7):619–25.

Absolute and Relative Contraindications to Pulmonary Resection
Effect of Lung Cancer Surgery Guidelines on Medical Practice

Farid M. Shamji, MBBS, FRCS(C), FACS

KEYWORDS

- Operability and resectability • Complete and incomplete resection
- Absolute and relative contraindications • Interdisciplinary care

KEY POINTS

- Clinical and radiological determinants of the intrathoracic and extrathoracic spread of lung cancer in guiding treatment.
- The absolute and relative contraindications to resection for lung cancer.

INTRODUCTION

Surgical treatment of primary lung cancer is based on sound clinical, surgical, oncological, radiological, and pathologic principles.[1] Operation still remains the most effective treatment of non–small cell lung cancer and chemotherapy for the small cell type. A successful operation requires complete resection. Incomplete resection results in local recurrence and incurable metastatic cascade thereof. Complete resection R0 means that the primary tumor has been completely removed, no macroscopic tumor is left behind, all microscopic margins are normal, systematic lymph node dissection has been performed for therapeutic benefit and staging, and the highest mediastinal lymph node at R2 or L2 is normal. It is considered incomplete resection when, after definitive pathologic examination, there is a finding of microscopic residual disease R1 or macroscopic residual disease R2.[2]

Pointers in the practical surgical management of primary lung cancer are:

1. The terms operability and resectability are not synonymous, and indiscriminate use of the terms should be avoided. Operability refers to the patient characteristics that permit a safe operation according to the adequacy of cardiopulmonary function and physiologic health. Resectability refers to the tumor characteristics and stage, taking into consideration the results of imaging studies, diagnostic biopsy, and mediastinal nodal staging. Observing these points helps to avoid misrepresentations and unnecessary expectations of surgical treatment, especially when the chest is explored and found to have a tumor, the resection of which is technically impossible, therapeutically pointless, or, at worse, incomplete (**Box 1**).

2. The multidisciplinary thoracic oncology team is obligated to look at the determinants of treatment based on clinical presentation, surgical risk, histology, staging investigations, and surgical assessment of mediastinal lymph nodes.

3. Surgical assessment of the mediastinum in relation to lymphatic drainage from each lung and each lobe to the bronchopulmonary N1 lymph nodes and mediastinal N2 and N3 lymph nodes is essential. Equally important is the recognition

Division of Thoracic Surgery, General Campus, The Ottawa Hospital, 501 Smyth Road, Ottawa, Ontario K1H 8L6, Canada
E-mail address: fshamji@ottawahospital.on.ca

Thorac Surg Clin 23 (2013) 247–255
http://dx.doi.org/10.1016/j.thorsurg.2013.01.010
1547-4127/13/$ – see front matter © 2013 Elsevier Inc. All rights reserved.

Box 1
Four groupings of patients with lung cancer

Operable and resectable

Inoperable and resectable

Operable and unresectable

Inoperable and unresectable

---

of ipsilateral and contralateral lymphatic drainage in the thorax; contralateral lymph flow happens more from the left lung than the right side.[3–5] This recognition allows accurate preoperative staging of the mediastinum, which is necessary for selecting patients for a successful operation Cancer cells may travel from the mediastinal lymph nodes to:

a. Cervical nodes (common)

b. Retroperitoneal para-aortic nodes and adrenal gland[6] (infrequent)

c. Axilla and internal mammary chain (rarely, through lymphatic connections between lung, chest wall, breast, and axilla[7])

4. Resection of distant solitary metastases

Three sites of distant metastases have been recognized at initial presentation of primary non–small cell lung cancer, for which surgical intervention may be indicated for optimal control of the disease, in the absence of local intrathoracic spread:

a. Unilateral adrenal gland metastases on the same side as the primary lung cancer

This lymphatic spread is through connections from the lower lobe to the inferior posterior mediastinal and retroperitoneal paraortic lymph nodes connecting with the rich capsular lymphatics of the adrenal gland.[6,8]

b. Brain

Brain is infiltrated by hematogenous dissemination and only the solitary metastasis is considered for resection or radiosurgery.[9,10]

c. Scalene lymph node metastases and normal mediastinum (N1 or N3?)

This condition is known to occur in true superior sulcus tumor, without first involving mediastinal lymph nodes, by direct regional lymphatic spread. It occurs by apical tumor penetrating through the Sibson fascia.

5. Peripheral lung cancer invading chest wall and adjoining structures may be apical, lateral, posterior, or anterior. Superior sulcus tumor is located at the extreme apex of the lung growing within the confines of the bony thoracic inlet, which, at the time of first investigation, may have invaded directly[8]:

a. Adjacent chest wall (first, second, and perhaps third rib)

b. Lower trunk of the brachial nerve plexus or its C8 or T1 roots, stellate sympathetic ganglion

c. Adjoining thoracic spine at T1 and T2, by apical posterior tumor

d. Subclavian vessels, by apical anterior tumor

e. Scalene nodes, by direct regional lymphatic drainage

At other sites of chest wall invasion, anterior or lateral, there is a slight possibility of lymphatic spread to the axillary or internal mammary nodes when invading lung cancer accesses lymphatics in the overlying soft tissues.[7]

6. Clinical and radiological features of lung cancer dissemination, intrathoracic and extrathoracic, to be noted at initial presentation when a mass suspicious for lung cancer is detected (**Box 2**).[11]

7. Determinants of absolute and relative contraindications to definitive resection in primary lung cancer

Surgery remains the most effective treatment of primary non–small cell lung cancer. It must be selective and ensure complete resection, and it is rare and unpredictable to convert incomplete resection into complete resection with adjuvant therapy. Surgical treatment is not preferred for small cell lung cancer because it is often widespread at initial presentation. Chemotherapy is the treatment of choice for limited and extensive small cell lung cancer, whereas surgery is reserved for early very limited stage I T1aN0 and T1bN0, and possibly II disease, with either induction or adjuvant chemotherapy.[12,13]

Selection of patients for surgery requires disciplined consideration of all absolute and relative contraindications to pulmonary resection.[1] This principle identifies those patients who will have favorable outcome and avoids unnecessary operation in those who will not benefit.

ABSOLUTE CONTRAINDICATIONS TO DEFINITIVE PULMONARY RESECTION
Surgical Management not Possible Because of Tumor Dissemination

Greater than 50% of patients, when they first present for investigation, are found to have extrapulmonary intrathoracic extension of cancer or extrathoracic distal spread that makes them unsuitable for operation (**Box 2**).

Cervical lymph node metastases

Lymph nodes within the scalene fat pad, located just anterior to the omohyoid fascial covering on scalenus anterior muscle and phrenic nerve, are juxtaposed, just lateral between the deep jugular chain of cervical lymph nodes above and the mediastinal lymph nodes below. On the right side, metastatic spread occurs by lymph flow from the right paratracheal mediastinal nodes, and on the left side by way of anterior mediastinal nodes lying just beneath the left innominate vein.[4]

Lymphatic spread to the scalene nodes N3 may be ipsilateral, bilateral, or contralateral. Routine scalene node biopsy in lung cancer is not advised unless it is clinically palpable.

In the presence of cervical lymph node metastases, often with additional evidence of extrapulmonary intrathoracic dissemination, survival longer than 6 months is uncommon.

Box 2
Recognition of disseminated lung cancer

Palpable Cervical Nodes	Metastases
Clinical neurologic disturbance	Intracranial metastases
Abnormal imaging studies	Bulky mediastinum, lymphangitic carcinomatosis, pulmonopulmonary metastases, nodular pleural and/or pericardial thickening and effusion, superior vena cava obstruction
Unrelenting bone pain	Bone metastases
Worsening dysphagia	Esophageal compression by enlarged metastatic mediastinal lymph nodes
Unexplained hoarseness	Recurrent laryngeal nerve interrupted: left, in the subaortic window; right, in the thoracic inlet
Painful lump in the muscles of the limbs or torso	Metastases
Palpable painful chest wall mass	Lung cancer directly invading the adjacent chest wall and soft tissues
Swollen plethoric face and dilated veins in the neck and over the chest	Superior vena cava obstruction from encasement or compression by enlarged metastatic mediastinal lymph nodes
Noisy breathing of severe stridor and other bronchopulmonary symptoms	Proximal central lung cancer invading distal trachea or both main bronchi
Rapidly progressive weakness in the legs	Paraneoplastic manifestation of peripheral motor neuropathy
Acute back pain and leg weakness, urinary incontinence	Spine metastases with spinal cord compression or cauda equina syndrome
Abnormal bronchoscopy, advanced mediastinal lymphatic spread	Tracheal compression, invasion and obstruction of main bronchi, or an ulcerated and broadened main carina
Direct pericardial invasion	Paralyzed diaphragm, chest discomfort, and dyspnea caused by refractory atrial fibrillation and large pericardial effusion
Delayed recognition of superior sulcus tumor	Extensive invasion of lung cancer within the local confines of the bony thoracic inlet
Severe breathlessness	Large pleural or pericardial effusion, complete lung atelectasis, impending cardiac tamponade
Generalized malaise and fatigue, new bronchopulmonary symptoms, palpable cervical nodes, abnormal imaging studies	Malignant cachexia
New skin nodule and subcutaneous nodule	Metastases
Life-threatening hemoptysis	Centrally seated advanced lung cancer invading large pulmonary arterial branch or obstructing major bronchus with distal infection resulting in formation of abnormal fragile bronchial arterial circulation and rupture with ensuing profuse hemorrhage

Mediastinal lymph node metastases

More than 70% of the patients in whom surgical assessment of mediastinum has confirmed lymphatic dissemination have cryptic or overt systemic metastases, considered an incurable disease. Preoperative mediastinal nodal biopsy helps to avoid an unnecessary chest exploration in incurable cases and to identify those potentially curable by resection.

The routine use of this 45-minute outpatient staging procedure, by ruling out mediastinal nodal N2, N3 spread, permits resection of lung cancer in more than 95% of patients when the chest is explored; very different from the days when only 50% proved to be resectable.[14,15]

Familiarity with N1, N2, and N3 descriptors and the nodal map in the tumor-node-metastasis (TNM) staging system is essential in the multidisciplinary management of lung cancer.[2,5,16] The prognosis in N2 descriptor is often poor, and the role of surgery with or without induction treatment must be evaluated for its risks and benefits.[17] Operation is not recommended when:

- Multiple nodes are infiltrated by cancer
- Only the subcarinal node harbors cancer
- Enlarged malignant nodes, by extracapsular extension, densely adhere to the adjoining structures, compressing or encasing them
- Cancer in the lower lobe involves superior or inferior mediastinal nodes

N3 descriptor, taken to mean contralateral spread to the mediastinal or hilar lymph nodes, represents incurable cancer.

Lymphangitic carcinomatosis

This condition, recognized by its characteristic radiographic appearance, indicates the presence of diffuse pulmonary perivascular and peribronchial lymphatic permeation of cancer throughout the lung or lobe that harbors the primary tumor. It may be the only evidence of tumor spread and bronchoscopy may be normal. These patients rarely survive longer than 10 weeks from the time of diagnosis.

Brain metastases as a presenting feature

Patients with primary lung cancer may present with symptoms and signs of intracranial metastases. The commonest neurologic disturbances are hemiplegia, convulsions, personality change, confusion, speech defects, ataxia, persistent headache and visual disturbances, and occasionally coma from increased intracranial pressure.

The duration of neurologic symptoms before investigation is usually less than a month, and, in some, less than a week. The immediate threat to life by brain metastases demands expedient investigations and treatment first for the brain metastases and later for the primary site.

When faced with multiple brain metastases, pulmonary resection is ruled out. Even if brain is the only site of solitary metastases, pulmonary resection is still ruled out if intrathoracic spread of lung cancer is present.

Bone metastases

It is common to find bone metastases as the only evidence, at the time of first investigation, of disseminated cancer. The most common site of bone metastases from lung cancer is the ribs and the patient may complain of acute pain in relation to coughing from pathologic fracture. The next most common site is the spine and the patient may present with severe back pain and possibly with neurologic symptoms. Pelvic bone metastases alone are common in the ischium and iliac crest. Pathologic fracture occurring through unsuspected metastasis in the femur has been seen during investigation for respiratory symptoms. All patients die within a year of investigation and most die within 6 months.

Hepatic metastases as the only contraindication to surgical management

Patients may first present with enlarged nodular liver as the only clinical evidence of disseminated lung cancer. More often, liver involvement is detected on staging computed tomography (CT) scan or positron emission tomography scan. It is a sign of advanced incurable disease, fatal within 6 months of presentation.

Pulmonopulmonary metastases

It is common for patients, when they first present for investigation for suspected localized primary lung cancer, to have radiographic evidence of pulmonopulmonary metastases as the only evidence of dissemination. This dissemination may be in the same lobe, in different lobes of the same lung, or to the contralateral lung. These tumor deposits may be multiple or isolated, varying in size from 0.5 cm to 4 cm, and rarely miliary.

Metastatic spread within the same lobe is T3 descriptor, T4 if another ipsilateral lobe, and M1 if the contralateral lung is involved. Pulmonary resection should not be offered for T4 or M1 descriptors because survival is limited to less than 6 months.

Obstruction of the superior vena cava

At first presentation, between 4% and 7% of the patients have clinical features of superior vena cava obstruction. Obstruction results from direct extension of tumor into the mediastinum, compressing or encasing the vein; or by compression from malignant mediastinal nodes. In most cases the cancer is on the right side in the upper lobe. Most patients present within 3 months of venous obstruction. Clinical recognition is obvious; patients appear gravely ill with plethoric swollen faces and dilated subcutaneous collateral veins, and distended jugular veins.

Treatment is palliative with chemotherapy for small cell cancer and radiotherapy for non–small cell cancer. Most patients die within 1 year.

Dysphagia as the presenting symptom
Lung cancer spreading to the mediastinal lymph nodes results in nodal enlargement and midesophageal obstruction by compression. Most patients die within 1 year of investigation and treatment.

Mediastinal invasion and diaphragm paralysis as the only contraindication
Direct mediastinal spread paralyzing the diaphragm by interrupting the phrenic nerve on the pericardium and accompanied by echocardiographic or CT scan evidence of visceral pericardial invasion is an absolute contraindication to pulmonary resection.

Mediastinal invasion and recurrent laryngeal nerve palsy
Left recurrent laryngeal nerve is vulnerable in the subaortic aortopulmonary window where it leaves the left vagus nerve to loop around the aortic arch to ascend to the neck. At this location, it lies in close contact with the left main bronchus and lymph nodes. The nerve becomes interrupted by direct tumor extension from the left main bronchus or by metastases to the lymph nodes. Another site, at which direct invasion from left upper lung cancer causes left vocal cord paralysis, is along the intrathoracic course of left vagus nerve above the aortic arch. Hoarseness of voice, when present before treatment, rules out the possibility of pulmonary resection.

Right vocal cord paralysis may result from superior sulcus tumor extending into the root of the neck. At this point, the right recurrent laryngeal nerve is interrupted as it leaves the vagus nerve and loops around the proximal subclavian artery as the vagus nerve crosses in front of the artery.

Other sites of metastases
Cutaneous or subcutaneous metastases may occur alone or in conjunction with additional clinical evidence of spread. Cutaneous metastases are always small split-pea size, reddened, often painless, and grow quickly. Subcutaneous metastases are generally the size of a small grape when they are clinically recognized. These metastases are more often felt than seen.

Preoperative staging CT scan detects adrenal metastases in only 1% to 3% of cases; these are rarely palpable and almost always clinically silent. Metastatic spread is through either the blood stream or lymph flow. Hematogenous spread is either bilateral or unilateral to the adrenal gland on the side opposite to the primary lung cancer. Lymphatic spread tends to be unilateral on the same side as the primary lung tumor.[8] Pulmonary resection concomitant with adrenalectomy is discouraged when:

- Widespread dissemination is present
- Both adrenal glands are diseased
- N2 disease is present

Abnormal bronchoscopy unsuitable for surgery
Pulmonary resection is problematic in the absence of widespread dissemination when bronchoscopy is judged to be grossly abnormal:

- Main carina is invaded by proximal tumor extension
- Main carina is widened by malignant subcarinal lymph nodes
- Distal trachea is involved beyond the lateral wall on the right side in relation to a tumor in the right upper bronchus
- Trachea is compressed side to side and stiffened
- Both main bronchi are invaded
- Main bronchus is invaded to within 0.5 cm, or the left within 1.5 cm, of the main carina and confirmed with N2 disease
- Patient cannot tolerate standard pneumonectomy or carinal pneumonectomy

Surgical Management Contraindicated for Reasons Other than Metastases

Severe limitation of lung function
Compromised lung function, from subjective impression and objective measurements, may contraindicate operation on this ground alone because of prohibitively high operative risk,[1,18] even if the cancer is localized and potentially curable by surgery alone. The major consequence of pulmonary resection is the permanent loss of physiologic function that nearly always accompanies pulmonary resection that harbors the cancer. This loss of function is less in limited lung resection, more with lobectomy (about 15%), and significant with pneumonectomy (about 35%–45%). Lung resection permanently takes away both the functioning lung parenchyma and the accompanying pulmonary circulation to the

detriment of the functional capacity for the patient; alveolar gas exchange is reduced, right ventricle function may be impaired if the pulmonary vascular resistance is increased and fixed; and the resultant pulmonary hypertension causing right to left intracardiac shunting of blood through patent foramen ovale and fixed hypoxia. Lung function deteriorates further with the complication of postoperative pleuropulmonary sepsis.

The postoperative impairment of functional capacity is greater when the non-neoplastic lung disease compromising lung function is fixed and irreversible, as in severe emphysema, idiopathic pulmonary fibrosis, radiation-induced fibrosis, pneumoconiosis, advanced sarcoidosis, previous pulmonary resection, pulmonary hypertension, and diffuse cystic lung disease. The operative risk is concerning when the estimated postoperative forced expiratory volume in 1 second decreases to less than 1 L corrected for body weight.

The major and minor criteria defining a patient at high risk for surgery are listed in the ACOSOG Z4099/RTOG 1021 randomized phase III study of sublobar resection versus stereotactic body radiation therapy.

Categorization into major risk, intermediate risk, and minor risk in the selection of patients with lung cancer for surgery has been described by Armstrong and colleagues[1] in the British Thoracic Society guidelines published in *Thorax* in 2001.

Other nonmetastatic contraindications to pulmonary resection

Chronologic age alone cannot preclude surgical treatment. To consider an operation in any patient more than 80 years of age requires the patient to be in good physiologic condition, living independently with good social support, fully ambulant and active, mentally alert, and with good nutritional health.[1] The patient must not be either chronologically or physiologically old. The patient should not have critical stenosis in the coronary arterial, or carotid arterial circulation, or severe renal impairment. Otherwise, age constitutes an absolute contraindication to resection.

Some patients may not be suitable for surgical treatment because of frailty caused by cryptic metastasis and advanced age, permanent deficit from stroke, dementia, and advanced parkinsonism.

Nonsurgical Management in Special Circumstances

Primary lung cancer with extensive direct invasion of the adjoining chest wall

Patients may first present with extensive invasion of the adjoining chest wall from peripheral lung cancer that is outside the scope of multimodality therapy.

For example, superior sulcus tumor with unchecked growth within the bony thoracic inlet eventually becomes unresectable because of:

- Complete erosion of the highest 3 ribs
- Invasion into the overlying soft tissues medial to the posterior rib angle, forming a mass palpable in the scapula-vertebra interval
- Advanced thoracic vertebral body invasion and destruction at T1 to T3
- Central perineural tumor extension through the spinal foramina at C8 to T1, T1 to T2, and T2 to T3 with risk of losing spinal cord function by epidural compression
- Extensive brachial plexus invasion that is beyond the lower trunk and its roots

Deep lateral chest wall invasion from tumor in the posterior segment of upper lobe may cause a mass inseparable from the chest wall and palpable in the axilla, possibly with lymphatic spread.

Anterior chest wall invasion from tumor in the anterior segment of the upper lobe may invade the sternum and adjoining ribs, and extend to involve the overlying muscle and soft tissues.

The TNM descriptor for chest wall invasion is T3 when tumor is densely adherent to the chest wall involving parietal pleura and endothoracic fascia, and possibly destroying the inner cortex of the ribs; and T4 when it invades the vertebral body.[16] What is not clear from the new staging system is the prognosis in relation to the depth of chest wall invasion; the prognosis is probably worsened when any tumor invades deeply through the chest wall into the overlying soft tissues.[17] Should T3 or T4 tumor be considered? Should surgical resection be offered in this situation? There is no justifiable answer. Any T3 or T4 descriptor of parietes invasion that is associated with positive N2 nodal spread should not be considered for surgery with or without induction or adjuvant therapy; it is unlikely that there will be 2-year survivors, let alone 5-year survivors, if such treatment is recommended.[19]

Primary lung cancer with malignant pleural effusion

Pleural effusion may be detected by clinical examination alone when it is large and causing profound shortness of breath. In most instances, the effusion is small to moderate in size and detected only on imaging studies. Investigation for malignant cells by pleural fluid cytology is mandatory. If required, the pleural space may be drained slowly and completely to examine the pleural surfaces by CT scan and thoracoscopic pleural biopsies.

Pulmonary resection in the presence of pleural carcinomatosis is pointless; no patients survive longer than 6 months.

Primary lung cancer with pericardial effusion

Pericardial effusion found on CT scan or echocardiogram during initial assessment must be investigated for cause. Direct extension involving visceral pericardium or by metastatic spread may be responsible. Delay in management carries a risk of cardiac tamponade. Urgent diagnosis requires search for malignant cells in pericardial fluid or infiltration in pericardium by biopsy.

Histology of lung cancer that makes it unsuitable for surgical management

Bronchoalveolar cell carcinoma, now called adenocarcinoma in situ (AIS), is pure ground-glass opacity on CT scan measuring 3 cm or less and pure lepidic growth in resected specimens that no longer requires an operation. An invasive adenocarcinoma should be suspected to have developed in AIS when a solid lesion appears during yearly CT scan surveillance within the ground-glass opacity.[20,21] Pulmonary resection should not be contemplated when multiple scattered ground-glass opacities are seen to contain solid components and guaranteed for incomplete resection when more than 1 lobe is involved on the same side, or when both lungs are affected.

Small cell lung cancer that is beyond stage II should not be considered for resection with or without induction or adjuvant chemotherapy.

Lung cancer treated previously with curative radiotherapy

It is unwise to consider operation for resection of recurrent lung cancer for the fear of serious intraoperative technical difficulties and the resulting postoperative complications that may prove fatal.

Relative Contraindications to Definitive Pulmonary Resection

Primary non–small cell lung cancer with limited mediastinal nodal spread and absent distal spread

Pulmonary resection by lobectomy may be considered, before or after chemotherapy, when limited N2 mediastinal spread is found in an otherwise healthy patient without systemic dissemination.[10,22] Treatment is decided only after multidisciplinary discussion in selected cases of localized T1 or T2 cancer in:

- Right upper lobe (RUL) with 1 or 2 lymph node stations in the superior mediastinum at R4 with intranodal metastases and without fixation in the mediastinum, and normal station 7 subcarinal nodes.[14,15]

- Left upper lobe with intranodal spread to only the subaortic station 5 node without adherence to the adjoining structures.[23]

Superior sulcus tumor with spread to scalene lymph node only

Induction chemotherapy and radiation therapy and complete en bloc resection is the recommended treatment of superior sulcus tumor if:

- Mediastinal staging is normal
- Central extension of the tumor into the spinal canal is ruled out
- Extrathoracic spread is absent.

Supported by the evidence discussed earlier, direct thoracic spine invasion from apical posterior tumor does not rule out resection if there is partial destruction of the vertebral bodies and complete resection can be afforded. Vascular invasion in the thoracic inlet from apical anterior tumor is similarly not a contraindication to complete en bloc tumor resection and vascular reconstruction.[24] Furthermore, lymphatic spread to the scalene lymph node only and normal mediastinum should be considered to be regional spread and not N3. Operation is permitted provided complete infraomohyoid cervical lymph node dissection is included in en bloc tumor resection.[19]

Primary non–small cell lung cancer that is early and localized in the chest but has metastasized to only 1 adrenal gland

Adrenal gland metastases, found in 1% to 3% of the cases on routine staging CT scan, are almost always clinically silent and rarely clinically palpable. Dissemination is via blood stream or lymph flow. Blood-borne adrenal metastases tend to be bilateral or unilateral to the gland on the side opposite to the primary side, and often with systemic spread elsewhere. Unilateral spread is more likely from the lymphatic route, more often from lung cancer on the same side, and may be the only site of spread. Downward lymph flow from infiltrated posterior inferior mediastinal lymph nodes to the retroperitoneal para-aortic lymph nodes gives cancer cells access to the rich capsular lymphatic network of the adrenal gland on the same side as the primary lung tumor.[6,8]

Combined resection of isolated adrenal gland metastases and primary lung cancer can be considered if[25]:

- Mediastinal lymph nodes are normal
- Adrenal metastases are on the same side as the primary lung cancer
- No other sites of systemic dissemination

Lower lobe lung cancer with direct invasion of the hemidiaphragm

This finding frequently indicates an intraoperative condition. En bloc complete resection and diaphragm reconstruction are encouraged in this situation with favorable outcome.

Lung cancer with direct attachment to the pericardium with or without phrenic paresis

Direct encroachment on the pericardium, without visceral pericardial invasion, by lung cancer may be discovered on preoperative CT scan or during pulmonary resection. It is a feature of centrally located lung cancer arising in the right middle lobe or lower lobe on either side. En bloc resection of the tumor with involved pericardium and reconstruction is recommended.

RUL cancer with partial attachment to superior vena cava

This pattern of direct spread from lung cancer in the RUL is often seen on preoperative CT scan in the absence of superior vena cava obstruction. Sometimes, it is only discovered during operation. If recognized preoperatively, staging should be complete and favorable for complete en bloc R0 resection. The extent of superior vena cava resection required, partial or complete, depends on how much of the circumference of the vein is involved by tumor. Reconstruction is completed with primary repair when less than 50% of vein circumference needs to be excised or with autologous pericardial patch when 50% of vein circumference is excised; complete superior vena cava resection is replaced with prosthetic polytetrafluoroethylene ringed graft when the superior vena cava is encased in tumor mass.[24,26–28]

Multicentric mixed ground-glass opacities with solid components

It is common to find multiple lesions on CT scan in 1 lung or both lungs that have solid features in the background of ground-glass opacities. The solid component implies that an invasive adenocarcinoma has developed in an in situ adenocarcinoma (bronchioloalveolar cell carcinoma, AIS). The size of the solid component has prognostic implications: less than 5 mm means minimally invasive and greater than 5 mm is deep invasion.[6,15,27] Limited resection of all peripherally located lesions with solid component less than 5 mm is in order and stereotactic body radiation therapy (SBRT) for concomitant deep-seated lesions after the operation. A single lesion that has a large solid component and is deep seated within the lobe requires lobectomy and the simultaneous small peripheral ones limited resections. Pneumonectomy must be avoided in such situations even if the disease is confined to 1 lung only; it is just a matter of time before the disease becomes evident in the contralateral lung.

Bilateral single synchronous primary lung cancers

Synchronous bilateral non–small cell lung cancers may be encountered, either the same cell type but radiologically distinct or different cell types. For operation to be considered:

- Patient must be able to tolerate staged bilateral tumor resections
- Each cancer has independent favorable prognostic features
- Complete resection is possible
- Operate first on the side that seems to have guarded prognosis
- Resect only 1 tumor and SBRT for the other

Primary non–small cell lung cancer and solitary brain metastases

Before staged treatment of brain metastases first and pulmonary resection second can be considered, the prerequisites are[9]:

- Non–small cell cancer
- Localized and resectable in the lung, T1 or T2
- Proven normal mediastinal nodes
- No other sites of distal spread
- Patient is physiologically fit
- Tumor deposit in the brain is solitary and amenable to resection or radiosurgery
- Multidisciplinary discussion is necessary in planning

Primary lung cancer with superimposed empyema

Empyema complicating lung cancer develops from:

- Infected distal obstructive atelectasis
- Diagnostic thoracoscopy
- Diagnostic needle aspiration biopsy
- Inadvertent esophageal injury at cervical mediastinoscopy

Pulmonary resection should be delayed until pleural sepsis is resolved.

SUMMARY

It is crucial for thoracic surgeons to recognize that there are 3 types of surgeon: those who know how to operate, those who know when to operate, and those who know when not to operate. Surgeons must always strive to be all three.

REFERENCES

1. Armstrong P, Congleton J, Fountain SW, et al. Guidelines on the selection of patients with lung cancer for surgery. Thorax 2001;56:89–108.

2. Detterbeck FC, Boffa DJ, Tanoue LT. The new lung cancer staging system. Chest 2009;136:260–71.

3. Naruke T, Tsuchiya R, Kondo H, et al. Lymph node sampling in lung cancer: how should it be done? Eur J Cardiothorac Surg 1999;16:17–24.

4. Nohl-Oser HC. An investigation of the anatomy of the lymphatic drainage of the lungs as shown by the lymphatic spread of bronchial carcinoma. Ann R Coll Surg Engl 1972;51:157–76.

5. Rusch VW, Asamura H, Watanabe H, et al. The IASLC Lung Cancer Staging Project: a proposal for a new international lymph node map in the forthcoming seventh edition of the TNM classification for lung cancer. J Thorac Oncol 2009;4(5):568–77.

6. Meyer KK. Direct lymphatic connections from the lower lobes of the lung to the abdomen. J Thorac Surg 1958;35(6):726–32.

7. McKeown KC, Wilkinson KW. Tuberculous disease of the breast. Br J Surg 1952;39(157):420–9.

8. Karoly P. Do adrenal metastases from lung cancer develop by lymphogenous or hematogenous route? J Surg Oncol 1990;43:154–6.

9. Billing PS, Miller DL, Allen MS, et al. Surgical treatment of primary lung cancer with synchronous brain metastases. J Thorac Cardiovasc Surg 2001;122(3):548–53.

10. Cerfolio RJ, Maniscalco L, Bryant AS. The treatment of patients with stage IIIA non-small cell lung cancer from N2 disease: who returns to the surgical arena and who survives? Ann Thorac Surg 2008;86:912–20.

11. Hyde L, Hyde CI. Clinical manifestations of lung cancer. Chest 1974;65:299–306.

12. Shepherd FA, Ginsberg R, Patterson GA, et al. Is there ever a role for salvage operations in limited small-cell lung cancer? J Thorac Cardiovasc Surg 1991;101:196–200.

13. Waddell TK, Shepherd FA. Should aggressive surgery ever be part of the management of small cell lung cancer? Thorac Surg Clin 2004;14(2):271–81.

14. Pearson FG, Delarue NC, Ilves R, et al. Significance of positive superior mediastinal nodes identified at mediastinoscopy in patients with resectable cancer of the lung. J Thorac Cardiovasc Surg 1982;83:1–11.

15. Pearson FG, Nelems JM, Henderson RD, et al. The role of mediastinoscopy in the selection of treatment for bronchial carcinoma with involvement of superior mediastinal lymph nodes. J Thorac Cardiovasc Surg 1972;64(3):382–90.

16. Goldstraw P, Crowley J, Chansky K, et al. The IASLC lung cancer staging project: proposals for the revision of the TNM stage groupings in the forthcoming (seventh) edition of the TNM Classification of malignant tumours. J Thorac Oncol 2007;2(8):706–14.

17. Murren JR, Buzaid AC, Hait WN. Critical analysis of neoadjuvant therapy for stage IIIa non-small cell lung cancer. Am Rev Respir Dis 1991;143(4 Pt 1):889–94.

18. Donington J, Ferguson MK, Mazzone P, et al. ACCP/STS systematic review for evaluation and management for high-risk patients with stage I non-small cell lung cancer. Chest 2012;142(6):1620–35.

19. Ginsberg RJ, Martini N, Zaman M, et al. Influence of surgical resection and brachytherapy in the management of superior sulcus tumor. Ann Thorac Surg 1994;57:1440–5.

20. Naidich DP, Bankier AA, MacMahon H. Recommendations for the management of subsolid pulmonary nodules detected at CT: a statement from the Fleischner Society. Radiology 2013;266(1):304–17.

21. Travis WD, Brambilla E, Noguchi M, et al. International multidisciplinary classification of lung adenocarcinoma. J Thorac Oncol 2011;6(2):244–85.

22. Kappers I, van Sandick JW, Burgers SA, et al. Surgery after induction chemotherapy in stage IIIA-N2 non-small cell lung cancer: why pneumonectomy should be avoided. Lung Cancer 2009;68(2):222–7.

23. Patterson GA, Piazza D, Pearson FG, et al. Significance of metastatic disease in subaortic lymph nodes. Ann Thorac Surg 1987;43:155–9.

24. Dartvelle P. Extended operations for the treatment of lung cancer. Ann Thorac Surg 1997;63:12–9.

25. Kim SH, Brennan MF, Russo P, et al. The role of surgery in the treatment of clinically isolated adrenal metastasis. Cancer 1997;82(2):389–94.

26. Dartvelle P, Macchiarini P, Chapelier A. techniques of superior vena cava resection and reconstruction. Chest Surg Clin N Am 1995;5(2):345–58.

27. Spaggiari L, Magdeleinat P, Kondo H, et al. Results of superior vena cava resection for lung cancer: analysis of prognostic factors. Lung Cancer 2004;44:339–46.

28. Thomas P, Magnan PE, Moulin G, et al. Extended operation for lung cancer invading the superior vena cava. Eur J Cardiothorac Surg 1994;8:177–82.

Approach to the Patient with Multiple Lung Nodules

Joseph B. Shrager, MD

KEYWORDS

- Non–small cell lung cancer • Adenocarcinoma in situ • Minimally invasive adenocarcinoma
- Lepidic-predominant adenocarcinoma • Ground-glass opacity • Multifocal lung cancer
- Synchronous primary lung cancer

KEY POINTS

- Typical solid, invasive non–small cell lung cancer (NSCLC) behaves much more aggressively than lepidic-predominate adenocarcinoma with a small invasive focus, and thus these disease processes must be managed differently, in cases of both single and multiple tumors.
- Patients with pure ground-glass opacities (GGOs) less than 1 cm in diameter likely do not require surgical resection.
- Minimally invasive adenocarcinomas and pure GGOs less than 2 cm in diameter may be managed by sublobar resection, preferably anatomic segmentectomy.
- Patients with an invasive adenocarcinoma and as many as approximately 10 synchronous, pure GGOs should be approached by anatomic resection of the primary tumor, wedge resection of accessible, ipsilateral GGOs, and serial computed tomography follow-up.

INTRODUCTION

When Bob Ginsberg was at the peak of his practice, a patient with more than 1 pulmonary nodule in separate lobes would have been considered to harbor stage 4 disease with a presumed attendant extremely poor prognosis. That patient would therefore more than likely not have been considered for surgical resection. In recent years, however, data have accumulated that even with standard, solid, invasive, cigarette-smoking–associated non–small-cell lung cancer (NSCLC), a patient with a single malignant nodule in a separate lobe actually does not have such a dire prognosis with resection. Our staging system, in fact, has been changed to reflect this, rendering such a tumor T4 (potentially stage IIIB) rather than stage IV, and this does not even take into consideration the real possibility of the 2 tumors representing separate primaries. In short, many of these patients are now clearly candidates for surgical resection.

Furthermore, in the past decade entirely new types of NSCLC have emerged, namely minimally invasive adenocarcinoma (MIA) and adenocarcinoma in situ (AIS). The unique clinical behavior of these tumors has enormous importance for how we approach patients with multiple nodules of these subtypes. These adenocarcinomas, frequently occurring in nonsmokers, are very often multifocal at presentation, and yet early data on this tumor type would suggest that this multifocality should not dissuade us from operating on these tumors once one or more of the lesions appear to have developed an invasive phenotype.

This article reviews the data underlying the recommended approach to each of these tumor-types when they present with more than a single nodule, and discusses the overall clinical approach to patients with each of these types of multifocal tumors.

Division of Thoracic Surgery, VA Palo Alto Healthcare System, Stanford Medical Center, Stanford University School of Medicine, 300 Pasteur Drive, 2nd Floor, Falk Building, Stanford, CA 94305-5407, USA
E-mail address: shrager@stanford.edu

Thorac Surg Clin 23 (2013) 257–266
http://dx.doi.org/10.1016/j.thorsurg.2013.01.004
1547-4127/13/$ – see front matter © 2013 Elsevier Inc. All rights reserved.

HISTORICAL NOTES

- 1975: Martini and Melamed report the seminal series of 50 patients with synchronous and metachronous NSCLC, and propose criteria for differentiating metastases from separate primary tumors.[1]
- 1997: Revision of the of American Joint Cancer Committee/International Union Against Cancer (AJCC/UICC) International System for Staging Lung Cancer is published[2]; separate tumor in ipsilateral lobe is specifically classified as M1 and thus generally considered nonsurgical.
- 2007: Seventh edition of AJCC/UICC staging system is published[3]; separate tumor in ipsilateral lobe reclassified as T4 (IIIB if N0).
- 1995: Noguchi publishes his classification of small pulmonary adenocarcinomas that includes the first clear description of in situ tumors, with their extremely good prognosis.[4]
- 2011: Publication of joint International Association for the Study of Lung Cancer/American Thoracic Society/European Respiratory Society (IASLC/ATS/ERS) Classification of Lung Adenocarcinoma that eliminates term bronchioloalveolar carcinoma (BAC) and proposes 5 categories, including AIS and MIA (**Box 1**).[5]

THE PATIENT WITH MULTIPLE FOCI OF "SOLID" NSCLC

As suggested in the introduction, it is very important to differentiate between solid tumors and tumors that are in part nonsolid (or "ground glass"), when discussing the approach to multifocal lung cancer. First discussed are tumors that are predominately solid on CT imaging, upon which our current official staging system is based. These tumors are presumed to represent invasive NSCLC, with substantial potential for lymph node metastasis and distant metastasis; they may represent squamous cell carcinomas or invasive adenocarcinomas, and are highly associated with cigarette smoking.

Two Solid Tumors in Separate, Ipsilateral Lobes

Before the 2007 revision of the AJCC/IUCC lung cancer classification, tumors with an NSCLC in one lobe and a second tumor in a separate, ipsilateral lobe were classified as stage IV. However, this classification failed to take account of several important issues. First, it is usually not at all clear in these situations if the 2 tumors represent a single primary tumor with a site of metastasis within the lung, or whether they in fact represent 2 separate

> **Box 1**
> **The IASLC/ATS/ERS classification of lung adenocarcinoma**
>
> Preinvasive Lesions
>
> > Atypical adenomatous hyperplasia (AAH): a pure in situ tumor ≤5 mm diameter
> >
> > Adenocarcinoma in situ (AIS): a pure in situ tumor >5 mm and ≤3 cm
> >
> > > Mucinous (may also be invasive in some cases)
> > >
> > > Nonmucinous
> > >
> > > Mixed
>
> Minimally Invasive Adenocarcinoma: a lepidic-predominant tumor ≤3 cm with ≤5 mm invasive focus
>
> Invasive Adenocarcinoma
>
> > Lepidic predominant: a lepidic-predominant tumor with >5 mm invasive focus
> >
> > Acinar predominant
> >
> > Papillary predominant
> >
> > Micropapillary predominant
> >
> > Solid predominant with mucin
>
> Variants of Invasive Adenocarcinoma (4; not listed here)
>
> *Adapted from* Travis W, Brambilla E, Noguchi M, et al. International Association for the Study of Lung Cancer/American Thoracic Society/European Respiratory Society international multidisciplinary classification of lung adenocarcinoma. J Thorac Oncol 2011;6:244–85.

primary tumors. Although one can have a suspicion that the smaller lesion is a metastasis that has spread from the larger one if that smaller lesion has a well-circumscribed, "punched-out" appearance, this is far from being a reliable indicator. Even if a biopsy of each tumor suggests the same basic histology (eg, squamous or adenocarcinoma), they still may represent separate primary tumors. And of course a patient with a true metastasis to another lobe of the lung will have a far poorer prognosis than a patient with 2 separate primaries, at least 1 of which is likely to be a very early, stage I tumor with a very high cure rate.

For these reasons, many surgeons, even before the 2007 revision of the lung cancer classification that restaged tumors with a concurrent lesion in a different ipsilateral lobe as T4, would consider these patients for surgical resection. This approach was proved, in retrospect, to be appropriate by the survival curves used to create the 2007 revision.[6] These curves showed that a T4 tumor of this type had an approximately 13-month median survival and a 20% rate of 5-year survival, both substantially higher than seen with other tumor presentations defined as M1, and closer in outcome to other types of T4 tumors.

Whether pneumonectomy, given its greater rates of morbidity and mortality, is an appropriate resection to perform for T4 tumors of this type is a matter open for debate, and clearly this will depend on the overall fitness of the patient and his or her own feelings about proceeding with operation given the increased risks. Fortunately, however, this issue rarely presents itself, as it is far more common for one tumor to be of substantial size, with the second ipsilateral tumor being far smaller and/or more peripherally placed. With this anatomic arrangement, one can typically perform a lobectomy for the larger tumor and a sublobar resection for the smaller tumor. Often, if the second tumor is small (< ~2 cm) and peripheral enough, a wedge resection is adequate to manage it. It is not uncommon, however, to perform an upper lobectomy and a formal superior segmentectomy, a left lower lobectomy and lingulectomy, or similar procedures. The literature on lung cancer is full of articles suggesting that for a sub–2-cm, single, primary NSCLC, sublobar resection may be appropriate. Thus, in this situation whereby one must weigh the risks and potential benefits of pneumonectomy versus lobectomy plus sublobar resection, the author believes that sublobar resection comes out easily on the winning side of the argument for the second tumor.

It is critical to perform pathologic evaluation of the mediastinal lymph nodes in all of these cases of multifocal, solid NSCLC, regardless of the CT or positron emission tomography (PET)/CT findings within the lymph nodes. All busy thoracic surgeons have seen many cases of CT and PET/CT "negative" mediastinal lymph nodes that are positive on pathologic analysis. Published data bear this out, suggesting that even PET/CT has an approximately negative predictive value of only 87% for mediastinal nodal involvement.[7] The author is a strong advocate of operating on most patients with single NSCLC tumors amenable to lobectomy who bear limited N2 disease (after administering neoadjuvant chemotherapy). However, patients with T4 disease by virtue of tumors in separate ipsilateral lobes should be operated on only if they are proved to have noninvolved N2 lymph nodes. The choice between mediastinoscopy and endobronchial ultrasonography with transbronchial needle biopsies should be made according to which technique the surgeon feels most facile with; however, mediastinoscopy is likely more reliable for microscopic disease,[8] and has the added benefit of being able to be performed under the same anesthetic as the lung resection if the nodes are negative on frozen-section examination.

Several studies that can inform our clinical practice have reported good results in resecting selected patients with ipsilateral, synchronous, apparently solid tumors in different lobes. Some of the larger studies are mentioned here. Fukuse and colleagues[9] reported a 5-year survival rate of 21% with such patients. Okada and colleagues[10] reported a 23.4% 5-year survival, and noted that those with N0-N1 disease had statistically better survival than those with N2 disease. Vansteenkiste and colleagues[11] reported a 33% 5-year survival. Battafarano and colleagues[12] found a 66.5% 5-year survival for N0 patients. Voltolini and colleagues[13] found a 57% 5-year survival rate for N0 patients and 0% for N1-N2 patients, including both ipsilateral and contralateral synchronous tumors. Although the survival in this study was somewhat greater for those with unilateral than with bilateral tumors (43% vs 27%), this difference did not reach statistical significance. Fabian and colleagues[14] reported 5-year survival of 54% in mediastinoscopy-negative patients with ipsilateral synchronous tumors, and also found no significant survival difference whether the tumors were ipsilateral or bilateral.

When more than 2 solid tumors are present in separate ipsilateral lobes, even in the absence of nodal disease, it would seem that the likelihood that this represents metastatic rather than multiple separate primary disease rises dramatically. In this situation, it would be unusual to manage the patient with local therapy, and systemic therapy is the primary mode of treatment. Only if no distant or additional pulmonary disease develops over a reasonable time interval (approximately 18 months) might it be reasonable to approach a patient of this sort surgically or by some combination of surgery and stereotactic ablative radiation therapy (SABR).

Two, Solid, Contralateral Tumors

Although the current TNM classification system for NSCLC labels 2 contralateral tumors as M1a disease while labeling ipsilateral tumors in separate lobes T4, It is the author's opinion that the approaches to patients bearing these 2 presentations should not dramatically differ (**Fig. 1**). The basis for the staging system are survival curves that demonstrate close to 0% 5-year survival for separate tumor in contralateral lung versus 20% for separate tumors in different, ipsilateral lobes.[6] However, as alluded to earlier, single-institution studies, which perhaps one should lend less weight than the larger studies used to create the

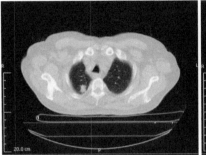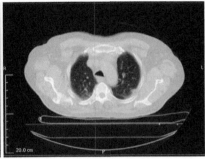

Fig. 1. Computed tomogram of a male patient with bilateral, solid NSCLCs. This patient, as recommended in the text, was assumed to have separate primary tumors. After a negative mediastinoscopy, he underwent thoracoscopic right upper lobectomy followed by lingula-sparing left upper lobectomy. His tumors were proved to be a stage IA (T1bN0M0) adenocarcinoma on the right and a stage IB (T2N0M0) squamous cell carcinoma on the left. He is alive without disease at 3.5 years postoperatively.

staging system, do show much better results than this for 2 synchronous, contralateral tumors. The studies by Voltolini and colleagues[13] and Fabian and colleagues[14] showed 5-year survivals for these patients (largely N0) of 27% to 50%, and no significant difference between this group and those with ipsilateral tumors. De Leyn and colleagues[15] reported a 5-year survival of 38% with resection of synchronous bilateral tumors. More recently, however, Shah and colleagues[16] reported a somewhat lower 3-year disease-free survival of 24% in this group of patients.

Given this information, in fit patients it would be inappropriate to deny surgical resection to patients with 2 contralateral, solid NSCLCs who demonstrate no mediastinal lymph node involvement and have suspected stage II disease on no more than one side. As with ipsilateral disease, sublobar resection is preferred for appropriate sized (<2 cm) and appropriately located (ie, well away from the nearest intersegmental plane) tumors, to reduce surgical morbidity and improve long-term quality of life. Also, as in patients with ipsilateral disease, pathologic evaluation of the mediastinal lymph nodes is critical: those with any mediastinal nodal involvement should not be considered surgical candidates.

THE PATIENT WITH MULTIPLE FOCI OF PREDOMINATELY "NONSOLID" NSCLC: THE LEPIDIC-PREDOMINANT ADENOCARCINOMA SPECTRUM

Recent years have witnessed a marked increase in the incidence of adenocarcinomas on the spectrum of what is now called AIS or lepidic-predominant adenocarcinoma. These tumors are either nonsolid (appearing as pure ground-glass opacity [GGO] on CT) or part-solid. About half of the patients who develop these are lifelong

nonsmokers and many others are light and/or remote cigarette smokers. Approximately half of these tumors bear a mutation in the epidermal growth factor receptor (EGFR).[5] These tumors have a tendency to occur in those of Asian descent, particularly Asian women, and for this reason much of the original work describing their pathologic and clinical characteristics has come from groups in Japan (see the article by Okada elsewhere in this issue for additional information on the topic).

For the purposes of this article on multifocal lung cancer, these lepidic-type adenocarcinomas are critically important because they very often present with multiple foci of involvement within the lung. If multiple foci are not visible at presentation, they not infrequently occur metachronously as one follows these patients.

Clinical Behavior of Single, Lepidic-Predominant Adenocarcinomas and Relationship to Pathology

To understand and manage multifocal lepidic-predominant adenocarcinoma, one must first understand the behavior of single adenocarcinomas of this type.

Noguchi and colleagues[4] were perhaps the first to recognize that tumors with a lepidic growth pattern (growth along alveolar septae) may remain completely noninvasive and thus have a virtually zero rate of metastasis. In their adenocarcinoma classification, they identified 2 noninvasive BAC (types A and B) and invasive BAC, the former having an approximately 100% 5-year survival rate and 0% rate of lymph node metastasis, and the latter approaching the behavior of typical, invasive NSCLC.

The recent international multidisciplinary classification of adenocarcinomas (see **Box 1**)[5] eliminated the term BAC because of its previous loose, nonspecific application to several very different radiologic, pathologic, and clinical situations, including both invasive and noninvasive tumors. This classification has instead introduced the terms atypical adenomatous hyperplasia (AAH) for a lesion less than or equal to 5 mm in size without invasion, AIS for a lesion less than or equal to 3 cm in size without invasion (corresponding to Noguchi types A and B, respectively), MIA for a lesion less than or equal to 3 cm in size that is lepidic predominant with an invasive focus less than 5 mm in size, and lepidic-predominant invasive adenocarcinoma for a lepidic-predominant tumor less than or equal to 3 cm in size with an invasive focus of more than 5 mm in size. A great deal of study has demonstrated that these tumors have an excellent prognosis up to and including the point of minimal invasion (<5 mm focus of invasion), whereas beyond that point they begin to behave similarly to standard, solid, invasive NSCLC and therefore must be treated as such.

By histology, then, it is clear that one can identify a subtype of lepidic-type adenocarcinoma with a small invasive focus that still has a very low rate of lymph node spread and recurrence/metastasis. Relevant data show that a lepidic tumor bearing a scar at least 5 mm in size,[17] an invasive focus at least 5 mm in size,[18] greater than 75% lepidic growth pattern,[19] or greater than 50% lepidic growth pattern[20] all are cured in nearly 100% of patients with resection.

Is sublobar resection appropriate for AIS/MIA?

It has been repeatedly demonstrated that sublobar resection has an extremely high cure rate for AIS and MIA (ie, up to a 5-mm invasive focus). Although this has not been established in prospective, randomized studies, the data (at least in Japanese patients) are compelling. When choosing sublobar resection based on intraoperative frozen sections showing no invasion or a focus of invasion of less than 5 mm, at least 4 groups have shown close to 100% cure rates.[21–23]

Perhaps even more importantly, it has become clear that preoperative imaging characteristics can be used to select AIS and MIA, which can then be safely treated by sublobar resection. It has been shown, for example, that when more than 50% of the 2-dimensional tumor volume on high-resolution CT is composed of ground glass, the 5-year cancer-specific survival is 100%[24]; that a tumor smaller than 1 cm with any ground glass within it has 0% incidence of nodal metastasis and 100% survival with resection[25]; and that a tumor smaller than 1.5 cm that is "mainly" ground glass has 100% survival with sublobar resection.[26] The maximum standard uptake value

on PET/CT has been shown to have an inverse correlation with the proportion of tumor that is lepidic/noninvasive,[27] but this appears to be less predictive than fine-cut CT appearance.[28] PET/CT will generally not show elevated fluorodeoxyglucose (FDG) activity in AIS, and it would not be expected to show substantially elevated FDG activity with a subcentimeter invasive focus, which is below its anatomic resolution. However, a negative PET/CT does make one feel more comfortable that there is no occult, larger invasive focus, and this finding is reassuring when one plans sublobar resection for such patients.

Which type of sublobar resection is appropriate (wedge vs segmentectomy)?

There are no randomized data available on the issue of wedge resection versus segmentectomy, in the case of either standard solid NSCLCs or lepidic-predominant tumors. Several nonrandomized studies do, however, suggest that segmentectomy provides a substantial benefit over wedge resection for typical, invasive NSCLC. To allude to just one of these, Sienel and colleagues[29] showed in well-matched groups of clinical stage IA patients who underwent either segmentectomy or wedge resection that the rate of locoregional recurrences markedly favored the segmentectomy group (55% vs 16%; $P = .001$) while the cancer-specific survival trended in the same direction (48% vs 71%; $P = .16$).

It must be noted, however, that most of the Japanese studies that report extremely high cure rates using sublobar resection for AIS and MIA less than 2 cm in size used, for the most part, wedge resections. One must admit, therefore, that for a predominantly ground-glass tumor with a suspected invasive focus of less than 5 mm, a wedge resection may ultimately prove to be adequate therapy.

Given the current absence of definitive data on this issue, the author's personal bias is to always perform a formal anatomic segmentectomy for predominantly ground-glass tumors that show any focus of higher density on CT. This approach allows dissection of the intersegmental lymph nodes (the first location that one would expect to find a lymph node metastasis). If the intersegmental or mediastinal lymph nodes are positive for malignancy, or if there is any concern about the parenchymal margin being at least as large as the tumor itself,[30] the procedure will be converted to a lobectomy in fit patients. Most pure GGOs less than 2 cm in diameter, containing no denser focus, can be adequately treated with a generous wedge resection. A 3-cm tumor seems to be reaching the point at which even segmentectomy cannot often be done with adequate parenchymal margins, and at that size the author will typically perform lobectomy.

Do pure ground-glass opacities even require resection?

Taking this issue of extent of resection still further, it can be reasonably asked whether small GGOs require any resection. Because only a subset appears to grow, because these grow and/or develop an invasive component only over the course of years, and because even with an invasive component up to 5 mm in size they seem to be highly curable, perhaps even by wedge resection, one wonders if there is any urgency to resect pure GGOs. Kondo and Monden[31] showed that 86% of all adenocarcinomas in their practice smaller than 1 cm in size were Noguchi type A or B (the types associated with 100% 5-year survival and 0% lymph node metastasis).[4] Furthermore, 100% of pure GGOs in this series were types A or B at the time of resection. Hiramatsu and colleagues[32] showed initial size over 1 cm to be the strongest risk factor for future growth of a GGO. Lastly, in the lung cancer CT screening experience accumulated over the past several years, thousands of subcentimeter nodules were followed that proved to be cancers—even solid nodules—and only rarely did these prove to be beyond stage I at the time of resection.

From these data, it is safe to conclude that a pure GGO less than 1 cm in size does not require resection. These likely AIS (or areas of AAH) can be followed with serial CT scans, and they may remain unchanged for many years. Scans can be done at a 6-month interval initially but lengthened to 1-year intervals thereafter. In the author's opinion, it is not yet clear that pure GGOs larger than 1 cm can be safely followed, although it may ultimately be proved safe to follow pure GGOs up to 2 cm in size. The concern is that as the size of the GGO increases, so does the risk that it will contain a focus of invasion, even an occult focus not seen as an area of increased density on CT. The author has encountered multiple patients in whom a larger focus of what was thought to be a pure GGO on CT has been proved to harbor invasive adenocarcinoma on final histology.

Approach to the Patient with Multiple Foci of Predominately Nonsolid NSCLC

Many patients with AIS and/or lepidic-predominant adenocarcinoma will present with multifocal disease. In fact, in experience practicing pulmonary surgery in an area with a very large population of Asian descent, the author finds that it is more the exception than the rule to find a patient with one tumor composed largely of ground glass that is not associated with at least 1 or 2 other GGOs elsewhere in the lungs. These other lesions are often quite small and not necessarily appreciated on an initial, cursory examination of the CT. The more carefully one looks at the scans, the more of these GGOs one tends to find. The most common situation seems to be a patient who presents with a single, dominant, part-solid tumor suspicious for representing an MIA, with other scattered, pure GGOs (**Fig. 2**).

It is clear that these scattered lesions do not behave as though they are metastases, but rather behave as multiple sites of premalignant (AIS) or very early malignant (MIA) lesions. This presentation must not be considered stage IV disease! Although very little has been published to date regarding this increasingly common clinical scenario, these few studies do suggest that these multifocal cases have an excellent prognosis that in the medium term is dependent on the stage of the dominant, resected, invasive carcinoma, and not on the pure GGOs (**Box 2**). Kim and colleagues[33] reported 23 patients with 1 part-solid lesion and multiple pure GGOs, of whom 5 patients had all lesions resected and 18 had some GGOs left in place. At a median follow-up of 40.3 months, survival was 100%, only 1 patient developed a new invasive adenocarcinoma, and none of the GGOs that were left in place (n = 16) grew or became invasive. Mun and Kohno[34] reported 27 patients with 91 GGOs or part-solid lesions resected. At 46 months' median follow-up there were no deaths, but new GGOs developed in 26% of patients. Tsutsui and colleagues[35] reported 23 patients with one invasive tumor and a mean of 8.5 synchronous pure GGOs. Seventy-four of the GGOs were resected, representing mainly AAH. One hundred and ten GGOs were not resected and followed by CT for a mean of almost 4 years, and none of these lesions grew during that interval. Disease-free survival was 87%.

The experience at Stanford (presented in abstract form at the Society of Thoracic Surgeons' Meeting in January 2013) is generally consistent with these findings. The author's group identified 43 patients with suspected multifocal AIS and 1 invasive lesion. The mean number of GGOs was 2.7 (range 1–7). The approach was to perform typically an anatomic resection of the invasive-appearing tumor, with wedge resection of accessible ipsilateral pure GGOs. With this approach, disease-free survival at a mean follow-up of 30 months has been 95%. Only 1 patient (2%) required intervention for a growing/invasive previously pure GGO lesion. However, 21% of patients did demonstrate growth of original GGOs during follow-up, and 42% of patients developed new GGOs.

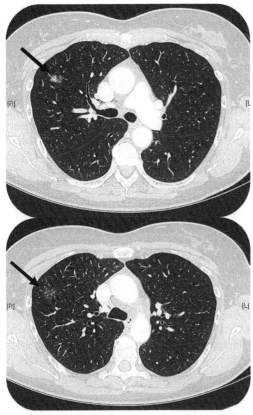

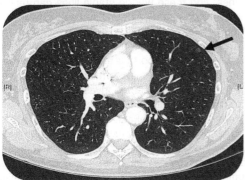

Fig. 2. Computed tomogram of a typical nonsmoking female patient with a single, part-solid tumor in the right upper lobe (*arrow, upper image*), and 4 (2 seen on these cuts) pure ground-glass opacities (GGOs) elsewhere in the lungs (*other arrows*). This patient underwent a thoracoscopic right upper lobectomy and was found to have a lepidic-predominant adenocarcinoma (the part-solid tumor) with a 7-mm invasive focus (stage IA; T1aN0M0) and a separate area of pure adenocarcinoma in situ (the pure GGO) in that lobe. At 4 years postoperatively she is well, and the left upper lobe GGO pictured (*arrow, lower image*) has grown by only 2 mm and remains free of any dense focus.

Box 2
Summary of publications reporting surgical results with multifocal lepidic-type adenocarcinomas

Kim et al,[33] 2010	n = 23 patients with synchronous tumors 1 bilobectomy/10 lobectomies/15 wedges performed 3.3-y overall survival 100%; invasive disease–free survival 95.7%
Mun and Kohno,[34] 2007	n = 27 patients with synchronous tumors 14 lobectomies/3 segmentectomies/12 wedges performed 3.9-y overall survival 100%; invasive disease–free survival 100%
Nakata et al,[36] 2004	n = 26 patients with synchronous tumors 32 lobectomies/8 segmentectomies/28 wedges performed 3-y overall survival 93%; invasive disease–free survival 79%
Gu et al,[37] 2012	n = 43 patients with synchronous tumors 32 lobectomies/2 segmentectomies/16 wedges performed 2.5-y overall survival 100%; invasive disease–free survival 95%
Tsutsui et al,[35] 2010	n = 20 patients with synchronous tumors 22 lobectomies/2 segmentectomies/3 wedges performed (initially) 4.9-y overall survival 90%; invasive disease–free survival unclear

All of these accumulating data would suggest that patients with an invasive, lepidic-predominant adenocarcinoma and a limited number of pure GGO lesions (perhaps <10) can be treated with a high rate of 5-year survival by resecting the most concerning tumor by the appropriate procedure (often segmentectomy) and simultaneously resecting small ipsilateral GGOs that are accessible to wedge resection. It seems unnecessary, based on the relatively slow rate of progression of unresected GGOs, to resect contralateral pure GGOs, or those that are too deeply seated within an ipsilateral lobe to be removed by wedge only.

On the other hand, a certain percentage (one might guess from the available literature approximately 20%) of patients will, over 2 to 5 years, have a lesion that will grow sufficiently and/or show signs of invasion, or develop new lesions, which will require additional treatment. For this reason it is optimal to treat the invasive lesion that one is addressing at the initial operation with a sublobar resection if possible, sparing lung tissue for the future, and to resect accessible ipsilateral lesions at the same time by wedge.

The mechanics of treating patients with multifocal lepidic-predominant tumors

To biopsy or not to biopsy? In the usual situation of a woman of Asian ancestry with several GGOs, 1 of which has developed a solid-appearing component suspicious for invasion, needle biopsy has not been generally required to proceed with resection. It would be highly unusual to find any diagnosis other than lepidic-type adenocarcinoma in someone presenting with this clinical scenario, so it is reasonable to proceed directly to surgical resection.

However, when the scenario is not as clear (eg, if there have been recent signs of lung infection, or if the CT appearance is not characteristic), it is reasonable to attempt transthoracic needle biopsy (TTNB) for the one dominant tumor. It is very important to understand that cytology from a TTNB will not provide information about whether the lesion is invasive or not; it will only identify whether adenocarcinoma cells are present. Thus, it is not necessarily indicated to resect a small, pure GGO that on biopsy is read out as "adenocarcinoma," because this may very well still be an in situ lesion with minimal chance of spread and, thus, not require resection (see earlier discussion). Extensiveness of resection (ie, wedge vs anatomic resection) also should not be chosen based on biopsy findings, but rather on thin-section CT and/or PET/CT criteria of invasiveness.

Lastly, as for all lesions suspicious for being an NSCLC, it must be remembered that a "nondiagnostic" biopsy does not rule out malignancy. The only nonmalignant findings on TTNB that do not mandate an additional diagnostic procedure are those that provide a specific benign diagnosis.

Intraoperative details of the author's experience *Tumor-localization techniques.* I have not found that tumor-localization procedures are a particular help in these cases (nor in other cases). Multiple such techniques have been described, whether based on lung surface marking, ultrasonography, hook-wire, radioactivity, and so forth, generally with reasonably good efficacy results reported. It is very difficult to know in these studies, however, if the lesions chosen for study actually required any localization technique in the first place. My opinion is that if one sets out to wedge-resect a tumor, the tumor should be palpable to the finger of the operating thoracoscopic surgeon (using video-assisted thoracoscopic surgery [VATS]) or the procedure should be done by thoracotomy. Although lepidic-type adenocarcinomas are admittedly softer than standard, solid NSCLC, lesions larger than 1 cm that are in the outer third of the lung amenable to wedge resection are almost always palpable thoracoscopically, and pure GGOs smaller than 1 cm likely do not require resection (see previously discussed data supporting this). I fear that nodules that are not palpable will not be able to be wedged with an adequate margin of resection—localizing procedure or no localizing procedure. I fear that occasionally, noncurative wedge resections with positive margins will result from attempted VATS-wedge of nonpalpable lesions—localizing procedure or not.

Wedge first if planning segment? If I am planning, based on a CT appearance of an MIA, to do a segmentectomy, I generally do not carry out wedge resection first. Frequently a preliminary wedge resection will need to cross intersegmental planes, and these wedge staple lines can render the eventual segmentectomy somewhat awkward to complete.

Technique of segmentectomy for the dominant tumor. It is very important that one adopts a relatively rigid protocol for performing segmentectomy for tumors with suspected invasion, and for what circumstances will dictate proceeding to a more extensive resection. First, it is critical to resect and obtain frozen sections on the intersegmental lymph node, and to either sample or completely resect (and freeze) all other N1 and N2 nodal stations. If any of these lymph nodes are positive for malignancy, I believe that one should convert the segmentectomy to a lobectomy in a patient with adequate pulmonary function to tolerate a lobectomy. Second, the parenchymal margin of resection should be at least as large as the diameter of the tumor.[31] If this is not possible to achieve, very strong consideration should be given to proceeding with lobectomy.

Management of ipsilateral pure GGOs. All ipsilateral pure GGOs that are amenable to wedge resection should be removed during the procedure. This recommendation is based on the data demonstrating that some of these lesions will grow slowly, others may arise, and a few will become invasive, requiring future local therapy. A redo surgical procedure in a previously operated chest will clearly be more difficult, if and when these grow to invasive lesions, than wedging out these lesions at the initial procedure if this can be accomplished. However, given the markedly increased morbidity of pneumonectomy over lobectomy plus wedge resections, I do not consider that a sub-2 cm, pure GGO that would require removal of a second lobe ipsilateral to the dominant tumor should be resected. Like all contralateral small, pure GGOs, this can be left in place and followed for growth or development of invasiveness with serial studies.

A role for stereotactic ablative radiotherapy? There may well prove to be a role for SABR in patients with multifocal lepidic-predominant adenocarcinomas. I would argue, as many surgeons would, that the data some radiation oncologists believe has shown equivalence of SABR to surgical resection for standard, solid, stage IA NSCLC is highly flawed. However, the ideal lesion for SABR, as for wedge resection, is an AIS or MIA, both of which have very little risk of harboring nodal metastases. Therefore in patients with elevated surgical risk, or who would be left with markedly reduced quality of life by additional pulmonary resection when a remaining GGO grows or becomes minimally invasive, it would be very reasonable to proceed with SABR as an alternative. Most often this will be when the now concerning lesion is ipsilateral, requiring a redo procedure, and/or when it is centrally placed in a lobe, requiring lobectomy for resection.

REFERENCES

1. Martini N, Melamed M. Multiple primary lung cancers. J Thorac Cardiovasc Surg 1975;70:606–12.
2. Mountain C. Revisions in the international system for staging lung cancer. Chest 1997;111:1710–7.
3. Goldstraw P, Crowley J, Chansky K, et al. The IASLC lung cancer staging project: proposals for the revision of the TNM stage groupings in the forthcoming (seventh) edition of the TNM classification of malignant tumours. J Thorac Oncol 2007;2:706–14.
4. Noguchi M, Morikawa A, Kawasaki M, et al. Small adenocarcinoma of the lung. Histologic characteristics and prognosis. Cancer 1995;75:2844–52.
5. Travis W, Brambilla E, Noguchi M, et al. International Association for the Study of Lung Cancer/American Thoracic Society/European Respiratory Society international multidisciplinary classification of lung adenocarcinoma. J Thorac Oncol 2011;6:244–85.
6. Postmus P, Brambilla E, Chansky K, et al. The IASLC lung cancer staging project: proposals for revision of the M descriptors in the forthcoming (seventh) edition of the TNM classification of lung cancer. J Thorac Oncol 2007;2:686–93.
7. Reed C, Harpole D, Posther K, et al. Results of the American College of Surgeons Oncology Group Z0050 trial: the utility of positron emission tomography in staging potentially operable non-small cell lung cancer. J Thorac Cardiovasc Surg 2003;126: 1943–51.
8. de Cabanyes Candela S, Detterbeck F. A systematic review of restaging after induction therapy for stage IIIa lung cancer: prediction of pathologic stage. J Thorac Oncol 2010;5:389–98.
9. Fukuse T, Hirata T, Tanaka F, et al. Prognosis of ipsilateral intrapulmonary metastases in resected non-small cell lung cancer. Eur J Cardiothorac Surg 1997;12:218–23.
10. Okada M, Tsubota N, Yoshimura M, et al. Evaluation of TMN classification for lung carcinoma with ipsilateral intrapulmonary metastasis. Ann Thorac Surg 1999;68:326–30.
11. Vansteenkiste J, De Belie B, Deneffe G, et al. Practical approach to patients presenting with multiple synchronous suspect lung lesions: a reflection on the current TNM classification based on 54 cases with complete follow-up. Lung Cancer 2001;34:169–75.
12. Battafarano R, Meyers B, Guthrie T, et al. Surgical resection of multifocal non-small cell lung cancer is associated with prolonged survival. Ann Thorac Surg 2002;74:988–93.
13. Voltolini L, Rapicetta C, Luzzi L, et al. Surgical treatment of synchronous multiple lung cancer located in a different lobe or lung: high survival in node-negative subgroup. Eur J Cardiothorac Surg 2010; 37:1198–204.
14. Fabian T, Bryant A, Mouhlas A, et al. Survival after resection of synchronous non-small cell lung cancer. J Thorac Cardiovasc Surg 2011;142:547–53.
15. De Leyn P, Moons J, Vansteenkiste J, et al. Survival after resection of synchronous bilateral lung cancer. Eur J Cardiothorac Surg 2008;34:1215–22.
16. Shah A, Barfield M, Kelsey C, et al. Outcomes after surgical management of synchronous bilateral primary lung cancers. Ann Thorac Surg 2012;93:1055–60.
17. Suzuki Y, Pagani F, Bolling S. Left thoracotomy for multiple-time redo mitral valve surgery using on-pump beating heart technique. Ann Thorac Surg 2008;86:466–71.
18. Terasaki H, Niki T, Matsuno Y, et al. Lung adenocarcinoma with mixed bronchioloalveolar and invasive components: clinicopathological features, subclassification by extent of invasive foci, and immunohistochemical characterization. Am J Surg Pathol 2003; 27:937–51.
19. Yokose T, Suzuki K, Nagai K, et al. Favorable and unfavorable morphological prognostic factors in peripheral adenocarcinoma of the lung 3 cm or less in diameter. Lung Cancer 2000;29:179–88.
20. Suzuki K, Asamura H, Kusumoto M, et al. "Early" peripheral lung cancer: prognostic significance of

ground glass opacity on thin-section computed tomographic scan. Ann Thorac Surg 2002;74:1635–9.

21. Koike T, Togashi K, Shirato T, et al. Limited resection for noninvasive bronchioloalveolar carcinoma diagnosed by intraoperative pathologic examination. Ann Thorac Surg 2009;88:1106–11.

22. Yamato Y, Tsuchida M, Watanabe T, et al. Early results of a prospective study of limited resection for bronchioloalveolar adenocarcinoma of the lung. Ann Thorac Surg 2001;71:971–4.

23. Watanabe S, Watanabe T, Arai K, et al. Results of wedge resection for focal bronchioloalveolar carcinoma showing pure ground-glass attenuation on computed tomography. Ann Thorac Surg 2002;73:1071–5.

24. Nakayama H, Yamada K, Saito H, et al. Sublobar resection for patients with peripheral small adenocarcinomas of the lung: surgical outcome is associated with features on computed tomographic imaging. Ann Thorac Surg 2007;84:1675–9.

25. Shi C, Zhang X, Han B, et al. A clinicopathological study of resected non-small cell lung cancers 2 cm or less in diameter: a prognostic assessment. Med Oncol 2011;28:1441–6.

26. Sugi K, Kobayashi S, Sudou M, et al. Long-term prognosis of video-assisted limited surgery for early lung cancer. Eur J Cardiothorac Surg 2010;37:456–60.

27. Liu S, Cheng H, Yao S, et al. The clinical application value of PET/CT in adenocarcinoma with bronchioloalveolar carcinoma features. Ann Nucl Med 2010;24:541–7.

28. Okada M, Tauchi S, Iwanaga K, et al. Associations among bronchioloalveolar carcinoma components, positron emission tomographic and computed tomographic findings, and malignant behavior in small lung adenocarcinomas. J Thorac Cardiovasc Surg 2007;133:1448–54.

29. Sienel W, Dango S, Kirschbaum A, et al. Sublobar resections in stage IA non-small cell lung cancer: segmentectomies result in significantly better cancer-related survival than wedge resections. Eur J Cardiothorac Surg 2008;33:728–34.

30. El-Sherif A, Fernando H, Santos R, et al. Margin and local recurrence after sublobar resection of non-small cell lung cancer. Ann Surg Oncol 2007;14:2400–5.

31. Kondo K, Monden Y. Lymphogenous and hematogenous metastasis of thymic epithelial tumors. Ann Thorac Surg 2003;76:1859–64.

32. Hiramatsu M, Inagaki T, Matsui Y, et al. Pulmonary ground-glass opacity (GGO) lesions-large size and a history of lung cancer are risk factors for growth. J Thorac Oncol 2008;3:1245–50.

33. Kim H, Choi Y, Kim J, et al. Management of multiple pure ground-glass opacity lesions in patients with bronchioloalveolar carcinoma. J Thorac Oncol 2010;5:206–10.

34. Mun M, Kohno T. Efficacy of thoracoscopic resection for multifocal bronchioloalveolar carcinoma showing pure ground-glass opacities of 20 mm or less in diameter. J Thorac Cardiovasc Surg 2007;134:877–82.

35. Tsutsui S, Ashizawa K, Minami K, et al. Multiple focal pure ground-glass opacities on high-resolution CT images: clinical significance in patients with lung cancer. AJR Am J Roentgenol 2010;195:131–8.

36. Nakata M, Sawada S, Yamashita M, et al. Surgical treatments for multiple primary adenocarcinoma of the lung. Ann Thorac Surg 2004;78:1194–9.

37. Gu B, Stephanie S, Hoang C, et al. A dominant, invasive adenocarcinoma associated with multifocal in situ lesions does not represent M1 disease and should be treated surgically. Abstract presented at Society of Thoracic Surgeons Meeting. Los Angeles, January 29, 2012.

Index

Note: Page numbers of article titles are in **boldface** type.

A

Absolute and relative contraindications to pulmonary resection: Effect of lung cancer surgery guidelines on medical practice, **247–255**
ADC. See *Adenocarcinoma.*
Adenocarcinoma
    and cytopathology, 164, 169, 170, 172
    lepidic-predominant, 258, 260–265
    subtyping of, 179–185
    and survival outcomes, 184
Adenocarcinoma in situ
    and sublobar resection, 261
    and subtyping of adenocarcinoma, 180, 181, 184
Adrenal gland
    non–small cell lung cancer metastasis to, 253
Advances in cytopathology for lung cancer: The impact and challenges of new technologies, **163–178**
AFB. See *Autofluorescence bronchoscopy.*
Air pollution
    and lung cancer, 117–119
AIS. See *Adenocarcinoma in situ.*
Anaerobic threshold
    and cardiopulmonary exercise testing, 235
Antimicrobials
    and suspicious pulmonary nodules, 147
Approach to the patient with multiple lung nodules, **257–266**
Arsenic
    and lung cancer, 118, 119
Asbestos
    and lung cancer, 118, 119
Autofluorescence bronchoscopy
    and imaging of carcinoma in situ, 154–156
    vs. white light bronchoscopy, 154, 155

B

BAC. See *Bronchioloalveolar carcinoma.*
Beryllium
    and lung cancer, 118, 119
Biomarkers
    for early detection of lung cancer, 214–216
    and EML4-ALK, 220
    and epidermal growth factor receptor, 217–220
    and epigenomics, 213
    and excision repair cross-complementation group 1, 220, 221
    and fusion proteins, 220

    and genomics, 212, 213
    and KRAS mutations, 220
    in lung cancer, 214–217
    and matrix-assisted laser desorption/ionization mass spectrometry, 214–217
    and mutational analysis of NSCLC, 217–221
    and non–small cell lung cancer, 216–221
    platforms in measurement of, 212–214
    and prediction of treatment response, 217–221
    and prognostication of lung cancer, 216–218
    and proteomics, 213, 214
    and ribonucleotide reductase messenger 1, 221
    and role in lung cancer screening, 136, 137
    and ROS1, 220
Biomarkers and molecular testing for early detection, diagnosis, and therapeutic prediction of lung cancer, **211–224**
Bone metastases
    as a contraindication to pulmonary resection, 250
Brain metastases
    as a contraindication to pulmonary resection, 250
    in non–small cell lung cancer, 254
Bronchioloalveolar carcinoma
    and lung cancer screening, 134, 135
    and subtyping of adenocarcinoma, 179–185
Bronchoscopy
    abnormal results as a contraindication to pulmonary resection, 251
    and diagnosis of lung lesions, 156–158
    and electromagnetic navigation, 157
    and imaging of lung lesions, 153–158
    vs. low-dose thoracic computed tomography, 156
    vs. positron emission tomography, 156
    principles of, 153, 154
    and radial ultrasound, 157, 158
    vs. transthoracic needle biopsy, 158

C

Cadmium
    and lung cancer, 118, 119
Carcinogens
    and cigarette smoking, 107, 108
Carcinoma in situ
    and autofluorescence bronchoscopy, 154–156
Cardiopulmonary exercise testing
    alternatives to, 239–242
    and anaerobic threshold, 235
    and cardiovascular limitation, 235